Autism and Child Psychopathology Series

Series Editor

Johnny L. Matson, Department of Psychology, Louisiana State University, Baton Rouge, LA, USA

More information about this series at http://www.springer.com/series/8665

Frederick Furniss • Asit B. Biswas

Self-Injurious Behavior in Individuals with Neurodevelopmental Conditions

Springer

Frederick Furniss
George Davies Centre
University of Leicester
Leicester, UK

Asit B. Biswas
University of Leicester
Leicester, UK

ISSN 2192-922X ISSN 2192-9238 (electronic)
Autism and Child Psychopathology Series
ISBN 978-3-030-36015-3 ISBN 978-3-030-36016-0 (eBook)
https://doi.org/10.1007/978-3-030-36016-0

This Springer imprint is published by the registered company Springer Nature Switzerland AG
The registered company address is: Gewerbestrasse 11, 6330 Cham, Switzerland

To Susan and Ajanta

Preface

This book provides an overview of current knowledge regarding the complex, and often chronic and highly distressing, issue of self-injury in people with neurodevelopmental conditions. The first three chapters sketch developments in thinking about self-injury from the beginning of modern psychiatry to the present day, survey what is known about the phenomenology and natural history of self-injury in people with neurodevelopmental conditions, and describe research on neurobiological processes involved in the development of self-injurious behaviors. At the end of Chap. 3, we outline a model of the interactions between environmental and neural processes involved in the initial development of self-injury and its potential progression to increasingly difficult-to-treat stages. The next three chapters discuss the use of this model as a basis for individualizing assessment and intervention according to the processes predominant in maintaining self-injury for each person. The final chapters deal with the issue of self-restraint among people who self-injure, explore why people with autism spectrum conditions may be at particular risk for self-injury, and look to current research with promise to improve our ability to prevent the development of self-injury and help people with established self-injurious behaviors.

Our title reflects an assumption that future research will identify many more microdeletions, single gene mutations, and other genetic correlates associated with neurodevelopmental conditions. We use the term "condition" rather than "disorder," mainly because many people living with these conditions prefer to regard them as such, but also to make it clear that the book does not deal with all the conditions categorized as "neurodevelopmental disorders" in DSM-5. We generally use "person-first" language, but in discussing their own experiences of self-injury have used the "identity-first" language currently preferred by many autistic adults in the UK. Chapters 4–7 include case studies intended to provide students in particular with a practical appreciation of how assessment and intervention may proceed with individual clients. The cases and assessment results presented are all completely hypothetical.

We hope that the book will be of interest to clinicians, clinical trainees, researchers and students in applied behavior analysis, clinical psychology, intellectual disability nursing, psychiatry, speech and language therapy, and other clinical, education, and social care professions. While standard safety precautions must always be followed, our constantly increasing knowledge regarding the reliability and validity of assessment and diagnostic procedures and the effects (both positive and untoward) of intervention methods will require ongoing changes in these procedures and methods. Professional guidelines and statutory regulations can also differ across communities, and practitioners must rely on their training, the current evidence base, their knowledge of the individual client/patient, and relevant professional and regulatory frameworks to ensure that each person receives optimal support. Practitioners licensed to prescribe or recommend medications or other therapeutic products should always consult the most current information provided by product manufacturers regarding recommended doses, method and duration of administration, and contraindications.

We are grateful to many colleagues, and to the people with whom we have worked, their families, and their support workers, for all they have taught us about the complexities of living with self-injury. We also thank Professor Johnny Matson, Editor of the *Autism and Child Psychopathology* book series, for his encouragement and support, and Judy Jones (Senior Editor) and Michelle Tam (Assistant Editor) at Springer for their valuable advice.

Leicester, UK — Frederick Furniss
Leicester, UK — Asit B. Biswas
July 2019

Contents

About the Authors

Frederick Furniss, MA, PhD, is an honorary clinical psychology teacher at the University of Leicester, UK. He has more than 35 years of experience as a clinical psychologist working with children and adults with neurodevelopmental conditions, including extensive experience of assessment and intervention with people engaging in severe self-injury in both community and residential care settings. His clinical and research interests include assessment and intervention with self-injurious, restricted, and repetitive behaviors and the relationships between cognitive and behavioral phenotypes in neurodevelopmental conditions.

Asit B. Biswas, MD, FRCPsych, MMedSci, DPM, is a Consultant Psychiatrist with the Leicestershire Partnership NHS Trust specializing in the assessment and management of autism, ADHD, and challenging behavior in people with intellectual disabilities, having worked with the UK National Health Service for more than 28 years. He is also an Honorary Associate Professor at the University of Leicester, UK, and was past Chair of the Specialty Advisory Committee (Intellectual Disability Faculty, Royal College of Psychiatrists) responsible for curriculum development, and design of assessment structures and training pathways, for both Core and Higher specialist training in the Psychiatry of Intellectual Disability for doctors working toward completion of training to work as Consultants in this subspecialty in the UK. He has previously held the role of Training Programme Director in Psychiatry of Learning Disability at the East Midlands deanery. His clinical and research interests include management of challenging behavior, such as self-injurious behavior and aggression, in people with intellectual disability, autism, and ADHD. He was a Principal Investigator for a recently completed project evaluating the clinical effectiveness and cost-effectiveness of Positive Behavior Support for people with learning disability and challenging behavior funded by the UK National Institute of Health Research. He is currently the Vice-Chair of the Intellectual Disability Psychiatry Faculty, Royal College of Psychiatrists, London.

Chapter 1
Conceptualization and Taxonomy of Self-Injurious Behavior

1.1 Introduction

Self-injurious behaviors such as headbanging are seen transiently in early infancy in a substantial number of typically developing children (Sallustro & Atwell, 1978). In people with a variety of neurodevelopmental, neurological, and psychiatric conditions, however, the prevalence and persistence of these behaviors are such as to constitute major concerns to the individuals, their families, and professionals involved in their care. Conceptually, such behaviors are often differentiated both from attempts at suicide and from the self-harm such as cutting or burning themselves which people with conditions involving congenital insensitivity to pain may experience. Yates (2004), for example, defines self-injurious behavior (SIB) as comprising non-accidental self-inflicted acts causing damage to or destruction of body tissue and carried out without suicidal ideation or intent. In this chapter, we review developments in the conceptualization of SIB throughout the nineteenth, twentieth, and twenty-first centuries together with attempts to develop taxonomic systems.

The *Diagnostic and Statistical Manual of Mental Disorders* of the American Psychiatric Association recognized "nonsuicidal self-injury" (NSSI) as a condition potentially distinct from "suicidal behavior disorder" in its fifth edition (DSM-5; American Psychiatric Association, 2013), in which both NSSI and suicidal behavior disorder were included as "conditions for further study." Trichotillomania (hair-pulling disorder) and excoriation (skin-picking disorder) are however classified by DSM-5 within obsessive-compulsive and related disorders, while pica (which is sometimes regarded as a form of SIB in people with neurodevelopmental conditions) is classified by DSM-5 as a distinct "feeding and eating disorder." Meanwhile, the self-injurious behaviors such as head-hitting which cause concern for many people with neurodevelopmental conditions (NDCs) remain outside of the DSM-5 diagnostic framework.

F. Furniss, A. B. Biswas, *Self-Injurious Behavior in Individuals with Neurodevelopmental Conditions*, Autism and Child Psychopathology Series,
https://doi.org/10.1007/978-3-030-36016-0_1

The utility for diagnosis and treatment of distinguishing between different types of self-injury, and the grounds for making such distinctions, thus remain topics for further research both for people with NDCs and for others. The very use of the term SIB may unhelpfully imply commonalities of etiology and causation between apparently diverse topographies of behavior engaged in by people experiencing different neurodevelopmental, neurological, and psychiatric conditions (Schroeder, Mulick, & Rojahn, 1980). On the other hand, the fact that many people with NDCs engage in multiple forms of SIB suggests the existence of at least some common causal factors underlying different topographies.

One of Skinner's (1950) concerns regarding the adoption of a theoretical focus in research on behavior was that when psychological theories were discredited or discarded, the data collected in the course of research guided by the hypotheses were often simply discarded together with the theory. The observations of astute clinicians may share the same fate when the model of care within which they practiced is superseded. Some useful insights into the dynamics of SIB may therefore still be gleaned by studying previous attempts to derive clinically useful categorizations of subtypes of SIB. This chapter briefly reviews developments in the conceptualization of SIB throughout the nineteenth, twentieth, and twenty-first centuries, together with attempts to develop taxonomic systems. As developments in research into a number of adult mental health conditions such as schizophrenia and bipolar disorder are increasingly leading to these also being conceptualized as NDCs, the chapter also briefly reviews arguments for and against considering SIB in persons with NDCs associated with childhood developmental disabilities as a phenomenon distinct from deliberate self-harm in people without such conditions.

1.2 Conceptualizing Non-suicidal Self-Injury in the Nineteenth Century

Although the numbers of private and charitable asylums and hospitals had expanded substantially for at least 100 years previously, the scientific study of self-harm (and of course many other mental health conditions) was stimulated by the development of public institutions for people with mental health problems in the mid-nineteenth century. The *American Journal of Insanity*, later to become the *American Journal of Psychiatry*, commenced publication in 1844, followed by the *Asylum Journal*, the predecessor of the *British Journal of Psychiatry,* in 1853. Even prior to these developments, however, medical practitioners had begun to differentiate between patients who engaged in self-harm with a view to suicide and those who did so without suicidal intent (Angelotta, 2015; Chaney, 2013). Clinical notes from the Bethlem Royal Hospital in 1853 recorded that one patient picked at his skin to the extent that sores had developed on his face, head, and legs, while another banged her head against walls and bit herself (Chaney, 2013). By the late nineteenth century, psychiatrists (we use this term to refer to medical practitioners working with the asylums irrespective of their background) such as Adam (1883) were also differentiating between harm self-inflicted by people experiencing psychosis and those who self-injured in the absence of psychosis (Angelotta, 2015). As the growth of the large public asylums gave psychiatrists opportunities to observe greater numbers of patients, they also noted numerous cases in which patients self-harmed by hitting their own heads or bodies with clenched fists, skin-picking, self-biting, or pulling out their own hair, and distinguished these cases of repetitive self-harm from both those involving single acts of major self-wounding and those which presented an episodic, remitting-relapsing, course (Angelotta, 2015).

The increased use of the term "self-mutilation," rather than the previously used "self-injury," to refer to such behaviors in the second half of the nineteenth century possibly reflects an increased focus on understanding the causes of such behaviors rather than simply describing them (Chaney, 2013). Nineteenth-century psychiatrists had noted that individuals often engaged in more than one type of self-harm (Chaney, 2013), perhaps suggesting that common causal factors might be involved in different behavioral topographies. Nevertheless, attempts were made to differentiate causation across different types of cases. Command hallucinations were proposed to be the cause in cases accompanied by psychosis, whereas self-injury in the absence of psychosis was suggested to be motivated by remorse or self-hatred, malingering and task avoidance, or a desire to elicit sympathy and attention from other people. It was considered that repetitive minor self-injury such as skin-picking in patients with "dementia" on the other hand might be accounted for simply by "nervous, fidgety, restless habits, generating a desire to be doing something" (Adam, 1892, quoted by Angelotta, 2015) or to originate from an irritable state of the skin. Griesinger (1864) ascribed a major role to "decreased sensibility..... anaesthesia or analgesia" (p. 539) in cases of self-mutilation, including those where other factors might be involved. Self-mutilation was frequently observed to be associated with melancolia, but was also argued to result from mania or impaired impulse control or aggression which was directed toward the self in the absence of an external target (Chaney, 2013). Howden (1882), describing a family in which several members had engaged in self-harm, noted its co-occurrence with somatic disorder and hypothesized an inherited cause.

In the course of the second half of the nineteenth century, psychiatrists had thus developed an implicit taxonomy of subtypes of self-injury (Fig. 1.1) in which behavioral topography was only partially correlated with causation. For those cases not accompanied by delusions or hallucinations, depressed mood, impaired impulse control, hypoalgesia or analgesia, and physical discomfort or irritation were all hypothesized to be contributing factors. As yet, however, differentiation of causality had rather few implications for treatment, in which care and supervision, sound nutrition, and opportunities for exercise and occupation were regarded as important elements. An exception was in the use of restraint. Asylum psychiatrists had observed that some of their patients had developed their own ways of physically preventing themselves from self-harming, and despite a general ethos toward minimizing use of restraint in the later nineteenth century, padded gloves and "strong dresses" were used either to physically prevent or to minimize the damage caused

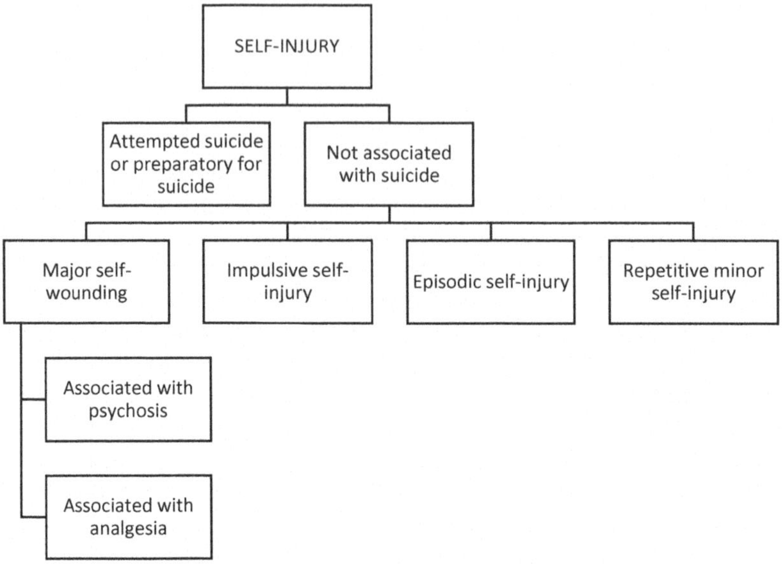

Fig. 1.1 An implicit taxonomy of self-injury in late nineteenth-century psychiatry

by various types of SIB; indeed, asylum medical notes sometimes recorded patients requesting the application of such restraints (Chaney, 2013). In some cases, it was observed that following a period of time in which restraints were applied, the patient ceased self-injury when they were removed, suggesting that the self-injury might have been a habit, developed in a context of poor impulse control, which could be cured by a period of physical prevention.

By the turn of the century, however, new theoretical frameworks in psychiatry began to contribute to the understanding of self-harm. The eclectic conceptual framework of the nineteenth century, which had grown from the clinical work of the asylum psychiatrists, and which had drawn freely on concepts from a variety of fields of study, began to be replaced by coherent psychological theories which emphasized the importance of unconscious motivation.

1.3 Conceptualizing Non-suicidal Self-Injury in the Twentieth Century

In 1899, the Section of Psychology of the British Medical Association held its Annual Meeting in Portsmouth, UK. The number of papers submitted for presentation was so great, and the discussions following presentations so lively, that several papers had to be "taken as read" because of lack of time or absence of the authors (Section of Psychology, British Medical Association, 1899). Among these was a paper by T.H. Hyslop, the Superintendent of the Bethlem Royal Hospital in London, on the subject of "Double Consciousness" (Hyslop, 1899). Although there had long been controversy as to the extent to which certain mental operations could take place without consciousness (Davies, 1873), and interest in the phenomena seen in hypnotic states (Section of Psychology, 1880), Hyslop's paper reflected the growing influence of the idea that there could exist organized systems of motive which were inaccessible to everyday waking consciousness. A person might therefore engage in self-injury for reasons of which they themselves were unaware or might unconsciously restrain themselves so as to avoid causing excessive self-harm from behaviors engaged in deliberately (Chaney, 2013). The rapid development and dissemination of these new psychological theories are illustrated by the fact that when Pernet (1915) presented two cases of dermatitis factitia (skin lesions which were believed to have been caused by the patients themselves) to the Dermatological Section of the Royal Society of Medicine, there appears to have been broad agreement on the importance of unconscious mental processes in their causation; the debate concerned whether these were best understood in terms of the Freudian theory of repression or though French psychiatrist Pierre Janet's concepts of coexistent dual personalities.

Janet himself (1906) continued to argue that "subconscious phenomena" motivated impulsive behaviors including self-injury in only a proportion of cases. In others, he asserted, the fundamental cause of the self-injury was a state of depression; impulsive behaviors such as self-injury (or, in other cases, impulsive drinking, eating, or exercise) became linked to the state of depression as "accidental phenomena" when the patient discovered that the stimulation of engaging in the behavior temporarily lifted their depressed mood. In some cases, Janet observed, the impulsive behaviors linked to the underlying depressive state changed over the years. An originally bulimic patient, for example, might later develop an impulsive need to walk. Generally, however, a patient would increasingly engage in one particular form of impulsive behavior, unable in their depressed mood to explore alternative and less damaging sources of stimulation.

Despite Janet's caution that "We must not think that all the impulsions in the various neuroses and psychoses have always the same mechanism" (Janet, 1906, p. 2), the elegance, simplicity, and explanatory power of the new psychological hypotheses of subconscious phenomena represented an exciting advance on the ad hoc, multidisciplinary explanations of earlier psychiatrists. Psychoanalytic case reports from the earlier years of the twentieth century continued however to reflect that view that self-injury could be multiply motivated both within and across cases, with inability to cope with mental distress following childhood psychosexual trauma, masochism, sexual relief, the castration complex, and a need for consideration from others all hypothesized to play a role (Angelotta, 2015). The work of Karl Menninger (1933, 1935, 1938) however provided a further extension and rationalization of the psychoanalytic approach. In a classic exposition of the application of late Freudian theory to self-injury, Menninger argued that diverse forms of self-injury (and other problems) resulted from the conflict between the death and life instincts. Menninger's account proposed a single mechanism underlying suicide, self-injury, and a range of other clinical problems (and lifestyle choices), with differing outcomes dependent on the balance between instinctive and repressing forces. Although Menninger differentiated suicide, "chronic suicide" (including asceticism, alcoholism, and psychosis), "focal suicide" (including self-injury, malingering, impotence, and frigidity), and "organic suicide" (organic illness), all were explained by the same underlying process. Self-injury represented a crude defense against actual suicide in which the suicidal impulse was concentrated upon one part of the body as a substitute for the whole.

Menninger's work provided a unified account of a range of clinical phenomena which psychiatrists up to and including Janet had believed to be etiologically diverse and re-established a proposed continuum between suicide and self-injury. It also provided a theoretical explanation of an aspect of self-injury noted by earlier clinicians, namely, the subjective sense of relief from distress described by some patients as accompanying the act of self-harm, which could now be understood in terms of the achievement of a compromise between instinctive and repressing forces. Even before Menninger published his most comprehensive exposition of this unified theory of suicide and self-injury in his book *Man Against Himself* (1938), other psychiatrists (e.g., Zilboorg, 1937) began to observe that his hypothesis of a single fundamental dynamic underlying self-injury and suicide might be inadequate to explain the diversity of clinical presentations seen in people who engaged in self-injury. Although the influence of Menninger's work probably reduced interest in self-injury as a clinical issue in itself, epidemiological studies of the phenomenology of suicide and "attempted suicide" continued to raise questions as to the utility of the hypothesis of a single causal process. Hendin (1950), for example, found differences in mean age and gender balance between cases of attempted suicide seen at the Bellevue Psychiatric Hospital in New York and cases of actual suicide recorded by the City Department of Health, and through in-depth evaluation of 100 cases of attempted suicide noted apparent differences in "intent to die" between subgroups of patients with differing presentations. Hendin (1951) later expanded on these findings to propose a differential diagnosis of suicidal patients, based on "dynamic-motivational" factors but linked to clinical phenomenology. Critically, he differentiated five subgroups within the patients he studied. In three of these subgroups, there was high intent to die: patients with psychosis, for whom guilt was a major factor motivating suicide attempts which were often repeated, neurotic patients in whom there was a "turning back on the self" of aggressive drives following the loss of an object relationship which had previously satisfied those needs, and "passive" and "dependent" patients who made suicide attempts following the loss of a significant relationship, often in later middle age. In two other subgroups however, "emotionally immature" patients or those with "character disorders," Hendin noted minimal or low intent to die and interpersonal motivations of "spite" or forcing affection from others. Although the number of subgroups identified varied, subsequent studies of suicide and attempted suicide (e.g., Dorpat & Boswell, 1963) continued to identify a group of patients who harmed themselves with no intent to die and who self-injured with primarily interpersonal motives.

By the second half of the twentieth century, therefore, professional interest in NSSI as a clinical issue distinct from attempted suicide was renewed. Although much psychiatric research during this period focused on self-cutting, large-scale studies of psychiatric patients continued to confirm that patients engaged in a range of self-injurious behaviors. Phillips and Alkan (1961), for example, surveyed all patients in a large psychiatric hospital and found that over 4% engaged in self-injury, with most women who self-injured being reported to scratch, dig, or pick at their skin, while most male self-injurers were found to hit themselves. The latter years of the twentieth century and the start of the twenty-first saw a series of initiatives toward establishing self-injury as a distinct diagnostic category. Pattison and Kahan (1983) reviewed 56 published case reports of deliberate self-harm and argued for identification of a distinct syndrome characterized by onset in late adolescence; engagement in multiple forms of nonlethal self-harm in repeated episodes over extended time periods; associated psychological experiences of despair, anxiety, aggression, and cognitive constriction; and predisposing factors including lack of social support and alcohol or drug abuse. Muehlenkamp (2005) critically reviewed the evidence for self-injury as a phenomenon distinct from suicide and borderline personality disorder and proposed that it be considered a distinct syndrome, noting however that the etiology of SIB remained largely unknown and that research suggested the existence of differing subgroups of persons engaging in SIB.

1.4 Self-Injury in People with Neurodevelopmental Conditions

The psychiatrists of the nineteenth century were well aware that some patients with NDCs engaged in self-injury. Ireland (1872), in an article on "The classification and prognosis of idiocy," described a boy of 11 who experienced epilepsy and intellectual disabilities (IDs) and who struck his hand against walls and, when angry, bit his hand and hit his head. Self-injury in people with NDCs does not appear however to have stimulated scientific interest to the same extent as SIB in people without such conditions. This relative neglect may have resulted from the assumption that difficulties in volitional control and sensory insensitivity were sufficient explanations of self-injury in persons with NDCs. In the UK, prominent medical professionals working with people with NDCs such as Bucknill (1873) and Ireland (1886) were also more interested in promoting the adoption in the UK of the progressive educational approaches developed in continental Europe and the USA than in investigating the causes of emotional and behavioral difficulties. Further, the early psychiatrists were aware of the limitations of their methods in understanding the behavior of patients with intellectual and communication difficulties.

The development of scientific interest in SIB in people with NDCs in the twentieth century was, perhaps paradoxically, stimulated by the development of the new psychologies of unconscious motivation. The assumption that an understanding of the motives of a person's behavior could not be simply based on his or her self-report of those motives provided a new perspective for understanding SIB in people who could not provide such self-reports. In the early years of the century, Potter (1927) proposed that rhythmic slapping or biting of body parts by adults and children with severe IDs represented a form of "extragenital erotism," while more severe self-biting and self-hitting was a manifestation of masochism. In the latter case also however, Potter differentiated between rhythmic stereotyped SIB and that associated with "emotional outbreak." Zuk (1960) on the other hand argued that in children and adults with IDs, SIB resulted from aggressive impulses directed toward external sources of frustration rather than against the self. Zuk proposed that in situations of inaccessibility of the source of frustration, or fear of retaliation, aggressive impulses were directed against the nearest object, the person's own body, which was perceived as an external object owing to breakdown of the identification of the ego and the body.

By the middle of the twentieth century however, intrapsychic accounts of the causation of SIB were challenged by two new streams of empirical evidence. The first originated from reports that children with a disorder of uric acid metabolism engaged in severe SIB of a specific form, namely, biting of their own fingers and/or lips (Nyhan, 1965). Within a few years, Nyhan (1972), noting that children with Cornelia de Lange syndrome also engaged in SIB involving self-biting and skin-picking, had coined the term "behavioral phenotype" and suggested that SIB might be studied in nonhuman animal models, proposing that these behaviors might ultimately be accounted for by changes in neuroanatomical development in people with these syndromes. Almost simultaneously, single-case experiments began to demonstrate that rates of SIB were highly sensitive to changes in the social environment (Smolev, 1971). As early as the late 1950s and early 1960s, researchers had reported interventions in which the behavior of children without NDCs had been modified by changing the reactions of caring adults to the children's behavior (Williams, 1959; Zimmerman & Zimmerman, 1962). Others had shown that children with NDCs showed patterns of learning similar to those of children without such conditions in operant conditioning procedures (Orlando & Bijou, 1960). The first application of these approaches to SIB in a child with an NDC was reported by Wolf, Risley, and Mees (1963), who reported reduction to near-zero frequency of episodes of head-banging, self-scratching, and pulling of his own hair engaged in by a preschool boy, who was described as having an autism spectrum condition (ASC), following the introduction of an intervention of "time-out from positive reinforcement." The intervention involved placing the boy in a room on his own for a fixed period of time if he engaged in "tantrums" involving these self-injurious behaviors. Although the child rarely engaged in these forms of SIB after 2.5 months of the intervention, the frequency of episodes of less severe SIB such as face-slapping was reduced to near-zero levels only after a further 3 months of time-out. Approximately 1 year later, the boy entered a nursery school setting and began to react to attempts to engage him in play or activity by slapping his face; a time-out intervention was reinstated, and his face-slapping was reduced to zero levels after only three implementations of the time-out procedure (Wolf, Risley, Johnston, Harris, & Allen, 1967).

Throughout the remainder of the twentieth century and the years to date of the twenty-first, the conceptualizations of SIB as an aspect of the behavioral phenotype of specific syndromes, or alternatively as an operant behavior shaped and maintained by social reinforcement, have been highly influential in stimulating empirical research into SIB in people with NDCs and developments in psychosocial and pharmacological interventions (Huisman et al., 2018; Minshawi, Hurwitz, Morriss, & McDougle, 2015). Progress in understanding the etiology of SIB and developing a classificatory framework to guide treatment selection in individual cases has however been limited. Since the genetic abnormalities associated with several NDCs have been identified, and specific topographies of SIB are prominent in some of these conditions, there was early optimism that it would be possible to identify, and then disrupt, the chain of biological processes leading from the genetic abnormality to the behavior (Nyhan, 1972). The Lesch-Nyhan syndrome (LNS), for example, is associated with mutations of the *HPRT1* gene on the X chromosome, which cause absence or severe underproduction of hypoxanthine-guanine phosphoribosyltransferase (HPRT), an enzyme which enables cells to recycle purines, which are major building blocks for ribonucleic acid and deoxyribonucleic acid. This deficiency, for unknown reasons, is associated with reduced levels in the striatum of the neurotransmitter dopamine and the dopamine transporter protein, which returns dopamine which has been released into synapses to the presynaptic neuron. The striatum is involved in control of motor movements, and people with LNS experience severe motor handicaps comprising generalized dystonia and (for some) choreoathetosis. Although it often later progresses to include biting of the hands and fingers and self-hitting, the SIB experienced by people with LNS typically appears initially in the form of self-biting of the lips, often developing shortly after the eruption of teeth, suggesting a possible developmental relationship with the motor difficulties characteristic of LNS. However, it is not clear whether the SIB experienced by people with LNS is associated with reduced numbers (or reduced branching) of dopaminergic neurons or with hypersensitivity of dopamine receptors resulting from this dopaminergic deficiency, and pharmacological attempts both to increase dopamine production and to block the activity of dopamine receptors in people with LNS have produced variable effects on both motor difficulties and SIB (Bell, Kolobova, Crapper, & Ernst, 2016). As research progresses, even in the case of this apparently straightforward monogenic condition, it is becoming increasingly apparent that HPRT deficiency may produce a complex range of effects including dysregulation of transcription factor genes relevant to neuronal differentiation and development not only of dopamine receptors but also receptors for several other neurotransmitters (Torres & Puig, 2015).

In contrast to these attempts to delineate syndrome-specific causal pathways to the development of SIB, operant theorists have developed general, cross-syndrome models for the development of SIB. These typically propose that SIB develops from early repetitive behaviors through a process in which those behaviors first develop homeostatic functions in regulating overall degree of stimulation and are then shaped into SIB through socially or automatically mediated operant reinforcement (Guess & Carr, 1991; Kennedy, 2002). It is proposed that the severity of SIB increases through a process of shaping in which carers progressively reinforce increasingly severe forms of the behavior by ceasing to respond to milder forms but reinstating their response to the more severe and/or frequent behavior which occurs in the ensuing extinction burst (Oliver & Head, 1990).

Observational studies of the development of SIB in young children (Hall, Oliver, & Murphy, 2001; Oliver, Hall, & Murphy, 2005) have shown that children whose SIB increased with age were more likely to engage in SIB when levels of social contact with carers was low and that probability of social interaction decreased before episodes of SIB and increased during and following SIB, supporting the operant account of its development. In another study with younger children (aged between 14 and 32 months at the start of the study), Richman and Lindauer (2005) further observed that emergent "proto-SIB" was topographically related to pre-existing stereotyped behaviors and that for five children proto-SIB developed into actually injurious SIB, providing further support for the operant model. The principal support for the validity of the operant model of SIB is however the reported effectiveness of behavioral interventions based on the model. In a review of behavioral treatment of SIB published between 1964 and 2000, Kahng, Iwata, and Lewin (2002) noted that most interventions produced reductions in SIB of at least 80% from baseline to the end of treatment, with a mean reduction of 83.7%. The behavioral perspective replaces the classification of SIB based on its topography with one based on the functions of the behaviors, and intervention is matched to the assessed function of the behavior (Carr, 1977). The foundation for the application of this principle was provided when Iwata, Dorsey, Slifer, Bauman, and Richman (1982) described a method for assessing behavioral function prior to treatment planning. Iwata et al.'s (1982) methodology of "experimental functional analysis" (EFA) involves briefly placing the person engaging in SIB into a variety of highly structured social situations, each of which is designed to evoke high rates of problem behavior maintained by specific functions. In a review of applications of EFA in 152 cases of SIB in persons with developmental disabilities, Iwata et al. (1994) reported that social-negative reinforcement (e.g., escape from task demands) maintained SIB in 38.1% of the sample, social-positive reinforcement (e.g., securing attention from carers) maintained SIB for 26.3%, automatic (sensory) reinforcement accounted for 25.7% of cases, and SIB in 5.3% of cases was found to be maintained by multiple controlling variables. A subsequent review of 277 empirical studies, including 235 participants for whom SIB was the behavior assessed, similarly reported that a maintaining reinforcer was identified in almost 95% of cases (Hanley, Iwata, & McCord, 2003), while Hagopian, Rooker, Jessel, and DeLeon (2013) reported a further case series of people with IDs for whom EFA identified an operant function for challenging behaviors (including but not limited to SIB) in over 93% of cases.

The high proportion of cases in which operant functions of SIB are identified though EFAs has strengthened confidence in the ability of the operant model to account for the majority of cases in which SIB is observed (Iwata et al., 1994). Certainly, together with studies demonstrating social influences on SIB experienced by people with specific NDCs such as fragile X syndrome (Hall, Hustyi, & Barnett, 2018; Kurtz, Chin, Robinson, O'Connor, & Hagopian, 2015) and Smith-Magenis syndrome (Hodnett, Scheithauer, Call, Mevers, & Miller, 2018), these studies have established that the social environment is a major influence on SIB in many cases.

Despite this, and the high success rates of interventions based on the operant model, such interventions however rarely completely eliminate SIB, and the overall effectiveness of the interventions has not increased since the 1960s (DeLeon, Rodriguez-Catter, & Cataldo, 2002; Kahng et al., 2002). Further, questions remain regarding the high percentage of cases in which operant functions are identified through EFAs. Firstly, "automatic reinforcement," which is identified as the maintaining factor for SIB in over a quarter of cases (Iwata et al., 1994), is typically held to be the cause of SIB not only if SIB is most frequent in an "alone" condition (i.e., when the participant is observed when alone and without any means to occupy themselves) but also if rates of SIB are high across all conditions of the EFA (Hagopian et al., 1997). Secondly, operant-based interventions are successful in a substantially lower proportion of such cases than in cases where a social function of SIB has been identified (Iwata et al., 1994). Thirdly, in children under 5, cases in which automatic reinforcement is inferred because of high levels of SIB across all conditions, together with those in which no maintaining consequence is identified, account for over 50% of cases (Kurtz et al., 2003).

1.5 Understanding Self-Injury: Perspectives for the New Century

In retrospect, it appears that our understanding of SIB developed from the clinical empiricism and phenomenological categorizations of the nineteenth century into a phase of theoretical models (psychodynamic, biological, and operant) and functional classification in the twentieth. In the early years of this century, the indications that each of these models of SIB, despite their explanatory power, elegance, and clinical significance, may yet be incomplete has led to a renewed interest in direct study of the early development of SIB. A number of studies have now shown that substantial numbers of young children with and without NDCs show SIB or proto-SIB (Dimian et al., 2017; Kurtz, Chin, Huete, & Cataldo, 2012; MacLean & Dornbush, 2012; MacLean, Tervo, Hoch, Tervo, & Symons, 2010; Murphy, Hall, Oliver, & Kissi-Debra, 1999), that tissue-damaging SIB typically emerges before 25 months and at a comparable age to proto-SIB, that headbanging or hitting is commonly the first topography observed, and that many young children with IDs show these behaviors transiently (Baghdadli et al., 2008; Berkson, 2002; Berkson, Tupa, & Sherman, 2001; Chadwick, Kusel, Cuddy, & Taylor, 2005; Kurtz et al., 2003, 2012; Richman & Lindauer, 2005). Berkson (2002) and Kurtz et al. (2012) have reported that SIB was often first seen in association with tantrums following frustration or rapid situational transitions, but in cases in which social functions of the behavior are observed, these are predominantly positive, in contrast to the negative reinforcement processes frequently observed with older children (Iwata et al., 1994). Kurtz et al. (2012) have noted that many children start to engage in SIB at or before 1 year of age and rapidly begin to engage in multiple SIB topographies.

This resurgence of interest in the developmental phenomenology of SIB has raised new questions regarding the limitations of current theoretical models and led to renewed interest in categorical definition. Kurtz et al. (2012) noted that only 37% of their sample of 32 young children who had recently begun to engage in SIB also engaged in stereotyped behaviors and suggested that the operant model proposing development of SIB from early repetitive behaviors through a process involving socially or automatically mediated operant reinforcement (Guess & Carr, 1991; Kennedy, 2002; Oliver & Head, 1990) may reflect only one of several developmental pathways for the emergence of SIB. We (Furniss & Biswas, 2012) have suggested that the early age and dynamics of the emergence of SIB demonstrated by recent research are consistent with the proposal of Romanczyk and Matthews (1998) and Schroeder, Reese, Hellings, Loupe, and Tessel (1999) that one such pathway may be Pavlovian conditioning of aggression which is originally elicited by aversive stimulation (including pain caused by previous acts of SIB) or denial of expected reinforcement, but which may become conditioned to a variety of stimuli associated with such situations and then be both shaped and maintained by operant processes and elicited by environmental stimuli associated with SIB-related arousal via Pavlovian processes.

This developing awareness that there may be several pathways for the development of SIB has been accompanied by a renewed interest in defining subtypes of SIB. For individuals with NDCs, Mace and Mauk (1995) had suggested that SIB could be classified as operant, possibly biologic, or mixed operant and possibly biologic. They proposed four subtypes of "possibly biologic" SIB, comprising SIB with extreme tissue damage, repetitive or stereotyped SIB, high rate SIB with agitation when SIB is interrupted, and SIB co-occurring with agitation. From the operant perspective, SIB was generally classified functionally according to the reinforcement processes identified or hypothesized as maintaining the behavior, leading to a broad classification of SIB as socially or automatically reinforced SIB. Hagopian and his colleagues (Hagopian & Frank-Crawford, 2018; Hagopian, Rooker, & Yenokyan, 2018; Hagopian, Rooker, & Zarcone, 2015; Hagopian, Rooker, Zarcone, Bonner, & Arevalo, 2017) have now proposed however that "automatically reinforced" SIB can be differentiated into three subtypes, one characterized by high rates of occurrence in conditions with minimal external stimulation but low rates in enriched environments, one characterized by high rates of occurrence across high and low stimulation conditions, and one characterized by the presence of self-restraint, and have demonstrated that the first subtype is more amenable to reinforcement-based intervention than the second. Meanwhile, research comparing the prevalence and phenomenology of SIB across NDCs has shown that although in some genetic syndromes (e.g., Smith-Magenis syndrome) the prevalences of multiple topographies of SIB are elevated by comparison with people with IDs of heterogeneous etiology, people with other NDCs are at significantly elevated risk for only some specific topographies of SIB, e.g., self-scratching in Prader-Willi syndrome (Arron, Oliver, Moss, Berg, & Burbidge, 2011). Such findings, together with findings that the behavioral and affective correlates of SIB also differ across syndromes (Arron et al., 2011), raise the possibility that causal mechanisms and developmental pathways to SIB may differ between NDCs.

Current perspectives on the nature and causes of SIB are therefore challenging the utility of attempts to develop unified accounts of the development of SIB across different NDCs and have re-emphasized the need for detailed study of the development and phenomenology of SIB in each condition (Oliver, 2017). Nevertheless, throughout almost two centuries of scientific study, clinicians and researchers have repeatedly arrived at certain broad conclusions. The first is that a meaningful distinction in terms of phenomenology and causation can be made between SIB and suicide and attempted suicide. The second is that the extremely severe but infrequent episodes of SIB sometimes associated with psychosis can likewise be meaningfully differentiated from other forms of SIB. The third conclusion is that those other forms of SIB comprise at least three subtypes; one is repetitive, stereotyped SIB which can be relatively easily interrupted by providing stimulation or environmental enrichment, and one appears "compulsive" in the sense that it is also very frequent but is difficult to interrupt and persistent across varying levels of alternative stimulation. The third subtype of SIB appears "impulsive" insofar as the person engages in SIB in response to interpersonal challenges or other stressors but seems unable to inhibit the SIB when faced with those challenges even if the overall level of external motivation for their SIB has been reduced.

This outline categorization of SIB clearly mirrors the descriptive classification of SIB in persons without NDCs as major, stereotypic, compulsive, and impulsive (Favazza, 2012) and raises the issue of whether SIB in people with and without NDCs can usefully be approached within a common conceptual framework. The salience of this question has increased as developmental studies have shown that at least some people with psychiatric disorders associated with SIB, such as bipolar disorder (MacPherson, Weinstein, & West, 2018), show trajectories of cognitive development suggesting a neurodevelopmental component to the disorder (Bora & Özerdem, 2017). Studies such as those of Nock and Prinstein (2004, 2005) have shown that functional classification of SIB according to source (social vs. automatic) and type (positive vs. negative) of reinforcement, drawing on the operant perspective, can be applied in studying SIB in people without NDCs, and Crapper and Ernst (2015) have argued for increased efforts to understand commonalities in causation of SIB in people with and without NDCs. It does indeed seem very likely that in the longer term, common causal factors will be identified in the development of SIB in people with and without NDCs. Currently however divergences in research approaches used between people with and without NDCs, including definitions of SIB, sub-population studies, and degree of reliance on self-reporting versus observational or third-party reports of situational correlates of SIB, make it difficult to effectively integrate research findings across groups. In the remainder of this volume, we shall therefore focus almost entirely on research into SIB in people with NDCs.

References

Adam, J. (1883). Cases of self-mutilation by the Insane. *Journal of Mental Science, 29*(126), 213–219. https://doi.org/10.1192/bjp.29.126.213

American Psychiatric Association. (2013). *Diagnostic and statistical manual of mental disorders* (5th ed.). Washington, DC: American Psychiatric Association.

Angelotta, C. (2015). Defining and refining self-harm: A historical perspective on nonsuicidal self-injury. *Journal of Nervous and Mental Disease, 203*(2), 75–80. https://doi.org/10.1097/NMD.0000000000000243

Arron, K., Oliver, C., Moss, J., Berg, K., & Burbidge, C. (2011). The prevalence and phenomenology of self-injurious and aggressive behaviour in genetic syndromes. *Journal of Intellectual Disability Research, 55*(2), 109–120. https://doi.org/10.1111/j.1365-2788.2010.01337.x

Baghdadli, A., Picot, M. C., Pry, R., Michelon, C., Burzstejn, C., Lazartigues, A., & Aussilloux, C. (2008). What factors are related to a negative outcome of self-injurious behaviour during childhood in pervasive developmental disorders? *Journal of Applied Research in Intellectual Disabilities, 21*(2), 142–149. https://doi.org/10.1111/j.1468-3148.2007.00389.x

Bell, S., Kolobova, I., Crapper, L., & Ernst, C. (2016). Lesch-Nyhan syndrome: Models, theories, and therapies. *Molecular Syndromology, 7*(6), 302–311. https://doi.org/10.1159/000449296

Berkson, G. (2002). Early development of stereotyped and self-injurious behaviors: II. Age trends. *American Journal on Mental Retardation, 107*(6), 468–477. https://doi.org/10.1352/0895-8017(2002)107<0468:EDOSAS>2.0.CO;2

Berkson, G., Tupa, M., & Sherman, L. (2001). Early development of stereotyped and self-injurious behaviors: I. incidence. *American Journal on Mental Retardation, 106*(6), 539–547. https://doi.org/10.1352/0895-8017(2001)106<0539:EDOSAS>2.0.CO;2

Bora, E., & Özerdem, A. (2017). Meta-analysis of longitudinal studies of cognition in bipolar disorder: Comparison with healthy controls and schizophrenia. *Psychological Medicine, 47*(16), 2753–2766. https://doi.org/10.1017/S0033291717001490

Bucknill, J. (1873). Address on idiocy. *Journal of Mental Science, 19*(86), 169–183. https://doi.org/10.1192/bjp.19.86.169

Carr, E. G. (1977). The motivation of self-injurious behavior: A review of some hypotheses. *Psychological Bulletin, 84*(4), 800–816. https://doi.org/10.1037/0033-2909.84.4.800

Chadwick, O., Kusel, Y., Cuddy, M., & Taylor, E. (2005). Psychiatric diagnoses and behaviour problems from childhood to early adolescence in young people with severe intellectual disabilities. *Psychological Medicine, 35*(5), 751–760. https://doi.org/10.1017/S0033291704003733

Chaney, S. (2013). *Self-mutilation and psychiatry: Impulse, identity and the unconscious in british explanations of self-inflicted injury, c. 1864–1914*. PhD thesis. London: University College London. Retrieved from http://discovery.ucl.ac.uk/1389021/

Crapper, L., & Ernst, C. (2015). Comparative analysis of self-injury in people with psychopathology or neurodevelopmental disorders. *Pediatric Clinics of North America, 62*(3), 619–631. https://doi.org/10.1016/j.pcl.2015.03.001

Davies, W. (1873). Consciousness and "Unconscious Cerebration". *Journal of Mental Science, 19(86)*, 202–217. https://doi.org/10.1192/bjp.19.86.202

DeLeon, I. G., Rodriguez-Catter, V., & Cataldo, M. F. (2002). Treatment: current standards of care and their research implications. In S. R. Schroeder, M. L. Oster-Granite, & T. Thompson (Eds.), *Self-injurious behavior: Gene-brain-behavior relationships* (pp. 81–91). Washington, DC: American Psychological Association.

Dimian, A. F., Botteron, K. N., Dager, S. R., Elison, J. T., Estes, A. M., Pruett, J. R., ... Wolff, J. J. (2017). Potential risk factors for the development of self-injurious behavior among infants at risk for autism spectrum disorder. *Journal of Autism and Developmental Disorders, 47*(5), 1403–1415. https://doi.org/10.1007/s10803-017-3057-9

Dorpat, T. L., & Boswell, J. W. (1963). An evaluation of suicidal intent in suicide attempts. *Comprehensive Psychiatry, 4*(2), 117–125. https://doi.org/10.1016/S0010-440X(63)80093-0

Favazza, A. R. (2012). Nonsuicidal self-injury: How categorization guides treatment. *Current Psychiatry, 11*(3), 21–25+A. Retrieved from https://www.mdedge.com/psychiatry/article/66298/nonsuicidal-self-injury-how-categorization-guides-treatment

Furniss, F., & Biswas, A. B. (2012). Recent research on aetiology, development and phenomenology of self-injurious behaviour in people with intellectual disabilities: A systematic review and implications for treatment. *Journal of Intellectual Disability Research, 56*(5), 453–475. https://doi.org/10.1111/j.1365-2788.2012.01534.x

Griesinger, W. (1864). German Psychiatrie; an Introductory Lecture, read at the opening of the Psychiatric Clinique, in Zürich (Summer Session, 1863). *Journal of Mental Science, 9(48)*, 531–547. https://doi.org/10.1192/bjp.9.48.531

Guess, D., & Carr, E. (1991). Emergence and maintenance of stereotypy and self-injury. *American Journal on Mental Retardation, 96*(3), 299–319.

Hagopian, L. P., Fisher, W. W., Thompson, R. H., Owen-Deschryver, J., Iwata, B. A., & Wacker, D. P. (1997). Toward the development of structured criteria for interpretation of functional analysis data. *Journal of Applied Behavior Analysis, 30*(2), 313–326. https://doi.org/10.1901/jaba.1997.30-313

Hagopian, L. P., & Frank-Crawford, M. A. (2018). Classification of self-injurious behaviour across the continuum of relative environmental–biological influence. *Journal of Intellectual Disability Research, 62*(12), 1108–1113. https://doi.org/10.1111/jir.12430

Hagopian, L. P., Rooker, G. W., Jessel, J., & DeLeon, I. G. (2013). Initial functional analysis outcomes and modifications in pursuit of differentiation: A summary of 176 inpatient cases. *Journal of Applied Behavior Analysis, 46*(1), 88–100. https://doi.org/10.1002/jaba.25

Hagopian, L. P., Rooker, G. W., & Yenokyan, G. (2018). Identifying predictive behavioral markers: A demonstration using automatically reinforced self-injurious behavior. *Journal of Applied Behavior Analysis, 51*(3), 443–465. https://doi.org/10.1002/jaba.477

Hagopian, L. P., Rooker, G. W., & Zarcone, J. R. (2015). Delineating subtypes of self-injurious behavior maintained by automatic reinforcement. *Journal of Applied Behavior Analysis, 48*(3), 523–543. https://doi.org/10.1002/jaba.236

Hagopian, L. P., Rooker, G. W., Zarcone, J. R., Bonner, A. C., & Arevalo, A. R. (2017). Further analysis of subtypes of automatically reinforced SIB: A replication and quantitative analysis of published datasets. *Journal of Applied Behavior Analysis, 50*(1), 48–66. https://doi.org/10.1002/jaba.368

Hall, S., Oliver, C., & Murphy, G. (2001). Early development of self-injurious behavior: An empirical study. *American Journal on Mental Retardation, 106*(2), 189–199+201+204. https://doi.org/10.1352/0895-8017(2001)106<0189:EDOSIB>2.0.CO;2

Hall, S. S., Hustyi, K. M., & Barnett, R. P. (2018). Examining the influence of social-environmental variables on self-injurious behaviour in adolescent boys with fragile X syndrome. *Journal of Intellectual Disability Research, 62*(12), 1072–1085. https://doi.org/10.1111/jir.12489

Hanley, G. P., Iwata, B. A., & McCord, B. E. (2003). Functional analysis of problem behavior: A review. *Journal of Applied Behavior Analysis, 36*(2), 147–185. https://doi.org/10.1901/jaba.2003.36-147

Hendin, H. (1950). Attempted suicide: A psychiatric and statistical study. *The Psychiatric Quarterly, 24*(1), 39–46. https://doi.org/10.1007/BF01813023

Hendin, H. (1951). Psychodynamic motivational factors in suicide. *The Psychiatric Quarterly, 25*(1-4), 672–678. https://doi.org/10.1007/BF01584312

Hodnett, J., Scheithauer, M., Call, N. A., Mevers, J. L., & Miller, S. J. (2018). Using a functional analysis followed by differential reinforcement and extinction to reduce challenging behaviors in children with Smith-Magenis syndrome. *American Journal on Intellectual and Developmental Disabilities, 123*(6), 558–573. https://doi.org/10.1352/1944-7558-123.6.558

Howden, J. (1882). Notes of a Case—Mania followed by Hyperesthesia and Osteomalacia, Singular family tendency to excessive constipation and self-mutilation. *Journal of Mental Science, 28*(121), 49–56. https://doi.org/10.1192/S0368315X00230284

Huisman, S., Mulder, P., Kuijk, J., Kerstholt, M., van Eeghen, A., Leenders, A., … Hennekam, R. (2018). Self-injurious behavior. *Neuroscience and Biobehavioral Reviews, 84*, 483–491. https://doi.org/10.1016/j.neubiorev.2017.02.027

Hyslop, T. B. (1899). On "Double Consciousness". *British Medical Journal, 2*(2021), 782–786.

Ireland, W. (1872). On the classification and prognosis of idiocy. *Journal of Mental Science, 18*(83), 333–354. https://doi.org/10.1192/bjp.18.83.333

Ireland, W. (1886). On the admission of idiotic and imbecile children into lunatic asylums. *Journal of Mental Science, 32*(138), 182–193. https://doi.org/10.1192/bjp.32.138.182

Iwata, B. A., Dorsey, M. F., Slifer, K. J., Bauman, K. E., & Richman, G. S. (1982). Toward a functional analysis of self-injury. *Analysis and Intervention in Developmental Disabilities, 2*(1), 3–20. https://doi.org/10.1016/0270-4684(82)90003-9

Iwata, B. A., Pace, G. M., Dorsey, M. F., Zarcone, J. R., Vollmer, T. R., Smith, R. G., … Willis, K. D. (1994). The functions of self-injurious behavior: An experimental-epidemiological analysis. *Journal of Applied Behavior Analysis, 27*(2), 215–240. https://doi.org/10.1901/jaba.1994.27-215

Janet, P. (1906). On the pathogenesis of some impulsions. *Journal of Abnormal Psychology, 1*(*1*), 1–17. https://doi.org/10.1037/h0069930

Kahng, S., Iwata, B. A., & Lewin, A. B. (2002). Behavioral treatment of self-injury, 1964 to 2000. *American Journal on Mental Retardation, 107*(3), 212–221+234. https://doi.org/10.1352/0895-8017(2002)107<0212:BTOSIT>2.0.CO;2

Kennedy, C. H. (2002). Evolution of stereotypy into self-injury. In S. R. Schroeder, M. L. Oster-Granite, & T. Thompson (Eds.), *Self-injurious behavior: gene-brain-behavior relationships* (pp. 133–143). Washington, DC: American Psychological Association.

Kurtz, P. F., Chin, M. D., Huete, J. M., & Cataldo, M. F. (2012). Identification of emerging self-injurious behavior in young children: A preliminary study. *Journal of Mental Health Research in Intellectual Disabilities, 5*(3-4), 260–285. https://doi.org/10.1080/19315864.2011.600809

Kurtz, P. F., Chin, M. D., Huete, J. M., Tarbox, R. S. F., O'Connor, J. T., Paclawskyj, T. R., & Rush, K. S. (2003). Functional analysis and treatment of self-injurious behavior in young children: A summary of 30 cases. *Journal of Applied Behavior Analysis, 36*(2), 205–219. https://doi.org/10.1901/jaba.2003.36-205

Kurtz, P. F., Chin, M. D., Robinson, A. N., O'Connor, J. T., & Hagopian, L. P. (2015). Functional analysis and treatment of problem behavior exhibited by children with fragile X syndrome. *Research in Developmental Disabilities, 43-44*, 150–166. https://doi.org/10.1016/j.ridd.2015.06.010

Mace, F. C., & Mauk, J. E. (1995). Bio-behavioral diagnosis and treatment of self-injury. *Mental Retardation and Developmental Disabilities Research Reviews, 1*(2), 104–110. https://doi.org/10.1002/mrdd.1410010206

MacLean, W. E., Jr., Tervo, R. C., Hoch, J., Tervo, M., & Symons, F. J. (2010). Self-injury among a community cohort of young children at risk for intellectual and developmental disabilities. *Journal of Pediatrics, 157*(6), 979–983. https://doi.org/10.1016/j.jpeds.2010.05.052

MacLean, W. E., & Dornbush, K. (2012). Self-injury in a statewide sample of young children with developmental disabilities. *Journal of Mental Health Research in Intellectual Disabilities, 5*(3-4), 236–245. https://doi.org/10.1080/19315864.2011.590627

MacPherson, H. A., Weinstein, S. M., & West, A. E. (2018). Non-suicidal self-injury in pediatric bipolar disorder: Clinical correlates and impact on psychosocial treatment outcomes. *Journal of Abnormal Child Psychology, 46*(4), 857–870. https://doi.org/10.1007/s10802-017-0331-4

Menninger, K. A. (1933). Psychoanalytic aspects of suicide. *International Journal of Psychoanalysis, 14*, 376–390.

Menninger, K. A. (1935). A psychoanalytic study of the significance of self-mutilations. *Psychoanalytic Quarterly, 4*(3), 408–466. https://doi.org/10.1080/21674086.1935.11925248

Menninger, K. A. (1938). *Man against himself.* New York: Harcourt Brace & Company.

Minshawi, N. F., Hurwitz, S., Morriss, D., & McDougle, C. J. (2015). Multidisciplinary assessment and treatment of self-injurious behavior in autism spectrum disorder and intellectual

disability: Integration of psychological and biological theory and approach. *Journal of Autism and Developmental Disorders, 45*(6), 1541–1568. https://doi.org/10.1007/s10803-014-2307-3
Muehlenkamp, J. J. (2005). Self-injurious behavior as a separate clinical syndrome. *American Journal of Orthopsychiatry, 75*(2), 324–333. https://doi.org/10.1037/0002-9432.75.2.324
Murphy, G., Hall, S., Oliver, C., & Kissi-Debra, R. (1999). Identification of early self-injurious behaviour in young children with intellectual disability. *Journal of Intellectual Disability Research, 43*(3), 149–163. https://doi.org/10.1046/j.1365-2788.1999.00183.x
Nock, M. K., & Prinstein, M. J. (2004). A functional approach to the assessment of self-mutilative behavior. *Journal of Consulting and Clinical Psychology, 72*(5), 885–890. https://doi.org/10.1037/0022-006X.72.5.885
Nock, M. K., & Prinstein, M. J. (2005). Contextual features and behavioral functions of self-mutilation among adolescents. *Journal of Abnormal Psychology, 114*(1), 140–146. https://doi.org/10.1037/0021-843X.114.1.140
Nyhan, W. L. (1965). A disorder of uric acid metabolism and cerebral function in childhood. *Arthritis & Rheumatism, 8*(4), 659–664. https://doi.org/10.1002/art.1780080425
Nyhan, W. L. (1972). Behavioral phenotypes in organic genetic disease: Presidential address to the Society for Pediatric Research, May 1, 1971. *Pediatric Research, 6*(1), 1–9. https://doi.org/10.1203/00006450-197201000-00001
Oliver, C. (2017). The importance of knowing when to be precise. *Journal of Intellectual Disability Research, 61*(12), 1079–1082. https://doi.org/10.1111/jir.12446
Oliver, C., Hall, S., & Murphy, G. (2005). The early development of self-injurious behaviour: Evaluating the role of social reinforcement. *Journal of Intellectual Disability Research, 49*(8), 591–599. https://doi.org/10.1111/j.1365-2788.2005.00694.x
Oliver, C., & Head, D. (1990). Self-injurious behaviour in people with learning disabilities: Determinants and interventions. *International Review of Psychiatry, 2*(1), 101–116. https://doi.org/10.3109/09540269009028276
Orlando, R., & Bijou, S. W. (1960). Single and multiple schedules of reinforcement in developmentally retarded children. *Journal of the Experimental Analysis of Behavior, 3*(4), 339–348. https://doi.org/10.1901/jeab.1960.3-339
Pattison, E. M., & Kahan, J. (1983). The deliberate self-harm syndrome. *American Journal of Psychiatry, 140*(7), 867–872. https://doi.org/10.1176/ajp.140.7.867
Pernet, G. (1915). Two cases of dermatitis factitia. *Journal of the Royal Society of Medicine, 8*(Dermatolological_Section), 89–91. https://doi.org/10.1177/003591571500800349
Phillips, R. H., & Alkan, M. (1961). Some aspects of self-mutilation in the general population of a large psychiatric hospital. *The Psychiatric Quarterly, 35*(3), 421–423. https://doi.org/10.1007/BF01573610
Potter, H. W. (1927). An introductory study of the erotic behavior of idiots. *Journal of Nervous and Mental Disease, 65*(5), 497–507. https://doi.org/10.1097/00005053-192705000-00004
Richman, D. M., & Lindauer, S. E. (2005). Longitudinal assessment of stereotypic, proto-injurious, and self-injurious behavior exhibited by young children with developmental delays. *American Journal on Mental Retardation, 110*(6), 439–450+497. https://doi.org/10.1352/0895-8017(2005)110[439:LAOSPA]2.0.CO;2
Romanczyk, R. G., & Matthews, A. L. (1998). Physiological state as antecedent: utilization in functional analysis. In J. K. Luiselli & M. J. Cameron (Eds.), *Antecedent control: Innovative approaches to behavioral support* (pp. 115–138). Baltimore: Paul H. Brookes.
Sallustro, F., & Atwell, C. W. (1978). Body rocking, head banging, and head rolling in normal children. *The Journal of Pediatrics, 93*(4), 704–708. https://doi.org/10.1016/S0022-3476(78)80922-6
Schroeder, S. R., Mulick, J. A., & Rojahn, J. (1980). The definition, taxonomy, epidemiology, and ecology of self-injurious behavior. *Journal of Autism and Developmental Disorders, 10(4)*, 417–432.
Schroeder, S. R., Reese, R. M., Hellings, J., Loupe, P., & Tessel, R. E. (1999). The cause of self-injurious behavior and their clinical applications. In N. A. Wieseler & R. H. Hanson (Eds.),

Challenging behavior of persons with mental health disorders and severe developmental disabilities (pp. 65–87). Washington, DC: American Association on Mental Retardation.
Section of Psychology. (1880). Discussion on sleep and hypnotism. *Journal of Mental Science, 26*(115), 471–474.
Section of Psychology. (1899). British Medical Association Annual Meeting, Portsmouth, 1899. *Journal of Mental Science, 45*(191), 841–843.
Skinner, B. F. (1950). Are theories of learning necessary? *Psychological Review, 57*(4), 193–216. https://doi.org/10.1037/h0054367
Smolev, S. R. (1971). Use of operant techniques for the modification of self-injurious behavior. *American Journal of Mental Deficiency, 76*(3), 295–305.
Torres, R. J., & Puig, J. G. (2015). Hypoxanthine deregulates genes involved in early neuronal development. Implications in Lesch-Nyhan disease pathogenesis. *Journal of Inherited Metabolic Disease, 38*(6), 1109–1118. https://doi.org/10.1007/s10545-015-9854-4
Williams, C. D. (1959). The elimination of tantrum behavior by extinction procedures. *Journal of Abnormal and Social Psychology, 59*(2), 269. https://doi.org/10.1037/h0046688
Wolf, M., Risley, T., Johnston, M., Harris, F., & Allen, E. (1967). Application of operant conditioning procedures to the behavior problems of an autistic child: A follow-up and extension. *Behaviour Research and Therapy, 5*(2), 103–111. https://doi.org/10.1016/0005-7967(67)90004-6
Wolf, M., Risley, T., & Mees, H. (1963). Application of operant conditioning procedures to the behaviour problems of an autistic child. *Behaviour Research and Therapy, 1*(2-4), 305–312. https://doi.org/10.1016/0005-7967(63)90045-7
Yates, T. M. (2004). The developmental psychopathology of self-injurious behavior: Compensatory regulation in posttraumatic adaptation. *Clinical Psychology Review, 24*(1), 35–74. https://doi.org/10.1016/j.cpr.2003.10.001
Zilboorg, G. (1937). Considerations on suicide, with particular reference to that of the young. *American Journal of Orthopsychiatry, 7*(1), 15–31. https://doi.org/10.1111/j.1939-0025.1937.tb05556.x
Zimmerman, E. H., & Zimmerman, J. (1962). The alteration of behavior in a special classroom situation. *Journal of the Experimental Analysis of Behavior, 5*(1), 59–60. https://doi.org/10.1901/jeab.1962.5-59
Zuk, G. H. (1960). Psychodynamic implications of self-injury in defective children and adults. *Journal of Clinical Psychology, 16*(1), 58–60. https://doi.org/10.1002/1097-4679(196001)16:1<58::AID-JCLP2270160123>3.0.CO;2-6

Chapter 2
Phenomenology and Natural History of Self-Injurious Behavior

2.1 Introduction

A key test of any model for understanding the self-injurious behavior (SIB) experienced by people with neurodevelopmental conditions (NDCs) is how well it fits with the observed phenomenology, incidence and prevalence, and natural history of SIB. A major problem with research in this area is that most has been conducted with people with intellectual disabilities (IDs) or autism spectrum conditions (ASCs) for whom diagnoses of other possible NDCs were either not known or not reported. It is thus very possible that findings reported relate overall trends from people with a diversity of NDCs, in each of which SIB may present with a differing phenomenology and natural history. Only recently, since the development of the concept of behavioral phenotypes, have studies of SIB for people with specific NDCs, and studies explicitly attempting to compare phenomenology and natural history across NDCs, begun to be undertaken.

In this chapter we also consider evidence regarding risk markers or factors for development of SIB, with particular reference to distinguishing those specifically related to SIB from those more broadly associated with behavioral difficulties in general, and also distinguishing risk factors for initial development of SIB from those predictive of chronicity of the disorder once developed. Once again, a limitation is that much research has relied on samples of people with IDs or ASCs without regard to diagnosis of other possible NDCs. In this case the problem is even more difficult in that identification of risk factors for SIB requires studies with relatively large samples, which are difficult to conduct with people with relatively uncommon NDCs. In this chapter we also consider how the operant model of SIB may account for the relationship between SIB and possible risk factors, including, pain, sleep disturbance, and mood disorder, and also briefly introduce other models of these relationships which will be explored further in Chap. 3.

F. Furniss, A. B. Biswas, *Self-Injurious Behavior in Individuals with Neurodevelopmental Conditions*, Autism and Child Psychopathology Series,
https://doi.org/10.1007/978-3-030-36016-0_2

2.2 Overall Prevalence of Self-Injurious Behavior

In large-scale population-based community surveys, SIB of sufficient severity to cause tissue damage, or to require specialist support and intervention, or to be a moderate or severe problem, is reported in between 4 and 12% of children with severe IDs, depending on age (Oliver, Murphy, & Corbett, 1987; Ruddick, Davies, Bacarese-Hamilton, & Oliver, 2015), between 10 and 11% of children with ASCs (Lecavalier, 2006), and in almost 5% of adults with IDs (Collacott, Cooper, Branford, & McGrother, 1998; Cooper et al., 2009). Other studies of people with ASCs have however reported much higher prevalence rates, with several studies of children and adolescents reporting prevalence rates of around 50% (Baghdadli, Pascal, Grisi, & Aussilloux, 2003; Duerden et al., 2012; McTiernan, Leader, Healy, & Mannion, 2011). Richards, Oliver, Nelson, and Moss (2012) reported a prevalence of 50% in a sample primarily composed of children with ASCs, but with ages ranging from 4 to 39, and Shattuck et al. (2007) reported a prevalence of 46.1% in a large sample mainly comprised of adolescents and young adults. Effective comparison of prevalence rates between studies is generally limited by differences in sampling, definition of SIB, and variation in measures used. Further studies of SIB prevalence with population-based samples of people with ASCs are needed, since several of the studies above used clinical samples. It does however seem that by comparison with people with IDs, people with ASCs either are at greater risk of experiencing SIB to any degree or are at greater risk of experiencing SIB of sufficient severity and/or frequency as to cause serious concern.

2.3 Incidence and Persistence of Self-Injurious Behavior

Only a handful of longitudinal studies have been conducted to examine the incidence and persistence of SIB, and of these, some have used relatively small samples or have followed up participants over relatively brief time periods. In Berkson's pioneering study of the development of SIB in 39 children receiving early intervention for developmental delay (Berkson, 2002; Berkson, Tupa, & Sherman, 2001), incidence of SIB (over 1–3 years) was 1.3%, but 23% of all children engaging in SIB did so only transiently. Children with an older biological sibling diagnosed with an ASC are regarded as themselves at high risk of being diagnosed with an ASC and therefore at relatively high risk also of developing SIB. In Dimian et al.'s (2017) sample of 235 such children, the cumulative incidence estimate for SIB between 12 and 24 months was 22%. Davies and Oliver (2016) reported a cumulative 1-year incidence of 4.7% among children with severe IDs aged 2–12 years, while Murphy, Hall, Oliver, and Kissi-Debra (1999) estimated the 1-year incidence of SIB in their sample of children under 11 with ASCs and/or severe IDs to be 3%. Cooper et al. (2009) found a 2-year incidence rate of only 0.6% in adults with IDs. Baghdadli et al. (2008) however found an incidence rate of 15.6% over 3 years in their group of children with ASCs aged 2–7 at first assessment, and Richards, Moss, Nelson, and Oliver (2016) reported an incidence estimate of 17.5% over a period of just over 3 years in a group of 40 people with ASCs (those not showing SIB at initial assessment from a group of 67 people with a median age of 10 years at that assessment). It is possible therefore that the incidence of SIB in later childhood is elevated among people with ASCs by comparison with those with IDs.

With regard to persistence vs. remission of SIB once established, Dimian et al. (2017) found that 48% of children engaging in SIB at age 12 months continued to do so at 24 months, with 52% no longer reported to engage in SIB at 24 months. Baghdadli et al. (2008) found that only 51% of children with ASCs aged 2–7 showing SIB continued to do so 3 years later, and Davies and Oliver (2016) reported 58% persistence in their sample of children with severe IDs over a period of 15–18 months, rather consistent with the persistence rate of just under 50% at 5-year follow-up for children originally aged 4–11 reported by Chadwick, Kusel, Cuddy, and Taylor (2005). Richards et al. (2016) however reported a persistence rate of 77.8% in their sample of children with ASCs. Studies of samples including or comprised of adults show high persistence rates of 62% over 2 years (Cooper et al., 2009), 71% over 7 years (Emerson et al., 2001b), and 84% over 20 years (Taylor, Oliver, & Murphy, 2011), while Totsika, Toogood, Hastings, and Lewis (2008) reported that 47% of a group of adults with IDs who showed "serious" or "serious but controlled" SIB continued to present SIB at this level of severity 11 years later. In a group of older children and adults with ASCs, Shattuck et al. (2007) reported that the prevalence of SIB reduced from 46.1 to 36.5% over a period of 4.5 years, but did not report the persistence rate for those who entered the study with SIB. Baghdadli and colleagues (Rattaz, Michelon, & Baghdadli, 2015; Rattaz, Michelon, Munir, & Baghdadli, 2018) followed up their group of children with ASCs into adolescence and early adulthood. Unfortunately, the method of assessing presence of SIB changed from the earlier two to the later studies, but the prevalence of SIB, which had been 49% at age 5 and 33% at age 8, was found to be 35.8% at age 15 and 34% at age 20.6 years.

2.4 Etiology and Early Development of Self-Injurious Behavior

Studies of preschool children show that a high proportion of children with NDCs engage in SIB from a young age. Although Berkson et al. (2001) identified SIB in only 4.6% of young children using early intervention services, MacLean, Tervo, Hoch, Tervo, and Symons (2010) and Hoch et al. (2016) found prevalences of 32% and 59%, respectively, in clinical samples of young children with developmental disabilities (DDs), while Murphy et al. (1999) observed potentially self-injurious topographies (presented with low frequencies) in 90% of children not identified as showing SIB by teachers. Many children however engage in SIB on a less than daily basis (MacLean et al. 2010). Both actually injurious SIB and "proto-SIB" (i.e., potentially self-injurious topographies not causing tissue damage) typically emerge before or at the age of 25 months (Berkson et al., 2001; Dominick, Davis, Lainhart, Tager-Flusberg, & Folstein, 2007; Kurtz et al., 2003; Richman & Lindauer, 2005). In contrast to findings from older children and adults, studies of SIB in young children have not found presence and extent of SIB to be related to gender, sensory impairment, diagnosis and severity of autism, or percentage time engaged in stereotyped behavior (MacLean et al., 2010; Murphy et al., 1999). Developmental level and mobility have been found to be negatively associated with extent, but not presence vs. absence, of SIB (MacLean et al. 2010; Murphy et al. 1999). The small numbers of participants in many studies to date of SIB in young children will clearly limit their power to detect factors associated with the presence and severity of SIB. In a study drawing on data from 257 children representing all those aged between 18 and 72 months in a US state who had been assessed for eligibility for a program for children with intellectual and developmental disabilities (IDDs), MacLean and Dornbush (2012) however found a prevalence of SIB of 19.1%, but again found that groups of children engaging and not engaging in SIB did not differ in gender balance, chronological or developmental age, rates of visual or hearing impairment, mobility, or diagnosis of autism. Presence of SIB was not associated with presence of unusual/repetitive habits, but was associated with engaging in behaviors hurtful to others.

A substantial number of young children without diagnosed NDCs and showing no signs of delayed development also engage in stereotyped behaviors (STBs) and SIB, and there has been renewed interest in understanding how the developmental trajectories of STBs and SIBs in these children differ from those in children with NDCs. Hoch et al. (2016) compared the parent-reported prevalences of STBs and SIBs in preschoolers who had been referred for assessment because of concerns regarding developmental delay with those for a group of children with no known developmental concerns. Parents reported the occurrence of SIB in 59.1% of the children with developmental delay and 28.5% of the "typically developing" group. Gender, age group, and developmental level were not associated with SIB. No parent of a typically developing child described their child's SIB as other than a "mild" problem, whereas many parents of children with developmental delay rated their child's SIB as a moderate to severe problem. The most commonly reported topography of SIB for the children with developmental delay was hitting themselves against a surface or object, whereas for the typically developing group, it was rubbing or scratching themselves.

Dimian et al. (2017) collected data on parent-reported STBs and SIB, together with assessments of developmental level and adaptive behavior, from their sample of 235 children at risk for developing an ASC at ages 12 and 24 months. At age 24 months, 47 of the children (20%) met clinical best-estimate criteria for presence of an ASC. Of the whole "at-risk" group, approximately 39% were reported to engage in SIB at the age of 12 months. By 24 months this figure had fallen to 32%. Of the children reported to engage in SIB at age 12 months, 48% continued to do so at 24 months, while 31 additional children had begun to engage in SIB. For those children who engaged in SIB at both 12 and 24 months of age, the number of different topographies of SIB they engaged in reduced for 47%, remained stable for 26%, and increased for 28%. At age 12 months, the topographies of SIB most frequently reported for the children, both of which were reported for over 40 participants, were hitting themselves against a surface and pulling at their own skin or hair. Hitting themselves with objects, self-rubbing or scratching, hitting themselves with a hand or other body part, and inserting fingers into body orifices were all reported for 10 or more participants. At 24 months hitting self against a surface was still the form of SIB most commonly reported by parents, with over 30 children engaging in this topography. Pulling at their own skin or hair had become less commonly reported, but more than ten children engaged in this behavior, self-hitting, inserting fingers or objects, and rubbing/scratching. Fewer children were reported to hit themselves with objects, but more (over ten) were reported to bite themselves and to engage in skin-picking.

Berkson et al. (2001) and Richman and Lindauer (2005) reported that when actually injurious behavior is observed very early (between 12 and 15 months), it often takes the forms of eye-poking or hand-mouthing. However, consistent with the findings of Dimian et al. (2017), for many children headbanging or hitting is the first SIB or proto-SIB seen, developing at around 18–24 months (Berkson, 2002; Berkson et al., 2001; Kurtz et al., 2003; Richman & Lindauer, 2005). Headbanging resulting in injury may present only transiently (Berkson et al., 2001), but headbanging and hitting self were the most frequently recorded primary self-injurious behavior topographies in the sample of MacLean and Dornbush (2012).

Recent research has also attempted to directly evaluate the theory that STBs may be precursors to SIB. In a longitudinal study of preschoolers assessed as being at risk for developmental delay (including genetic NDCs) or ASCs, Rojahn, Barnard-Brak, Medeiros, and Schroeder (2016) contacted parents of 160 children aged 4–44 months at the beginning of the study at 3 time points over a period of approximately 1 year and collected parent reports of the frequency and severity of a number of STBs and SIBs using the Behavior Problems Inventory (BPI-01; Rojahn, Matson, Lott, Esbensen, & Smalls, 2001). Evaluation of the relationship between STB and SIB using latent growth modelling suggested that a model in which earlier STBs (with age and cognitive development score as covariates) predicted later SIB fitted the data better than a model in which SIB predicted stereotypy, but not significantly better than a model in which STBs and SIB were regarded as correlated. Richman and Lindauer (2005) observed the emergence of proto-SIB comprising head-hitting and/or headbanging during their study and reported that at least four of the seven topographies observed were apparently related to a pre-existing STB. Proto-SIB was observed to begin to cause tissue damage during the study in five children, at a mean age of 25 months. However, repeated functional analyses suggested a social function for the behaviors in the case of only one child, who had entered the study displaying actually injurious SIB. In studies of slightly older children by Hall, Oliver, and Murphy (2001) and Oliver, Hall, and Murphy (2005) however, naturalistic observation suggested that positive social reinforcement contingencies were operating on the SIB of three of the four children who showed increasing levels of

SIB throughout the study. Children whose SIB increased over time showed elevated probabilities of SIB under conditions of reduced social contact and patterns of decreasing probability of social interaction before SIB and increases in such contact during and following SIB. Kurtz et al. (2003) found evidence for social functions of SIB in 50% of their cases. Petty, Allen, and Oliver (2009) examined the role of social reinforcement in the transition from proto-SIB to SIB in slightly older children already showing injurious SIB. Employing experimental and descriptive functional analyses of the SIB, proto-SIB, aggressive/destructive, repetitive, and "proto-imperative" (e.g., crying, pushing another's hand away) behaviors of six children with IDs, Petty et al. identified a social function for the SIB of five children. For four children SIB was a member of a functionally equivalent class (or classes) of response with aggressive/destructive and/or proto-imperative behaviors, but in only one case was proto-SIB also a member of the class. Temporal analyses demonstrated that proto-imperative, aggressive/destructive, and proto-SIB behaviors were significant precursors to SIB for six, four, and two children, respectively. There is therefore evidence that for some children stereotyped behaviors can evolve into SIB and also that for some children social reinforcement can strengthen existing SIB. The operant model clearly does not however provide a complete account of the early emergence of SIB. Only one of Richman and Lindauer's (2005) participants showed behaviors sensitive to social reinforcement processes during the period in which proto-SIB and SIB were developing and that participant already showed SIB at the beginning of the study. Petty et al. (2009) identified socially reinforced co-functional repetitive and proto-SIB behaviors in three children, consistent with the hypothesis of shaping of repetitive behaviors into proto-SIB, but co-functional SIB and proto-SIB in one child only.

Recent research has thus shown that substantial numbers of young children who have IDs or ASCs or are viewed as being at risk for later diagnosis of these conditions show SIB or proto-SIB (Dimian et al., 2017; Hoch et al., 2016; MacLean & Dornbush, 2012; MacLean et al., 2010; Murphy et al., 1999; Rojahn et al., 2016). Further, it seems that for many children SIB typically develops before 25 months, that headbanging (or otherwise hitting self against a surface) or head-hitting is often seen at a young age, and that many young children with DDs or ASCs show these behaviors transiently (Baghdadli et al., 2008; Berkson, 2002; Berkson et al., 2001; Chadwick et al., 2005; Dimian et al., 2017; Kurtz et al., 2003; MacLean & Dornbush, 2012; Richman & Lindauer, 2005).

Much of the research reviewed above supports the hypothesis that social reinforcement processes may strengthen SIB in some cases once tissue-damaging behavior has occurred and that such processes may also shape repetitive behaviors into proto-SIB. In cases in which social functions of the behavior are observed, these are predominantly positive, in contrast to the negative reinforcement processes frequently observed with older children (Iwata et al., 1994). Kurtz, Huete, Cataldo and Chin (2012) however noted that only 37% of their sample of 32 young children who had recently begun to engage in SIB also engaged in stereotyped behaviors and suggested that the operant model proposing development of SIB from early repetitive behaviors may reflect only one of several developmental pathways for the emergence of SIB. The very early age at which SIB develops in many children has however, to date, severely limited the ability of researchers to observe the initial emergence of SIB or to measure factors predictive of incidence of SIB. Berkson (2002) reported that SIB was often first seen in association with tantrums following frustration or rapid situational transitions. Bijam-Schulte, Janssen & Stolk (1996) interviewed the parents of 59 children and adults with IDs who engaged in SIB regarding their recollections of the emergence of the behavior. Although in many cases the parents were describing events which had happened many years in the past, 17 of the people with IDs were between 6 and 15 years old at the time of the study. When questioned about behaviors which might have been precursors of their son or daughter's SIB, or had been in some sense "replaced" by the SIB, 18 parents (or parental couples) recalled such a precursor. For half of these people, the apparent precursor was a stereotyped behavior; for the other nine, precursors included "crying fits" and "shouting." The people engaging in SIB were compared with a small control group ($n = 13$) of people matched for age, ability, and gender balance, but not currently engaging in SIB; group membership was associated with parental recollection of their child as being fearful or feeling threatened in many situations.

Although relevant data are scarce, therefore, it is possible that early SIB emerges through at least two alternative processes in different children, evolving in some by operant shaping of STBs into self-injurious forms, and in the second originating in temper outbursts evoked by frustration or rapid transitions. It seems likely however that whatever its origin, social reinforcement plays an important role in the further development of SIB. Whether there are alternative pathways in the early development of SIB, and whether different early pathways are associated with differences in long-term outcome, remains a fascinating issue for further research.

2.5 Risk Factors, Risk Markers, and Correlates for Self-Injurious Behavior

A substantial number of studies have now been undertaken in which the prevalence of SIB has been examined in relatively large clinically referred or population-based samples of children and adults with NDCs, and factors associated with the presence of SIB have been studied. Although such studies in principle have the potential to identify possible risk markers and risk factors for development of SIB, methodological issues have to date severely limited their utility in this regard. The most fundamental of these limitations is that most studies have used samples of children or adults whose ages are such that the research on early development of SIB would suggest that many will have developed SIB many years before the associated variables were measured. It is of course possible that these variables may nevertheless constitute risk markers or risk factors. It is also however possible that they represent factors associated with the chronicity of SIB once established rather than risk markers or factors for its initial development. Although identification of factors associated with chronicity may be of value, it clearly does not equate with identification of risk factors in the commonly accepted sense of factors which enable clinicians to identify individuals likely to develop a problem before it is clinically recognizable (Devine & Symons, 2013). Methodological issues such as heterogeneity of samples with regard to diagnoses; differences in definitions of SIB, especially with regard to criteria related to severity of impact; the high correlations often observed between putative risk markers/factors (e.g., between overall intellectual ability and levels of communication skill); and differences in approaches to reporting relative risk (Devine & Symons, 2013) have also constrained the drawing of definitive conclusions from the relatively large numbers of studies conducted. Finally, although there have been some attempts to differentiate between behaviors with regard to risk markers/factors (e.g., Davies & Oliver, 2016), most research has focused on SIB alone. Such a focus ignores the high degree of co-occurrence with SIB of other behavioral issues such as aggression to others, leaving open the possibility that the factors identified may be potential risk markers/factors for behavioral disturbance in general rather than SIB in particular. This possibility may not limit the usefulness of identifying such factors as possible correlates of persistence of SIB, but may limit their relevance to understanding its development.

With these caveats in mind, we will now briefly review the literature concerned.

2.6 Personal Risk Markers or Factors Associated with Self-Injury

2.6.1 Ability

Recent research has confirmed that the prevalence (and, where measured, frequency and severity) of SIB is associated with overall severity of ID in both children and adults and in people with ASCs and in those with IDs of heterogeneous cause (Barnard-Brak, Rojahn, Richman, Chesnut, & Wei, 2015; Cooper et al., 2009; Crocker et al., 2006; Deb, Thomas, & Bright, 2001; Folch et al., 2018; Kurzius-Spencer et al., 2018; Lundqvist, 2013; McTiernan et al., 2011; Oliver, Petty, Ruddick, & Bacarese-Hamilton, 2012; Rattaz et al., 2018; Richman et al., 2013; Saloviita, 2000; Soke et al., 2016, 2017, 2018a; Tsiouris, Kim, Brown, & Cohen, 2011). This association is generally found irrespective of whether severity of ID is measured in terms of intelligence quotient(IQ) or adaptive behavior, and the occasional failures to find the association (e.g., Davies & Oliver, 2016) probably result from participant samples with limited variability in ability. The association however may not hold in persons with some specific genetic syndromes (Arron, Oliver, Moss, Berg, & Burbidge, 2011). Attempts to isolate the relative contributions of communication, daily living, and socialization skills have produced less consistent results. Among studies using multiple regression and/or multivariable logistic regression analyses to examine the effects of these variables, both (lower) daily living skills (Baghdadli et al., 2003; Chadwick, Piroth, Walker, Bernard, & Taylor, 2000; Emerson et al., 2001a) and communication skills (Emerson et al., 2001a; Rattaz et al., 2015, 2018) have been found to predict SIB. Studies reporting individual associations between these variables and SIB in adults and children with ASCs and/or IDs have reported associations with poorer communication skills (Deb et al., 2001; Lowe et al., 2007; Maskey, Warnell, Parr, Le Couteur, & McConachie, 2013; Richards et al., 2012), poorer self-help skills (Richards et al., 2012), and lower socialization skills (Lowe et al., 2007), while (severe) SIB has also been reported not to be associated with any of these factors (Chadwick, Kusel, & Cuddy, 2008). Some of the variability in these results may result from variation in definitions of SIB, especially with respect to severity and frequency. In a rare study of the development of SIB in older teenagers and adults who presented apparently newly developed SIB 8 years after moving from an institution, Nøttestad and Linaker (2001) found that these persons had more severe disabilities and poorer communication and self-care skills (at baseline) than a group who had remained free from SIB.

As noted earlier, in younger (age 6 and below) children with developmental delays, overall developmental quotient and language skills are often found not be associated with measures of SIB (Hoch et al., 2016; MacLean & Dornbush, 2012; MacLean et al., 2010). The study of infants at risk of developing ASCs described above (Dimian et al., 2017) did however find that lower developmental quotient (DQ) at 12 months was predictive of the emergence (or persistence) of SIB at 24 months, although most of these children were showing typical developmental progress and only 19.9% met diagnostic criteria for an ASC by 24 months of age. Some clarification of this apparent conflict regarding the relationship between ability and risk for SIB may be provided by a study by Medeiros, Kozlowski, Beighley, Rojahn, and Matson (2012). Medeiros et al. evaluated the relationship between DQ and measures of SIB (and also aggressive/destructive behavior and STB) in three groups of toddlers (ages 17–36 months) referred to an early intervention service. For children evaluated as meeting diagnostic criteria for autistic disorder or pervasive developmental disorder-not otherwise specified (PDD-NOS), according to the *Diagnostic and Statistical Manual of Mental Disorders*, Fourth Edition, Text Revision (DSM-IV-TR; American Psychiatric Association, 2000), there was no significant relationship between DQ and score on a measure of SIB, whereas for children with developmental delay not associated with an ASC, DQ was negatively associated with SIB score. Further analyses showed negative relationships between SIB and adaptive functioning, personal-social development, and cognitive development, for the children without ASCs, and a positive relationship between communication skills and SIB for the group meeting criteria for autistic disorder, while for children meeting criteria for PDD-NOS, no relationship was found between any developmental domain and SIB. Variability in findings regarding the relationship between DQ and SIB in very young children may therefore result from variability in the numbers of participants with particular ASCs across studies. Further support for this possibility is offered by a study of young (6 years of age or younger) children with ASCs which found a positive relationship between child IQ and current SIB (Soke et al., 2018b).

2.6.2 Age

Chadwick et al. (2000, 2008) found no relationship between age and presence of SIB in children and adolescents with IDs. In a study of children and young adults with seven specific genetic syndromes, Arron et al. (2011) found no effect of age within any genetic group, as was also the case in a study of children and adults with ASCs (Richards et al., 2012). Studies of large population-based samples of children and adults with IDs, and of young children with ASCs, have found relatively weak negative associations between age and SIB (Emerson et al., 2001a; Lowe et al., 2007; Soke et al., 2017), while in studies of adults, Cooper et al. (2009) found no difference in mean ages of participants with and without SIB, and Deb et al. (2001) found no effect of age cohort on prevalence of SIB. Both Crocker et al. (2006) and Cohen et al. (2010) however found reductions in SIB in people aged 60 and over by comparison with younger ages, and Tsiouris et al. (2011) calculated that in their large sample scores on the New York State Institute for Basic Research in Developmental Disabilities Modified Overt Aggression Scale (IBR-MOAS; Cohen et al., 2010), "physical aggression against self" domain decreased by 14% as age increased by about one standard deviation (14 years). Both a large multinational study of a sample of people with IDs aged from 2 to 93 years using a dimensional measure of SIB (Barnard-Brak et al., 2015) and a study of a large national sample of adults with IDs using a categorical measure (Folch et al., 2018) have also found overall severity or prevalence of SIB to decrease with age.

In a 5-year follow-up of children aged 4–11 at original assessment, Chadwick et al. (2005) found no relationship between age and persistence/remission of SIB, and Taylor et al. (2011) also found no such relationship in their 19-year follow-up of children and adults. Emerson et al. (2001b) and Totsika et al. (2008) however both found younger age to be predictive of persistence of SIB, consistent with a decline in SIB with increasing age. A methodologically stringent review of studies reporting prevalences of SIB across age bands for people with IDs (Davies & Oliver, 2013) concluded that the prevalence of SIB increases with age until mid-adulthood and then declines. The authors noted however that cross-sectional studies potentially confounded effects of individual age and cohort (i.e., changes within individual lifetimes and changes across generations) and also that the apparent decline in SIB with age might reflect differential mortality effects rather than individual behavior change.

2.6.3 Gender

Studies of children with severe IDs (e.g., Davies & Oliver, 2016) generally find no association between participant gender and SIB. For adults, on the other hand, while both large-scale population-based studies (e.g., Cooper et al., 2009; Folch et al., 2018; Lundqvist, 2013; Tsiouris et al., 2011) and those in clinical samples (Tenneij

& Koot, 2008) have generally found no association between gender and presence of SIB, three large-scale community-based studies (Cohen et al., 2010; Crocker et al., 2006; Deb et al., 2001) have found SIB to be more prevalent and/or severe in women. One of these studies (Cohen et al., 2010) reported that this effect was most marked for women with ASCs, and a further study with a clinical sample (Saloviita, 2000) reported that the effect of gender was seen only in participants with ASCs. Studies of children with ASCs (or of mixed-age samples including many children) have however reported either no gender effect or nonsignificant trends for SIB to be more prevalent and/or severe in girls than in boys (Duerden et al., 2012; Kozlowski & Matson, 2012; MacLean & Dornbush, 2012; Richards et al., 2012; Soke et al., 2016, 2017). Soke et al. (2018b) however, although finding no association of gender with currently reported SIB in their group of young children with ASCs, did find that a reported history of SIB which was currently reported as slight or non-occurring was more common in boys than girls.

2.6.4 Sensory and Motor Impairments

In a large community-based total population study, Cooper et al. (2009) reported an association (with other variables controlled) of SIB with visual impairment, a finding also emerging from univariate analyses in a study of children and adults with profound IDs and serious motor problems (Poppes, van der Putten, & Vlaskamp, 2010). Emerson et al. (2001a) found (more restricted) mobility to predict SIB in a logistic regression analysis, while Nøttestad and Linaker (2001) found severe impairments of both mobility and hearing to predict new cases of SIB. Poppes, van der Putten, Post, and Vlaskamp (2016) found hearing problems to be associated with SIB in children and adults with profound intellectual and multiple disabilities. Studies of young children with developmental delays have however not found SIB to be associated with hearing or mobility or visual impairment (MacLean & Dornbush, 2012; MacLean et al., 2010).

2.6.5 Stereotyped Behaviors

Presence of SIB is associated with STB (Emerson et al., 2001a; González et al., 2009; Matson & Rivet, 2008b; Rojahn et al., 2016; Saloviita, 2000). Indeed, in a large study of young people (aged 4 years to 18 years 11 months) attending special schools for children with severe IDs, Oliver et al. (2012) found that in logistic regression models also including adaptive functioning and presence vs. absence of speech as predictor variables, high-frequency repetitive and/or ritualistic behavior was the only factor associated with high-frequency SIB in children with severe IDs, although adaptive behavior was an additional predictor of the presence of SIB of any severity. Having confirmed the association between repetitive behavior and SIB using a structural equation modeling approach with a large multinational sample of children and adults with IDs, Barnard-Brak et al. (2015) however further reported that mixed-modeling techniques revealed two subgroups within their sample. In one subgroup (comprising 69% of their overall sample), STB was strongly associated with SIB, whereas in the second group, STB was not associated with SIB, with the second group being older, and overall engaging in less SIB and STB, than the first. In the "at risk for ASC" infants studied by Dimian et al. (2017), 39% of whom were already engaging in SIB at 12 months, SIB at 12 months predicted SIB at 24 months, but STB at 12 months was not predictive of SIB at 24 months when SIB at 12 months was included in the model. In their sample of children and adults with ASCs, Richards et al. (2012) also found no difference between people who did and did not self-injure in scores on the stereotyped behavior subscale of the Repetitive Behaviour Questionnaire (RBQ; Moss, Oliver, Arron, Burbidge, & Berg, 2009) nor on any of the other subscales of the RBQ (compulsive behavior, insistence on sameness, restricted preferences, and repetitive language). Richman et al. (2013) however did find that STB was associated with SIB, even when measures of ability and degree of ASC characteristics were controlled for. Richman et al.'s (2013) sample included a relatively high proportion of more able individuals, so it may be that for people with ASCs, the relationship between STB and SIB only becomes apparent in groups for whom other risk markers for SIB (such as lower ability) are less prevalent.

2.6.6 Autism Spectrum Conditions

Studies controlling for ability have yielded mixed results on the issue of whether a diagnosis of an ASC is independently associated with SIB, with Cooper et al. (2009) and Emerson et al. (2001a) finding no association, but Cohen et al. (2010) and Tsiouris et al. (2011) reporting an association between scores on the IBR-MOAS "physical aggression against self" domain and presence of an ASC diagnosis. Studies using dimensional measures of the severity of features of autism have however found such measures to predict the presence and/or severity of SIB in samples of people with ASCs together with IDs (Baghdadli et al., 2003; Rattaz et al., 2015, 2018; Richards et al., 2012), in population-based samples of people with IDs (Lowe et al., 2007), and in samples of children and adults with fragile X syndrome and Down syndrome (Richards et al., 2012). Several studies comparing matched groups of adults with IDs with and without ASCs have reported higher scores on measures of SIB for participants with ASCs (Lundqvist, 2013; Matson & Rivet, 2008b; Rojahn, Wilkins, Matson, & Boisjoli, 2010; Smith & Matson, 2010) or found that participants with more severe features of autism score higher on measures of SIB than those with few or no features of an ASC (Matson & Rivet, 2008a). In a matched group comparison of adults with ID and ASCs and those with ID alone, Bodfish, Symons, Parker, and Lewis (2000) found no association between the presence of ASC and SIB and also found that participants with ASCs did not show more topographies of SIB than those with ID alone, but did find that the SIB of participants with ASCs was rated as more severe. Similar results have emerged from studies comparing young children with ASCs with those with developmental delays, including those not associated with genetic conditions or accompanied by seizures or severe sight or hearing loss (Fodstad, Rojahn, & Matson, 2012; Kozlowski & Matson, 2012; Soke et al., 2018a), although not all studies report these effects (MacLean & Dornbush, 2012; MacLean et al., 2010). Overall, it appears likely that whether or not a categorical diagnosis of an ASC is associated with presence vs. absence of SIB, there are relationships between presence/severity of characteristics associated with ASCs and extent/severity of SIB (Richards et al. 2012). Nonetheless, Richman et al. (2013) failed to find any such association in a large sample of children and younger adults with ASCs, as did Soke et al. (2017) in a large sample of children with ASCs. Richman et al. (2013) however also reported an unusual positive correlation between severity of features of ASC and IQ in their sample, which may be related to the fact that well over 50% of their participants had IQs of 85 or over.

Other studies have attempted to define which aspects of the ASC behavioral phenotype are associated with SIB. Duerden et al. (2012) used hierarchical regression to investigate atypical sensory processing, non-verbal IQ, functional communication ability, social communication and functioning, age, insistence on sameness, and rituals and compulsions, as predictors of SIB in children with ages between 21 months and 19 years. With variables entered into the regression analysis in the order listed above, atypical sensory processing, insistence on sameness, IQ, and social communication and functioning were significantly associated with SIB, explaining 12%, 10%, 4%, and 3%, respectively, of variance in scores on a composite measure of SIB. These findings were largely replicated in a study of over 2000 young people with ASCs aged 4–17 which also found SIB to be associated with anxiety (Dempsey, Dempsey, Guffey, Minard, & Goin-Kochel, 2016). Soke et al. (2017), despite finding no association between scores on an overall measure of ASC intensity and SIB in a sample of over 5000 young children with ASCs, did find an association between reported abnormalities in sensory processing and SIB both in that group and in a sample of over 8000 8-year-olds with ASCs. Soke et al. (2018b) further replicated this finding in a group of almost 700 children with ASCs.

People with a number of genetic syndromes may show more or less marked features of the ASC phenotype, and it is possible that different aspects of the phenotype may be associated with risk for SIB in different syndromes. Richards et al. (2012) compared scores on the subscales of the Social Communication Questionnaire—Lifetime version (Berument, Rutter, Lord, Pickles, & Bailey, 1999), a measure of aspects of ASC behaviors, for people who did and did not self-injure. For people with fragile X syndrome, total SCQ score and score on the SCQ social interaction subscale differed for people who did and did not self-injure, whereas for people with Down syndrome, SCQ total score and scores on all three subscales (communication, repetitive behavior, and social interaction) were higher for people who engaged in SIB.

2.6.7 Low Mood

As noted in Chap. 1, the idea that self-injury may be associated with low mood or depression has a long history. Empirical findings on this issue have been mixed. Tsiouris et al. (2011) found no association of depression with SIB, but argued that depression may have been underdiagnosed in their sample. The Mood, Interest, and Pleasure Questionnaire (MIPQ) and its short form (MIPQ-S; Ross & Oliver, 2003) are informant-based rating scales for assessing affect in people with severe IDs and are comprised of two subscales, "mood" and "interest and pleasure." Ross and Oliver (2002) administered the MIPQ to 53 individuals with severe and profound IDs and compared the 12 participants with highest, and 12 participants with lowest, MIPQ scores on the reported presence vs. absence and severity of 5 topographies of challenging behavior including SIB. They found no difference between the groups in reported prevalence or severity of SIB. Richards et al. (2012) found that compared with people with ASCs who did not self-injure, those who engaged in SIB had significantly lower scores, indicating lower affect, on both subscales of the MIPQ-S. The effect sizes for both comparisons however suggested weak effects. Turygin, Matson, MacMillan, and Konst (2013) found that scores on measures of depression and SIB were significantly correlated in a group of adults with IDs living in residential services, but that the association was greater for those diagnosed with an ASC. As with aspects of the ASC phenotype, the association of low mood with SIB may vary across genetic syndromes. Using the MIPQ-S, Arron et al. (2011) found that lowered mood was associated with SIB in participants with Angelman syndrome, while reduced interest and pleasure was associated with SIB in participants with Cornelia de Lange, fragile X, and Prader-Willi syndromes. Ross and Oliver (2002) suggested that lowered mood might be a contributing factor to, or a consequence of, persistent SIB. Bernstein, Visconti, Csorba, Radvanyi, and Rojahn (2015) examined these possibilities in a study involving 50 adults with IDs, again using the MIPQ-S, which was completed together with measures of SIB at an interval of 4–5 months. Scores on the interest/pleasure, but not mood, subscales of the MIPQ at the first assessment predicted SIB frequency and severity ratings between 4 and 5 months later, while the SIB frequency and severity ratings completed at the first assessment also predicted MIPQ-S interest/pleasure, but not mood, scores at the second assessment. Bernstein et al. (2015) observed that their findings may suggest that diminished interest in reinforcing stimuli might be associated with SIB.

2.6.8 Anxiety

Among toddlers referred to an early intervention program, both for those with an ASC diagnosis (Cervantes, Matson, Tureck, & Adams, 2013) and for those with developmental delays not associated with an ASC (Matson, Mahan, Sipes, & Kozlowski, 2010), children with no or minimal symptoms of anxiety showed lower levels of SIB (and aggressive/destructive behaviors and STB) than those with moderate or high levels of anxiety symptoms. The anxiety measure used (the anxiety/repetitive behavior factor from part two of the Baby and Infant Scale for Children with Autism Traits; Matson et al., 2009) however includes some items relating to repetitive behaviors associated with anxiety which may also be correlated with overall levels of STB. As noted earlier, Dempsey et al. (2016), in their study of over 2000 young people with ASCs, found SIB to be associated with anxiety, as did Soke et al. (2017) within 2 large samples of children with ASCs and Tsiouris et al. (2011) in a large sample of adults with IDs.

2.6.9 Impulsivity/Overactivity

A number of studies involving both children and adults have found presence of SIB to be associated with impulsivity and/or overactivity and/or attentional difficulties both for people with IDs of heterogeneous origin and for those with ASCs (Collacott et al., 1998; Cooper et al., 2009; Davies & Oliver, 2016; Richman et al., 2013; Rojahn, Matson, Naglieri, & Mayville, 2004; Tsiouris et al., 2011). Arron et al. (2011) found SIB to be associated with impulsivity/overactivity in participants with Cornelia de Lange, fragile X, Lowe, and Prader-Willi syndromes.

2.6.10 Sleep Problems and Pain

Several studies have found associations between SIB and disturbed or variable (nighttime) sleep in children and adults with IDs and/or ASCs, although the relationship appears to hold also for other behaviors including aggression to others (Brylewski & Wiggs, 1999; Cohen et al., 2018; Poppes et al., 2016; Soke et al., 2017, 2018b; Symons, Davis, & Thompson, 2000).

Studies of general expression of pain behavior have found this not to differ between children presenting and not presenting SIB, but to be more extensive in adults with chronic severe SIB than in those not presenting SIB (Breau et al., 2003; Symons, Harper, McGrath, Breau, & Bodfish, 2009). The possibility that discomfort and pain associated with gastrointestinal (GI) problems may be associated with SIB has attracted particular attention because of the high prevalence of such problems in children with ASCs (Ibrahim, Voigt, Katusic, Weaver, & Barbaresi, 2009) and in people with Cornelia de Lange syndrome (Oliver et al., 2013). In a large population-based sample of 8-year-olds with ASCs, Maenner et al. (2012) however found that the presence of medically documented GI problems was associated with reported sleep disturbance and oppositional behaviors, but not with SIB. Soke et al. (2017), in another large sample of young children with ASCs, also found no association of SIB with GI problems. Prosperi et al. (2017) studied 163 preschoolers with ASCs, 42 (26%) of whom were identified as experiencing GI symptoms.

Children with and without GI symptoms did not differ on a measure of severity of SIB; children with GI problems were however found to engage in a significantly greater number of SIB topographies than those without GI symptoms (at the $p \leq 0.05$ level), but the effect size associated with this difference was small. Soke et al. (2018b) did however find an association between GI problems and SIB in young children with ASCs, and Poppes et al. (2016) also found that bowel and abdominal problems were associated with SIB, with other relevant factors controlled for, in their sample of people with profound intellectual and multiple disabilities.

2.6.11 Physical Health Problems

In a study of 56 children under 5 years of age, Petty, Bacarese-Hamilton, Davies, and Oliver (2014) found that the association between parental ratings of the level of their children's eye, ear, dental, and skin problems and parental ratings of the severity of SIB approached significance with levels of developmental delay, overactivity/impulsivity, and STB controlled for.

2.6.12 Personal Risk Markers and Risk Factors for Self-Injurious Behavior: Summary

There is now a substantial body of evidence regarding personal risk markers (and potential risk factors) for SIB in children and adults with IDs and/or ASCs, including a number of studies which were population-based and/or had large numbers of participants. Despite some conflicting findings regarding many of the factors examined, and difficulties in cross-study comparisons caused by the use of different measures of SIB, some broad conclusions may be drawn. In general, people with more severe IDs, those who engage in higher levels of STBs, those with more marked features of an ASC, those who show generalized overactivity and/or impulsivity, and those experiencing high levels of anxiety are more likely to engage in SIB. However, there is also increasing evidence that even for the most robust overall risk markers for SIB, associations differ across NDCs or other groupings. Thus, for people with ASCs, the association between ability and risk for SIB appears to be less marked than is the case for people with IDs without ASCs.

Research into risk markers may be undertaken in the expectation that identification of risk markers will facilitate targeting of preventive interventions at individuals most at risk for developing SIB, and it may also be hoped that if markers prove to be risk factors, their identification will advance understanding of the etiology of SIB and lead to new possibilities for preventive intervention. Understanding the implications of this body of research remains complicated, however, for a number of reasons. As noted earlier, much of the research reviewed above has involved children aged 5 and upward and adults, i.e., people whose ages are well above that at which SIB typically emerges. Those studies which have involved young children have often failed to detect associations between SIB and characteristics such as ability which are generally found with older participants, consistent with the possibility that at least some of the risk markers identified must be viewed as markers for persistence of SIB rather than for its development. Further, many studies have focused on SIB alone, but people who engage in SIB also frequently engage in aggression directed at other people and property destruction (González et al., 2009; Matson & Rivet, 2008b; Rojahn et al., 2004; Tenneij, Didden, Stolker, & Koot, 2009; Tenneij & Koot, 2008), and research which consider these behaviors as well as SIB frequently find that personal characteristics such as ability (McTiernan et al., 2011), anxiety (Cervantes et al., 2013; Matson et al., 2010), diagnosis with an ASC (Tsiouris et al., 2011), STB (Oliver et al., 2012), and overactivity/impulsivity (Petty et al., 2014; Tsiouris et al., 2011) are associated with aggression toward others and/or property destruction as well as SIB. This does not diminish the potential practical value of such characteristics as markers for SIB risk, but does suggest that they are generalized markers for risk of behavior disturbance rather than being specific to SIB. Thirdly, not all studies have been able to consider all of the possible risk markers identified to date, but some of these risk markers are themselves strongly associated (e.g., presence of an ASC and anxiety; presence of an ASC and sleep disturbance; sleep disturbance and overactivity/impulsivity; chronic pain and sleep disturbance), meaning that some risk markers may be such only by virtue of such an association with another characteristic which may be a true risk factor. Talisa, Boyle, Crafa, and Kaufmann (2014), for example, examined factors associated with SIB in males with fragile X syndrome. Parents were asked whether their son had been diagnosed with or treated for a number of conditions including an ASC and anxiety. The highest proportion of participants experiencing SIB was found in those with an ASC and anxiety, while the subgroup with an ASC but no reported anxiety had a proportion of participants engaging in SIB similar to that of the subgroup with neither an ASC nor anxiety. Fourthly, only a few studies have attempted to quantify the change in risk for SIB associated with presence/absence or measurement unit of any putative risk factor (Devine & Symons, 2013). Finally, it will be apparent that the relationship between at least some identified risk markers and causal risk factors may be complex. From the perspective of the operant model of SIB, it can readily be seen how higher levels of self-help and communication skills might reduce risk for development and/or persistence of SIB by enabling people to achieve desired outcomes independently or by using language to persuade other people to provide them. Again, from the operant perspective, the presence of high levels of STBs might provide many opportunities for these behaviors to be inadvertently shaped into SIB. With a risk marker such as sleep disruption, it may be that sleep deprivation functions as an "establishing operation" (EO) which increases the aversiveness of events such as task demands and hence increases the probability of SIB which is reinforced by escape from such demands (O'Reilly, 1995). For each of these risk markers, therefore, a relatively straightforward account of how they might function as risk factors within an operant model of SIB is possible. In the case of pain, however, a much broader range of possible mechanisms relating SIB and pain have been hypothesized (Summers et al., 2017). Again, it is possible that painful conditions affect the motivational properties of environmental events; O'Reilly (1997), for example, demonstrated that the SIB of a 26-month-old girl diagnosed with Williams syndrome occurred at its highest levels when the girl was exposed to loud noises during periods when she had a middle ear infection and suggested that the ear infection acted as an EO increasing the aversiveness of noise. In this case, however, although O'Reilly demonstrated that levels of SIB were further increased when environmental noise was reduced contingent on self-injury, the combination of ear infection and high noise levels resulted in high levels of SIB even when the behavior did not result in escape from noise. Further, possible non-operant mechanisms by which pain originating from causes other than the SIB itself might lead to SIB have been suggested, including the possibility that pain signals resulting from SIB may engage inhibitory processes in the pain perception pathway, thereby increasing thresholds for pain perception from other body sites (Peebles & Price, 2012; Symons & Danov, 2005).

2.7 Personal Risk Markers or Factors for Emergence and Persistence of Self-Injury

The low numbers of incident cases of SIB in most studies have precluded analysis of predictors of the emergence of SIB. Davies and Oliver (2016) reported that among children with IDs, baseline levels of repetitive and restricted behaviors and interests predicted emergence of SIB at 15–18-month follow-up, but even this relatively large study (417 participants in total) identified only 29 incident cases of SIB. Some longitudinal studies have however reported baseline predictors of the presence of SIB at a later time point (whether persisting or emerging since the baseline measurement). Dimian et al. (2017) found that developmental quotient and presence of SIB at 12 months predicted presence of SIB at 24 months in their study of infants at risk for development of ASCs. Davies and Oliver (2016) found repetitive and restricted behaviors and interests to be the sole predictor of SIB at follow-up in their group of children with IDs. Baghdadli et al. (2008) reported that for their group of children with ASCs, severity of signs of ASCs and limited speech as assessed at mean age 4.9 years predicted presence of SIB at 3-year follow-up conducted when the children were 5–10 years of age. At adolescence (mean age 15 years), severity of signs of ASCs at the initial assessment remained a significant predictor of a high score on a measure of SIB, while object-related cognitive functioning at the initial assessment was a negative predictor (Rattaz et al., 2015). Chadwick et al. (2005) however found no associations between persistence vs. remission of SIB and measures of communication, daily living skills, socialization, or motor skills. Long-term follow-ups of adults with IDs have identified younger age, together with lower sociability (Totsika et al., 2008) and stability of SIB at initial assessment (Emerson et al., 2001b) as predictive of persistence of SIB.

2.8 Topographies and Persistence of Self-Injurious Behaviors

For both people with IDs and those with ASCs, self-scratching or picking or pulling, self-banging and hitting, and self-biting are established as the most common topographies of SIB at a young age (Berkson, 2002; Dimian et al., 2017; Hall et al., 2001; Kurtz et al., 2003; MacLean & Dornbush, 2012; Murphy et al., 1999; Richman & Lindauer, 2005) and remain so in childhood and adulthood (Emerson et al., 2001a; Folch et al., 2018; Poppes et al., 2010; Richards et al., 2016; Taylor et al., 2011).

Persistence rates in adulthood for the common individual topographies listed above are all over 60% (Emerson et al., 2001b; Taylor et al., 2011), and Emerson et al. (2001b) found head-directed SIB to be one of only three factors predictive of persistence of SIB in a logistic regression analysis.

2.9 Environmental Risk Factors for Self-Injury

The research reviewed in Sect. 2.6 of this chapter has identified a number of personal attributes which appear to be (at least) risk markers for the persistence of SIB. Nevertheless, studies which have used regression approaches to model the relationship between these personal attributes and SIB often note the relatively large proportion of variance remaining unexplained in these models. This issue appears to be particularly salient for studies of children with ASCs, where over 70% of variance was reported to be unexplained in the studies of Duerden et al. (2012) and Dempsey et al. (2016), and for studies of adults with IDs, where similarly high proportions of variance are unaccounted for (Folch et al., 2018; Richards, Davies, & Oliver, 2017). There are certainly potentially relevant individual characteristics such as child temperament (Duerden et al., 2012) whose relationship with SIB has yet to be investigated, and we return to this issue in Chap. 8. It might be expected, however, that these limitations on the explanatory power of models considering only individual characteristics would have stimulated research efforts focusing on possible environmental factors related to the development and/or persistence of SIB, particularly given the influence of the behavioral account of its development. However, although there is a substantial body of research demonstrating an association between behavior problems in children with IDs and ASCs and parental stress and mental health status (Zeedyk & Blacher, 2015, 2017), much of this has been conducted within a framework of assumptions regarding negative impacts of the child's problems on the mental health of other family members (Hastings, 2016).

Only relatively recently have researchers begun to consider the influence of the family environment on the trajectory of child behavior problems over time (Smith, Greenberg, & Mailick, 2014) and hence on the possibility that broader ecological factors which impact on the family environment might also indirectly influence that trajectory (Anderson, Roux, Kuo, & Shattuck, 2018).

Family socioeconomic disadvantage (SED) is generally considered to be a risk factor for mental health difficulties (including behavioral difficulties) in children without NDCs (Midouhas, Yogaratnam, Flouri, & Charman, 2013), while severely preterm birth is a risk factor for a range of cognitive and mental health difficulties in childhood (Johnson & Marlow, 2016). In two large samples from the USA, Soke et al. (2017) found SIB to be related to residence in a lower-income neighborhood in one sample and lower maternal education level and reliance on public (vs. private or other) health insurance in the other. In a further large group of children with ASCs, Soke et al. (2018b) have reported that younger age of the mother and caesarean delivery were associated with current SIB, while lower maternal age and lower gestational age were associated with a history of SIB in the child. Recently, Soke et al. (2019) have also reported that lower maternal educational achievement, maternal cigarette smoking in the period from 3 months prior to pregnancy until the end of pregnancy, and use of electronic monitoring of the fetus during labor are also associated with SIB in children with ASCs. Although these are indirect indicators, and some of these findings require replication, they suggest that family SED and perinatal or postnatal complications may be risk factors for development and/or persistence of SIB.

There has been little research on the relationship between family environment and SIB in young people with NDCs. Chadwick et al. (2008) evaluated the relationships between presence of severe SIB and reported lack of continuity in parental care and schooling, and ratings of expressed parental criticism, expressed parental warmth, and disciplinary practices (including self-reported parental loss of temper and physical chastisement), for adolescents with severe IDs. Of these factors, only expressed parental criticism was associated with SIB, with an odds ratio of 10.63, but the relationship did not meet the statistical significance level required by the number of relationships evaluated. However, lack of continuity in maternal care, expressed parental criticism, and aggressive parental discipline were all associated with an overall behavior problems score in separate univariate analyses, with aggressive parental disciplinary practices retaining significance in multivariate analysis. The factors of (low) parental warmth and (high) criticism considered by Chadwick et al. (2008), together with "emotional over-involvement," are among the domains typically assessed as constituting "expressed emotion" (EE). High levels of parental or carer EE have been shown to be associated with both internalizing and externalizing problems in children and adolescents. A systematic review by Romero-Gonzalez, Chandler, and Simonoff (2018) concluded that high levels of EE and/or criticism were also associated with behavior problems in adolescents with ASCs, but noted (as had Chadwick et al., 2008) that studies examining contemporaneous associations could not identify causal relationships. Romero-Gonzalez et al. (2018) also however identified several longitudinal studies which had found relationships between aspects of parent/carer EE and emotional or behavioral difficulties in people with ASCs. In a study of 149 mothers living together with an adolescent or adult with an ASC, Greenberg, Seltzer, Hong, and Orsmond (2006) found that high levels of maternal criticism predicted increases in the severity of internalizing and asocial behavior problems experienced by the person with an ASC 18 months later, even after controlling for initial levels of behavior problems and signs of autism. In a further follow-up of 118 families in this sample, extending the study period to 7 years, Baker, Smith, Greenberg, Seltzer, and Taylor (2011) showed that mean levels of criticism increased over time and that increases in criticism were associated with higher levels of problem behaviors at the end of the study, whereas changes in behavior problems were not associated with end-of-study levels of criticism. Bader and Barry (2014) reported a similar pattern of results in a 2-year longitudinal study involving children and young people with ASCs.

Several problems arise in evaluating the implications of these studies for understanding of the development of SIB. Firstly, they have used wide-range assessments of emotional and behavioral difficulties which typically provide overall scores for general constructs such as "externalizing behaviors" rather than detailed measures of specific behaviors such as SIB. Secondly, when these assessments do ask about SIB, responses regarding presence of SIB are often assessed as contributing to summary scores for a construct of "internalizing behaviors" which would also reflect signs of, for example, anxiety or social withdrawal. Thirdly, these studies typically rely on parents to rate the behaviors of their offspring, so the possibility cannot be discounted that levels of parental criticism might be related to parents' reports of these behaviors rather than to any objective rating of the behaviors themselves.

Nevertheless, these findings merit further attention for several reasons. Firstly, irrespective of the specific role played by parental EE, findings from research into parenting behaviors experienced by children with ASCs concur that baseline negative parental control increases the risk of later child internalizing problems (Dieleman, De Pauw, Soenens, Beyers, & Prinzie, 2017). Secondly, a number of diverse research streams have recently reported that in parents of children with ASCs, maternal psychological distress, physical health limitations, and lower life satisfaction are all risk factors for later child behavior problems (Totsika et al., 2013; Zaidman-Zait et al., 2014). Although it is possible that parental criticism/hostility does play a specific role beyond the factors of parental distress and parenting practices (Bader, Barry, & Hann, 2015), a broader picture is therefore emerging in which it appears that the family environment impacts significantly on the development of emotional and behavioral difficulties, in young people with ASCs and NDCs in which features of ASC are salient (Smith, Greenberg, Seltzer, & Hong, 2008; Smith, Hong, Greenberg, & Mailick, 2016), if not necessarily in children with other NDCs (Hastings, Daley, Burns, & Beck, 2006). Finally, for each of these streams of research, roles have also been identified in prospectively reducing later risk of child behavior problems for maternal well-being, warmth, and praise for the young person (Smith et al., 2016; Totsika et al., 2013; Woodman, Smith, Greenberg, & Mailick, 2016), suggesting obvious avenues for psychosocial interventions to improve behavioral outcome.

2.10 Phenomenology and Natural History of Self-Injurious Behavior: Summary and Conclusions

Approximately 1 child in 10 with an ID, up to 50% of children with ASCs, and about 1 in 20 adults with IDs engage in SIB of sufficient severity to cause tissue damage. Although a diagnosis of an ASC per se does not appear to be a risk factor for experiencing SIB, the severity of an ASC does increase risk, and several other defined NDCs are associated with much elevated risk of experiencing SIB. Studies of very young children with IDDs and/or ASCs, or those believed to be at risk for these conditions, show that SIB typically emerges before the age of 25 months and that the proportion of such children who engage in SIB at this age is much greater than the number who will continue to engage in SIB until the age of 11 and beyond. Hitting the self against a surface, hitting the self with a hand or other body part, and self-rubbing or scratching are prominent among the early emerging topographies. Studies of preschoolers often find, in contrast to the situation with older children, that ability, sensory impairments, diagnosis with an ASC, or degree of engagement in stereotyped behavior do not differentiate children who engage in SIB from those who do not, although it may be that the apparent lack of a relationship between SIB and ability overall results from differing patterns in this relationship between children with and without ASCs.

Many very young children who engage in SIB do so only transiently. Further, incidence rates appear to reduce dramatically, to around 3–5%, among children between the ages of 2 and 11, with a further reduction in adolescence and adulthood. However, one study of children with ASCs suggests that for these young people, the 3-year incidence rate remains over 17% in later childhood also (Richards et al., 2016). Throughout childhood, on the other hand, significant proportions of children who developed SIB in the preschool years cease to engage in the behavior, with remission rates of around 40–50% reported for both children with IDs and those with ASCs. It has been suggested by Richards et al. (2016) that for children with ASCs, this remission rate may at least partly reflect positive effects of clinical support for the young people and families concerned. However, Baghdadli et al. (2008) found no relationship between weekly hours of therapy and SIB outcome for their group of children with ASCs and found that psychoactive medication use at mean age 5 was a predictor of SIB presence at mean age 8. The issue of the relationship between early intervention and outcome for SIB clearly merits further research. On the basis of the results of research to date, however, a conservative hypothesis would be that a high proportion of children both with IDs and ASCs who have developed SIB at a young age stop engaging in the behavior during the early school years, but children with ASCs remain at relatively high risk of newly developing SIB in those years. This interpretation would be consistent with apparently puzzling reports from some studies involving children with ASCs of a positive relationship between developmental age and SIB, contrasting with the negative relationship generally found for people with IDs.

Owing to the early age at which SIB typically first emerges, and the relatively small numbers of incident cases which have been observed in studies to date, we know very little regarding risk factors for the initial emergence of SIB. Longitudinal studies in childhood suggest however that severity of signs of ASCs and specifically repetitive and restricted behaviors and interests are risk factors for a poor outcome of early SIB in terms of the persistence of the behavior into middle childhood. For adults with IDs, the incidence of SIB is very low, but if earlier developing SIB has continued into adulthood, it constitutes a highly persistent problem, although between 16 and 38% of those who engage in SIB are still able eventually to refrain from doing so. The proportion of those people who later "relapse" into SIB is however unknown. As is the case for its initial emergence, there appear to be no reliable risk markers for the persistence of SIB in adulthood beyond the stability with which the behavior is established.

There is now however a very substantial body of evidence on personal factors concurrently associated with the presence of SIB. As this research has largely been conducted with school-aged children and adults, the risk markers identified are probably best regarded as possible indicators of individuals for whom SIB is likely to persist. Lower ability is one such well-established risk marker for people with IDs, although it may not be so for people with some genetic NDCs or for young children with ASCs. Studies of the associations of STBs and features associated with ASCs with SIB have produced a complex pattern of results, partly at least no doubt dependent on the composition of groups studied and on the particular measures used. Three tentative conclusions however seem warranted. Firstly, the extent to which people show features associated with ASCs is a risk marker for persistent SIB, with STBs and "insistence on sameness" variably salient in this regard, probably dependent on the overall ability of the groups studied and whether participation has been limited to people diagnosed with ASCs. Secondly, there may be a defined subgroup of (generally older) people for whom engagement in STBs and SIB are not associated. Thirdly, the risk for SIB associated with ASCs is probably not defined solely by repetitive and restricted behaviors, but may also comprise abnormalities in sensory processing and anxiety. Sleep problems and impulsivity/overactivity have been found to be associated with SIB, but are probably associated with behavior disturbance in general rather than SIB in particular. Studies of the relationship between painful health problems and SIB have produced mixed results. Importantly for the prospects of secondary prevention of SIB, the personal characteristics associated with persistent SIB appear to differ across NDCs.

By comparison with personal characteristics, features of the social environment associated with persistence vs. remission of SIB have received little attention. Research, mainly carried out with the families of young people with ASCs, suggests that various features of the family environment including maternal well-being, maternal stress, and degree of maternal hostility/criticism directed toward the young person with an ASC contribute to determining behavioral outcomes. From a preventative perspective, these features of the family environment may well be a more promising target for psychosocial intervention than the individual risk factors identified to date.

Cooper et al. (2009) suggested that SIB might be considered a "remitting-relapsing" problem. Clinicians who have had the opportunity to work over a long period of time with individuals who engage in SIB will have encountered some who may engage in quite severe and frequent SIB over periods of months, but who also have long periods in which they engage in no SIB at all, or engage very occasionally and/or very gently in the behaviors (e.g., banging their heads against walls) which cause severe harm during their periods of "active" SIB. No study of older children or adults has yet conclusively determined what proportion of people in whom the behavior is reported as newly emerged or having ceased may represent such "remitting-relapsing" cases. Richards et al. (2016) in their 3-year follow-up of young people with ASCs did however compare people who showed "transient" SIB (i.e., those who were reported either to have started or to have ceased engaging in SIB at follow-up) with those who never engaged in SIB or for whom the behavior was persistent. Levels of impulsivity and impairment in social interaction differed across groups, but post hoc pairwise comparisons between groups found these differences to be significant only between the "SIB absent" and "SIB persistent" groups.

In the next chapter, we consider the neurobiology of SIB and present a model of the interactions between biological and social factors which account for its developmental course and correlates.

References

American Psychiatric Association. (2000). *Diagnostic and statistical manual of mental disorders.* (4th ed., text revision). Washington, DC: American Psychiatric Association. https://doi.org/10.1176/appi.books.9780890420249.dsm-iv-tr

Anderson, K. A., Roux, A. M., Kuo, A., & Shattuck, P. T. (2018). Social-ecological correlates in adult autism outcome studies: A scoping review. *Pediatrics, 141*, S306–S317. https://doi.org/10.1542/peds.2016-4300H

Arron, K., Oliver, C., Moss, J., Berg, K., & Burbidge, C. (2011). The prevalence and phenomenology of self-injurious and aggressive behaviour in genetic syndromes. *Journal of Intellectual Disability Research, 55*(2), 109–120. https://doi.org/10.1111/j.1365-2788.2010.01337.x

Bader, S. H., & Barry, T. D. (2014). A longitudinal examination of the relation between parental expressed emotion and externalizing behaviors in children and adolescents with autism spectrum disorder. *Journal of Autism and Developmental Disorders, 44*(11), 2820–2831. https://doi.org/10.1007/s10803-014-2142-6

Bader, S. H., Barry, T. D., & Hann, J. A. H. (2015). The relation between parental expressed emotion and externalizing behaviors in children and adolescents with an autism spectrum disorder. *Focus on Autism and Other Developmental Disabilities, 30*(1), 23–34. https://doi.org/10.1177/1088357614523065

Baghdadli, A., Pascal, C., Grisi, S., & Aussilloux, C. (2003). Risk factors for self-injurious behaviours among 222 young children with autistic disorders. *Journal of Intellectual Disability Research, 47*(8), 622–627. https://doi.org/10.1046/j.1365-2788.2003.00507.x

Baghdadli, A., Picot, M. C., Pry, R., Michelon, C., Burzstejn, C., Lazartigues, A., & Aussilloux, C. (2008). What factors are related to a negative outcome of self-injurious behaviour during childhood in pervasive developmental disorders? *Journal of Applied Research in Intellectual Disabilities, 21*(2), 142–149. https://doi.org/10.1111/j.1468-3148.2007.00389.x

Baker, J. K., Smith, L. E., Greenberg, J. S., Seltzer, M. M., & Taylor, J. L. (2011). Change in maternal criticism and behavior problems in adolescents and adults with autism across a 7-year period. *Journal of Abnormal Psychology, 120*(2), 465–475. https://doi.org/10.1037/a0021900

Barnard-Brak, L., Rojahn, J., Richman, D. M., Chesnut, S. R., & Wei, T. (2015). Stereotyped behaviors predicting self-injurious behavior in individuals with intellectual disabilities. *Research in Developmental Disabilities, 36*, 419–427. https://doi.org/10.1016/j.ridd.2014.08.017

Berkson, G. (2002). Early development of stereotyped and self-injurious behaviors: II. age trends. *American Journal on Mental Retardation, 107*(6), 468–477+493. https://doi.org/10.1352/0895-8017(2002)107<0468:EDOSAS>2.0.CO;2

Berkson, G., Tupa, M., & Sherman, L. (2001). Early development of stereotyped and self-injurious behaviors: I. incidence. *American Journal on Mental Retardation, 106*(6), 539–547. https://doi.org/10.1352/0895-8017(2001)106<0539:EDOSAS>2.0.CO;2

Bernstein, A. M., Visconti, K. J., Csorba, J., Radvanyi, K., & Rojahn, J. (2015). The relationship between challenging behaviours, mood and interest/pleasure in adults with severe and profound intellectual disabilities. *Journal of Intellectual Disability Research, 59*(11), 1033–1041. https://doi.org/10.1111/jir.12202

Berument, S., Rutter, M., Lord, C., Pickles, A., & Bailey, A. (1999). Autism screening questionnaire: Diagnostic validity. *British Journal of Psychiatry, 175*(5), 444–451. https://doi.org/10.1192/bjp.175.5.444

Bodfish, J. W., Symons, F. J., Parker, D. E., & Lewis, M. H. (2000). Varieties of repetitive behavior in autism: Comparisons to mental retardation. *Journal of Autism and Developmental Disorders, 30*(3), 237–243. https://doi.org/10.1023/A:1005596502855

Breau, L. M., Camfield, C. S., Symons, F. J., Bodfish, J. W., MacKay, A., Allen Finley, G., & McGrath, P. J. (2003). Relation between pain and self-injurious behavior in nonverbal children with severe cognitive impairments. *Journal of Pediatrics, 142*(5), 498–503. https://doi.org/10.1067/mpd.2003.163

Brylewski, J., & Wiggs, L. (1999). Sleep problems and daytime challenging behaviour in a community-based sample of adults with intellectual disability. *Journal of Intellectual Disability Research, 43*(6), 504–512. https://doi.org/10.1046/j.1365-2788.1999.00234.x

Cervantes, P., Matson, J. L., Tureck, K., & Adams, H. L. (2013). The relationship of comorbid anxiety symptom severity and challenging behaviors in infants and toddlers with autism spectrum disorder. *Research in Autism Spectrum Disorders, 7*(12), 1528–1534. https://doi.org/10.1016/j.rasd.2013.09.005

Chadwick, O., Kusel, Y., & Cuddy, M. (2008). Factors associated with the risk of behaviour problems in adolescents with severe intellectual disabilities. *Journal of Intellectual Disability Research, 52*(10), 864–876. https://doi.org/10.1111/j.1365-2788.2008.01102.x

Chadwick, O., Kusel, Y., Cuddy, M., & Taylor, E. (2005). Psychiatric diagnoses and behaviour problems from childhood to early adolescence in young people with severe intellectual disabilities. *Psychological Medicine, 35*(5), 751–760. https://doi.org/10.1017/S0033291704003733

Chadwick, O., Piroth, N., Walker, J., Bernard, S., & Taylor, E. (2000). Factors affecting the risk of behaviour problems in children with severe intellectual disability. *Journal of Intellectual Disability Research, 44*(2), 108–123. https://doi.org/10.1046/j.1365-2788.2000.00255.x

Cohen, I. L., Tsiouris, J. A., Flory, M. J., Kim, S., Freedland, R., Heaney, G., … Brown, W. T. (2010). A large scale study of the psychometric characteristics of the IBR modified overt aggression scale: Findings and evidence for increased self-destructive behaviors in adult females with autism spectrum disorder. *Journal of Autism and Developmental Disorders, 40*(5), 599–609. https://doi.org/10.1007/s10803-009-0908-z

Cohen, S., Fulcher, B. D., Rajaratnam, S. M. W., Conduit, R., Sullivan, J. P., St Hilaire, M. A., … Lockley, S. W. (2018). Sleep patterns predictive of daytime challenging behavior in individuals with low-functioning autism. *Autism Research, 11*(2), 391–403. https://doi.org/10.1002/aur.1899

Collacott, R., Cooper, S., Branford, D., & McGrother, C. (1998). Epidemiology of self-injurious behaviour in adults with learning disabilities. *British Journal of Psychiatry, 173*(5), 428–432. https://doi.org/10.1192/bjp.173.5.428

Cooper, S.-A., Smiley, E., Allan, L. M., Jackson, A., Finlayson, J., Mantry, D., & Morrison, J. (2009). Adults with intellectual disabilities: Prevalence, incidence and remission of self-injurious behaviour, and related factors. *Journal of Intellectual Disability Research, 53*(3), 200–216. https://doi.org/10.1111/j.1365-2788.2008.01060.x

Crocker, A. G., Mercier, C., Lachapelle, Y., Brunet, A., Morin, D., & Roy, M. (2006). Prevalence and types of aggressive behaviour among adults with intellectual disabilities. *Journal of Intellectual Disability Research, 50*(9), 652–661. https://doi.org/10.1111/j.1365-2788.2006.00815.x

Davies, L., & Oliver, C. (2013). The age related prevalence of aggression and self-injury in persons with an intellectual disability: A review. *Research in Developmental Disabilities, 34*(2), 764–775. https://doi.org/10.1016/j.ridd.2012.10.004

Davies, L. E., & Oliver, C. (2016). Self-injury, aggression and destruction in children with severe intellectual disability: Incidence, persistence and novel, predictive behavioural risk markers. *Research in Developmental Disabilities, 49-50*, 291–301. https://doi.org/10.1016/j.ridd.2015.12.003

Deb, S., Thomas, M., & Bright, C. (2001). Mental disorder in adults with intellectual disability. 2: The rate of behaviour disorders among a community-based population aged between 16 and 64 years. *Journal of Intellectual Disability Research, 45*(6), 506–514. https://doi.org/10.1046/j.1365-2788.2001.00373.x

Dempsey, J., Dempsey, A. G., Guffey, D., Minard, C. G., & Goin-Kochel, R. P. (2016). Brief report: Further examination of self-injurious behaviors in children and adolescents with autism spectrum disorders. *Journal of Autism and Developmental Disorders, 46*(5), 1872–1879. https://doi.org/10.1007/s10803-016-2704-x

Devine, D. P., & Symons, F. J. (2013). Biological vulnerability and risk for self-injury in intellectual and developmental disabilities. *International Review of Research in Developmental Disabilities, 44*, 37–67. https://doi.org/10.1016/B978-0-12-401662-0.00002-6

Dieleman, L. M., De Pauw, S. S. W., Soenens, B., Beyers, W., & Prinzie, P. (2017). Examining bidirectional relationships between parenting and child maladjustment in youth with autism spectrum disorder: A 9-year longitudinal study. *Development and Psychopathology, 29*(4), 1199–1213. https://doi.org/10.1017/S0954579416001243

Dimian, A. F., Botteron, K. N., Dager, S. R., Elison, J. T., Estes, A. M., Pruett, J. R., … Wolff, J. J. (2017). Potential risk factors for the development of self-injurious behavior among infants at risk for autism spectrum disorder. *Journal of Autism and Developmental Disorders, 47*(5), 1403–1415. https://doi.org/10.1007/s10803-017-3057-9

Dominick, K. C., Davis, N. O., Lainhart, J., Tager-Flusberg, H., & Folstein, S. (2007). Atypical behaviors in children with autism and children with a history of language impairment. *Research in Developmental Disabilities, 28*(2), 145–162. https://doi.org/10.1016/j.ridd.2006.02.003

Duerden, E. G., Oatley, H. K., Mak-Fan, K. M., McGrath, P. A., Taylor, M. J., Szatmari, P., & Roberts, S. W. (2012). Risk factors associated with self-injurious behaviors in children and adolescents with autism spectrum disorders. *Journal of Autism and Developmental Disorders, 42*(11), 2460–2470. https://doi.org/10.1007/s10803-012-1497-9

Emerson, E., Kiernan, C., Alborz, A., Reeves, D., Mason, H., Swarbrick, R., … Hatton, C. (2001a). The prevalence of challenging behaviors: A total population study. *Research in Developmental Disabilities, 22*(1), 77–93. https://doi.org/10.1016/S0891-4222(00)00061-5

Emerson, E., Kiernan, C., Alborz, A., Reeves, D., Mason, H., Swarbrick, R., … Hatton, C. (2001b). Predicting the persistence of severe self-injurious behavior. *Research in Developmental Disabilities, 22*(1), 67–75. https://doi.org/10.1016/S0891-4222(00)00062-7

Fodstad, J. C., Rojahn, J., & Matson, J. L. (2012). The emergence of challenging behaviors in at-risk toddlers with and without autism spectrum disorder: A cross-sectional study. *Journal of Developmental and Physical Disabilities, 24*(3), 217–234. https://doi.org/10.1007/s10882-011-9266-9

Folch, A., Cortés, M. J., Salvador-Carulla, L., Vicens, P., Irazábal, M., Muñoz, S., … Martínez-Leal, R. (2018). Risk factors and topographies for self-injurious behaviour in a sample of adults with intellectual developmental disorders. *Journal of Intellectual Disability Research, 62*(12), 1018–1029. https://doi.org/10.1111/jir.12487

González, M. L., Dixon, D. R., Rojahn, J., Esbensen, A. J., Matson, J. L., Terlonge, C., & Smith, K. R. (2009). The Behavior Problems Inventory: Reliability and factor validity in institutionalized adults with intellectual disabilities. *Journal of Applied Research in Intellectual Disabilities, 22*(3), 223–235. https://doi.org/10.1111/j.1468-3148.2008.00429.x

Greenberg, J. S., Seltzer, M. M., Hong, J., & Orsmond, G. I. (2006). Bidirectional effects of expressed emotion and behavior problems and symptoms in adolescents and adults with autism. *American Journal on Mental Retardation, 111*(4), 229–249. https://doi.org/10.1352/0895-8017(2006)111[229:BEOEEA]2.0.CO;2

Hall, S., Oliver, C., & Murphy, G. (2001). Early development of self-injurious behavior: An empirical study. *American Journal on Mental Retardation, 106*(2), 189–199+201+204. https://doi.org/10.1352/0895-8017(2001)106<0189:EDOSIB>2.0.CO;2

Hastings, R. P. (2016). Do children with intellectual and developmental disabilities have a negative impact on other family members? The case for rejecting a negative narrative. *International Review of Research in Developmental Disabilities, 50*, 165–194. https://doi.org/10.1016/bs.irrdd.2016.05.002

Hastings, R. P., Daley, D., Burns, C., & Beck, A. (2006). Maternal distress and expressed emotion: Cross-sectional and longitudinal relationships with behavior problems of children with intellectual disabilities. *American Journal on Mental Retardation, 111*(1), 48–61+75. https://doi.org/10.1352/0895-8017(2006)111[48:MDAEEC]2.0.CO;2

Hoch, J., Spofford, L., Dimian, A., Tervo, R., Maclean, W. E., & Symons, F. J. (2016). A direct comparison of self-injurious and stereotyped motor behavior between preschool-aged children with and without developmental delays. *Journal of Pediatric Psychology, 41*(5), 566–572. https://doi.org/10.1093/jpepsy/jsv102

Ibrahim, S. H., Voigt, R. G., Katusic, S. K., Weaver, A. L., & Barbaresi, W. J. (2009). Incidence of gastrointestinal symptoms in children with autism: A population-based study. *Pediatrics, 124*(2), 680–686. https://doi.org/10.1542/peds.2008-2933

Iwata, B. A., Pace, G. M., Dorsey, M. F., Zarcone, J. R., Vollmer, T. R., Smith, R. G., … Willis, K. D. (1994). The functions of self-injurious behavior: An experimental-epidemiological analysis. *Journal of Applied Behavior Analysis, 27*(2), 215–240. https://doi.org/10.1901/jaba.1994.27-215

Johnson, S., & Marlow, N. (2016). Charting the survival, health and development of extremely preterm infants: EPICure and beyond. *Paediatrics and Child Health (United Kingdom), 26*(11), 498–504. https://doi.org/10.1016/j.paed.2016.08.003

Kozlowski, A. M., & Matson, J. L. (2012). An examination of challenging behaviors in autistic disorder versus pervasive developmental disorder not otherwise specified: Significant differences and gender effects. *Research in Autism Spectrum Disorders, 6*(1), 319–325. https://doi.org/10.1016/j.rasd.2011.06.005

Kurtz, P. F., Chin, M. D., Huete, J. M., Tarbox, R. S. F., O'Connor, J. T., Paclawskyj, T. R., & Rush, K. S. (2003). Functional analysis and treatment of self-injurious behavior in young children: A summary of 30 cases. *Journal of Applied Behavior Analysis, 36*(2), 205–219. https://doi.org/10.1901/jaba.2003.36-205

Kurtz, P. F., Huete, J. M., Cataldo, M. F., & Chin, M. D. (2012). Identification of emerging self-injurious behavior in young children: A preliminary study. *Journal of Mental Health Research in Intellectual Disabilities, 5*, (3-4), 260–285. https://doi.org/10.1080/19315864.2011.600809

Kurzius-Spencer, M., Pettygrove, S., Christensen, D., Pedersen, A. L., Cunniff, C., Meaney, F. J., … Rice, S. (2018). Behavioral problems in children with autism spectrum disorder with and without co-occurring intellectual disability. *Research in Autism Spectrum Disorders, 56*, 61–71. https://doi.org/10.1016/j.rasd.2018.09.002

Lecavalier, L. (2006). Behavioral and emotional problems in young people with pervasive developmental disorders: Relative prevalence, effects of subject characteristics, and empirical classification. *Journal of Autism and Developmental Disorders, 36*(8), 1101–1114. https://doi.org/10.1007/s10803-006-0147-5

Lowe, K., Allen, D., Jones, E., Brophy, S., Moore, K., & James, W. (2007). Challenging behaviours: Prevalence and topographies. *Journal of Intellectual Disability Research, 51*(8), 625–636. https://doi.org/10.1111/j.1365-2788.2006.00948.x

Lundqvist, L. (2013). Prevalence and risk markers of behavior problems among adults with intellectual disabilities: A total population study in Örebro county, Sweden. *Research in Developmental Disabilities, 34*(4), 1346–1356. https://doi.org/10.1016/j.ridd.2013.01.010

MacLean, W. E., Jr., Tervo, R. C., Hoch, J., Tervo, M., & Symons, F. J. (2010). Self-injury among a community cohort of young children at risk for intellectual and developmental disabilities. *Journal of Pediatrics, 157*(6), 979–983. https://doi.org/10.1016/j.jpeds.2010.05.052

MacLean, W. E., & Dornbush, K. (2012). Self-injury in a statewide sample of young children with developmental disabilities. *Journal of Mental Health Research in Intellectual Disabilities, 5*(3-4), 236–245. https://doi.org/10.1080/19315864.2011.590627

Maenner, M. J., Arneson, C. L., Levy, S. E., Kirby, R. S., Nicholas, J. S., & Durkin, M. S. (2012). Brief report: Association between behavioral features and gastrointestinal problems among children with autism spectrum disorder. *Journal of Autism and Developmental Disorders, 42*(7), 1520–1525. https://doi.org/10.1007/s10803-011-1379-6

Maskey, M., Warnell, F., Parr, J. R., Le Couteur, A., & McConachie, H. (2013). Emotional and behavioural problems in children with autism spectrum disorder. *Journal of Autism and Developmental Disorders, 43*(4), 851–859. https://doi.org/10.1007/s10803-012-1622-9

Matson, J. L., Mahan, S., Sipes, M., & Kozlowski, A. M. (2010). Effects of symptoms of comorbid psychopathology on challenging behaviors among atypically developing infants and toddlers as assessed with the Baby and Infant Screen for Children with Autism Traits (BISCUIT). *Journal of Mental Health Research in Intellectual Disabilities, 3*(3), 164–176. https://doi.org/10.1080/19315864.2010.495920

Matson, J. L., & Rivet, T. T. (2008a). The effects of severity of autism and PDD-NOS symptoms on challenging behaviors in adults with intellectual disabilities. *Journal of Developmental and Physical Disabilities, 20*(1), 41–51. https://doi.org/10.1007/s10882-007-9078-0

Matson, J. L., & Rivet, T. T. (2008b). Characteristics of challenging behaviours in adults with autistic disorder, PDD-NOS, and intellectual disability. *Journal of Intellectual and Developmental Disability, 33*(4), 323–329. https://doi.org/10.1080/13668250802492600

Matson, J. L., Wilkins, J., Sevin, J. A., Knight, C., Boisjoli, J. A., & Sharp, B. (2009). Reliability and item content of the Baby and Infant screen for Children with aUtIsm Traits (BISCUIT): Parts 1-3. *Research in Autism Spectrum Disorders, 3*(2), 336–344. https://doi.org/10.1016/j.rasd.2008.08.001

McTiernan, A., Leader, G., Healy, O., & Mannion, A. (2011). Analysis of risk factors and early predictors of challenging behavior for children with autism spectrum disorder. *Research in Autism Spectrum Disorders, 5*(3), 1215–1222. https://doi.org/10.1016/j.rasd.2011.01.009

Medeiros, K., Kozlowski, A. M., Beighley, J. S., Rojahn, J., & Matson, J. L. (2012). The effects of developmental quotient and diagnostic criteria on challenging behaviors in toddlers with developmental disabilities. *Research in Developmental Disabilities, 33*(4), 1110–1116. https://doi.org/10.1016/j.ridd.2012.02.005

Midouhas, E., Yogaratnam, A., Flouri, E., & Charman, T. (2013). Psychopathology trajectories of children with autism spectrum disorder: The role of family poverty and parenting. *Journal of the American Academy of Child and Adolescent Psychiatry, 52*(10), 1057–1065. https://doi.org/10.1016/j.jaac.2013.07.011

Moss, J., Oliver, C., Arron, K., Burbidge, C., & Berg, K. (2009). The prevalence and phenomenology of repetitive behavior in genetic syndromes. *Journal of Autism and Developmental Disorders, 39*(4), 572–588. https://doi.org/10.1007/s10803-008-0655-6

Murphy, G., Hall, S., Oliver, C., & Kissi-Debra, R. (1999). Identification of early self-injurious behaviour in young children with intellectual disability. *Journal of Intellectual Disability Research, 43*(3), 149–163. https://doi.org/10.1046/j.1365-2788.1999.00183.x

Nøttestad, J. A., & Linaker, O. M. (2001). Self-injurious behaviour before and after deinstitutionalization. *Journal of Intellectual Disability Research, 45*(2), 121–129. https://doi.org/10.1046/j.1365-2788.2001.00332.x

Oliver, C., Adams, D., Allen, D., Bull, L., Heald, M., Moss, J., … Woodcock, K. (2013). Causal models of clinically significant behaviors in Angelman, Cornelia de Lange, Prader-Willi and Smith-Magenis syndromes. *International Review of Research in Developmental Disabilities, 44*, 167–211. https://doi.org/10.1016/B978-0-12-401662-0.00006-3

Oliver, C., Hall, S., & Murphy, G. (2005). The early development of self-injurious behaviour: Evaluating the role of social reinforcement. *Journal of Intellectual Disability Research, 49*(8), 591–599. https://doi.org/10.1111/j.1365-2788.2005.00694.x

Oliver, C., Murphy, G. H., & Corbett, J. A. (1987). Self-injurious behaviour in people with mental handicap: A total population study. *Journal of Mental Deficiency Research, 31*(2), 147–162. https://doi.org/10.1111/j.1365-2788.1987.tb01351.x

Oliver, C., Petty, J., Ruddick, L., & Bacarese-Hamilton, M. (2012). The association between repetitive, self-injurious and aggressive behavior in children with severe intellectual disability. *Journal of Autism and Developmental Disorders, 42*(6), 910–919. https://doi.org/10.1007/s10803-011-1320-z

O'Reilly, M. F. (1995). Functional analysis and treatment of escape-maintained aggression correlated with sleep deprivation. *Journal of Applied Behavior Analysis, 28*(2), 225–226. https://doi.org/10.1901/jaba.1995.28-225

O'Reilly, M. F. (1997). Functional analysis of episodic self-injury correlated with recurrent otitis media. *Journal of Applied Behavior Analysis, 30*(1), 165–167. https://doi.org/10.1901/jaba.1997.30-165

Peebles, K. A., & Price, T. J. (2012). Self-injurious behaviour in intellectual disability syndromes: Evidence for aberrant pain signalling as a contributing factor. *Journal of Intellectual Disability Research, 56*(5), 441–452. https://doi.org/10.1111/j.1365-2788.2011.01484.x

Petty, J., Allen, D., & Oliver, C. (2009). Relationship among challenging, repetitive, and communicative behaviors in children with severe intellectual disabilities. *American Journal on Intellectual and Developmental Disabilities, 114*(5), 356–368. https://doi.org/10.1352/1944-7558-114.5.356

Petty, J. L., Bacarese-Hamilton, M., Davies, L. E., & Oliver, C. (2014). Correlates of self-injurious, aggressive and destructive behaviour in children under five who are at risk of developmental delay. *Research in Developmental Disabilities, 35*(1), 36–45. https://doi.org/10.1016/j.ridd.2013.10.019

Poppes, P., van der Putten, A. J. J., Post, W. J., & Vlaskamp, C. (2016). Risk factors associated with challenging behaviour in people with profound intellectual and multiple disabilities. *Journal of Intellectual Disability Research, 60*(6), 537–552. https://doi.org/10.1111/jir.12268

Poppes, P., van der Putten, A. J. J., & Vlaskamp, C. (2010). Frequency and severity of challenging behaviour in people with profound intellectual and multiple disabilities. *Research in Developmental Disabilities, 31*(6), 1269–1275. https://doi.org/10.1016/j.ridd.2010.07.017

Prosperi, M., Santocchi, E., Balboni, G., Narzisi, A., Bozza, M., Fulceri, F., … Muratori, F. (2017). Behavioral phenotype of ASD preschoolers with gastrointestinal symptoms or food selectivity. *Journal of Autism and Developmental Disorders, 47*(11), 3574–3588. https://doi.org/10.1007/s10803-017-3271-5

Rattaz, C., Michelon, C., & Baghdadli, A. (2015). Symptom severity as a risk factor for self-injurious behaviours in adolescents with autism spectrum disorders. *Journal of Intellectual Disability Research, 59*(8), 730–740. https://doi.org/10.1111/jir.12177

Rattaz, C., Michelon, C., Munir, K., & Baghdadli, A. (2018). Challenging behaviours at early adulthood in autism spectrum disorders: Topography, risk factors and evolution. *Journal of Intellectual Disability Research, 62*(7), 637–649. https://doi.org/10.1111/jir.12503

Richards, C., Davies, L., & Oliver, C. (2017). Predictors of self-injurious behavior and self-restraint in autism spectrum disorder: Towards a hypothesis of impaired behavioral control. *Journal of Autism and Developmental Disorders, 47*(3), 701–713. https://doi.org/10.1007/s10803-016-3000-5

Richards, C., Moss, J., Nelson, L., & Oliver, C. (2016). Persistence of self-injurious behaviour in autism spectrum disorder over 3 years: A prospective cohort study of risk markers. *Journal of Neurodevelopmental Disorders, 8*(1). https://doi.org/10.1186/s11689-016-9153-x

Richards, C., Oliver, C., Nelson, L., & Moss, J. (2012). Self-injurious behaviour in individuals with autism spectrum disorder and intellectual disability. *Journal of Intellectual Disability Research, 56*(5), 476–489. https://doi.org/10.1111/j.1365-2788.2012.01537.x

Richman, D. M., Barnard-Brak, L., Bosch, A., Thompson, S., Grubb, L., & Abby, L. (2013). Predictors of self-injurious behaviour exhibited by individuals with autism spectrum disorder. *Journal of Intellectual Disability Research, 57*(5), 429–439. https://doi.org/10.1111/j.1365-2788.2012.01628.x

Richman, D. M., & Lindauer, S. E. (2005). Longitudinal assessment of stereotypic, proto-injurious, and self-injurious behavior exhibited by young children with developmental delays. *American Journal on Mental Retardation, 110*(6), 439–450+497. https://doi.org/10.1352/0895-8017(2005)110[439:LAOSPA]2.0.CO;2

Rojahn, J., Barnard-Brak, L., Medeiros, K., & Schroeder, S. R. (2016). Stereotyped behaviours as precursors of self-injurious behaviours: A longitudinal study with infants and toddlers at risk for developmental delay. *Journal of Intellectual Disability Research, 60*(2), 156–166. https://doi.org/10.1111/jir.12224

Rojahn, J., Matson, J. L., Lott, D., Esbensen, A. J., & Smalls, Y. (2001). The Behavior Problems Inventory: An instrument for the assessment of self-injury, stereotyped behavior, and aggression/destruction in individuals with developmental disabilities. *Journal of Autism and Developmental Disorders, 31*(6), 577–588. https://doi.org/10.1023/A:1013299028321

Rojahn, J., Matson, J. L., Naglieri, J. A., & Mayville, E. (2004). Relationships between psychiatric conditions and behavior problems among adults with mental retardation. *American Journal on Mental Retardation, 109*(1), 21–33+77. https://doi.org/10.1352/0895-8017(2004)109<21:RBPCAB>2.0.CO;2

Rojahn, J., Wilkins, J., Matson, J. L., & Boisjoli, J. (2010). A comparison of adults with intellectual disabilities with and without ASD on parallel measures of challenging behaviour: The Behavior Problems Inventory-01 (BPI-01) and Autism Spectrum Disorders-Behavior Problems for Intellectually Disabled Adults (ASD-BPA). *Journal of Applied Research in Intellectual Disabilities, 23*(2), 179–185. https://doi.org/10.1111/j.1468-3148.2009.00519.x

Romero-Gonzalez, M., Chandler, S., & Simonoff, E. (2018). The relationship of parental expressed emotion to co-occurring psychopathology in individuals with autism spectrum disorder: A systematic review. *Research in Developmental Disabilities, 72*, 152–165. https://doi.org/10.1016/j.ridd.2017.10.022

Ross, E., & Oliver, C. (2002). The relationship between levels of mood, interest, and pleasure and 'challenging behaviour' in adults with severe and profound intellectual disability. *Journal of Intellectual Disability Research, 46*(3), 191–197. https://doi.org/10.1046/j.1365-2788.2002.00397.x

Ross, E., & Oliver, C. (2003). Preliminary analysis of the psychometric properties of the Mood, Interest & Pleasure Questionnaire (MIPQ) for adults with severe and profound learning disabilities. *British Journal of Clinical Psychology, 42*(1), 81–93. https://doi.org/10.1348/014466503762842039

Ruddick, L., Davies, L., Bacarese-Hamilton, M., & Oliver, C. (2015). Self-injurious, aggressive and destructive behaviour in children with severe intellectual disability: Prevalence, service need and service receipt in the UK. *Research in Developmental Disabilities, 45-46*, 307–315. https://doi.org/10.1016/j.ridd.2015.07.019

Saloviita, T. (2000). The structure and correlates of self-injurious behavior in an institutional setting. *Research in Developmental Disabilities, 21*(6), 501–511. https://doi.org/10.1016/S0891-4222(00)00055-X

Schneider, M. J., Bijam-Schulte, A. M., Janssen, C. G. C., & Stolk, J. (1996). The origin of self-injurious behaviour of children with mental retardation. *British Journal of Developmental Disabilities, 42* (2), 136–148. https://doi.org/10.1179/bjdd.1996.012

Shattuck, P. T., Seltzer, M. M., Greenberg, J. S., Orsmond, G. I., Bolt, D., Kring, S., … Lord, C. (2007). Change in autism symptoms and maladaptive behaviors in adolescents and adults with an autism spectrum disorder. *Journal of Autism and Developmental Disorders, 37*(9), 1735–1747. https://doi.org/10.1007/s10803-006-0307-7

Smith, K. R. M., & Matson, J. L. (2010). Behavior problems: Differences among intellectually disabled adults with co-morbid autism spectrum disorders and epilepsy. *Research in Developmental Disabilities, 31*(5), 1062–1069. https://doi.org/10.1016/j.ridd.2010.04.003

Smith, L. E., Greenberg, J. S., & Mailick, M. R. (2014). The family context of autism spectrum disorders: Influence on the behavioral phenotype and quality of life. *Child and Adolescent Psychiatric Clinics of North America, 23*(1), 143–155. https://doi.org/10.1016/j.chc.2013.08.006

Smith, L. E., Greenberg, J. S., Seltzer, M. M., & Hong, J. (2008). Symptoms and behavior problems of adolescents and adults with autism: Effects of mother-child relationship quality, warmth, and praise. *American Journal on Mental Retardation, 113*(5), 387–402+419. https://doi.org/10.1352/2008.113:387-402

Smith, L. E., Hong, J., Greenberg, J. S., & Mailick, M. R. (2016). Change in the behavioral phenotype of adolescents and adults with FXS: Role of the family environment. *Journal of Autism and Developmental Disorders, 46*(5), 1824–1833. https://doi.org/10.1007/s10803-016-2714-8

Soke, G. N., Rosenberg, S. A., Hamman, R. F., Fingerlin, T., Robinson, C., Carpenter, L., … DiGuiseppi, C. (2016). Brief report: Prevalence of self-injurious behaviors among children with autism spectrum Disorder—A population-based study. *Journal of Autism and Developmental Disorders, 46*(11), 3607–3614. https://doi.org/10.1007/s10803-016-2879-1

Soke, G. N., Rosenberg, S. A., Hamman, R. F., Fingerlin, T., Rosenberg, C. R., Carpenter, L., … DiGuiseppi, C. (2017). Factors associated with self-injurious behaviors in children with autism spectrum disorder: Findings from two large national samples. *Journal of Autism and Developmental Disorders, 47*(2), 285–296. https://doi.org/10.1007/s10803-016-2951-x

Soke, G. N., Rosenberg, S. A., Hamman, R. F., Fingerlin, T. E., Rosenberg, C. R., Carpenter, L., … DiGuiseppi, C. (2019). Prenatal, perinatal, and neonatal factors associated with self-injurious behaviors in children with autism spectrum disorder. *Research in Autism Spectrum Disorders, 61*, 1–9. https://doi.org/10.1016/j.rasd.2019.01.007

Soke, G. N., Rosenberg, S. A., Rosenberg, C. R., Vasa, R. A., Lee, L., & Di Guiseppi, C. (2018a). Brief report: Self-injurious behaviors in preschool children with autism spectrum disorder compared to other developmental delays and disorders. *Journal of Autism and Developmental Disorders, 48*(7), 2558–2566. https://doi.org/10.1007/s10803-018-3490-4

Soke, G. N., Rosenberg, S. A., Rosenberg, C. R., Vasa, R. A., Lee, L., & Di Guiseppi, C. (2018b). Self-injurious behaviors in children with autism spectrum disorder enrolled in the study to explore early development. *Autism, 22*(5), 625–635. https://doi.org/10.1177/1362361316689330

Summers, J., Shahrami, A., Cali, S., D'Mello, C., Kako, M., Palikucin-Reljin, A., … Lunsky, Y. (2017). Self-injury in autism spectrum disorder and intellectual disability: Exploring the role of reactivity to pain and sensory input. *Brain Sciences, 7*(11). https://doi.org/10.3390/brainsci7110140

Symons, F. J., & Danov, S. E. (2005). A prospective clinical analysis of pain behavior and self-injurious behavior. *Pain, 117*(3), 473–477. https://doi.org/10.1016/j.pain.2005.07.010

Symons, F. J., Davis, M. L., & Thompson, T. (2000). Self-injurious behavior and sleep disturbance in adults with developmental disabilities. *Research in Developmental Disabilities, 21*(2), 115–123. https://doi.org/10.1016/S0891-4222(00)00028-7

Symons, F. J., Harper, V. N., McGrath, P. J., Breau, L. M., & Bodfish, J. W. (2009). Evidence of increased non-verbal behavioral signs of pain in adults with neurodevelopmental disorders and chronic self-injury. *Research in Developmental Disabilities, 30*(3), 521–528. https://doi.org/10.1016/j.ridd.2008.07.012

Talisa, V. B., Boyle, L., Crafa, D., & Kaufmann, W. E. (2014). Autism and anxiety in males with Fragile X syndrome: An exploratory analysis of neurobehavioral profiles from a parent survey. *American Journal of Medical Genetics, Part A, 164*(5), 1198–1203. https://doi.org/10.1002/ajmg.a.36468

Taylor, L., Oliver, C., & Murphy, G. (2011). The chronicity of self-injurious behaviour: A long-term follow-up of a total population study. *Journal of Applied Research in Intellectual Disabilities, 24*(2), 105–117. https://doi.org/10.1111/j.1468-3148.2010.00579.x

Tenneij, N. H., Didden, R., Stolker, J. J., & Koot, H. M. (2009). Markers for aggression in inpatient treatment facilities for adults with mild to borderline intellectual disability. *Research in Developmental Disabilities, 30*(6), 1248–1257. https://doi.org/10.1016/j.ridd.2009.04.006

Tenneij, N. H., & Koot, H. M. (2008). Incidence, types and characteristics of aggressive behaviour in treatment facilities for adults with mild intellectual disability and severe challenging behaviour. *Journal of Intellectual Disability Research, 52*(2), 114–124. https://doi.org/10.1111/j.1365-2788.2007.00968.x

Totsika, V., Hastings, R. P., Emerson, E., Lancaster, G. A., Berridge, D. M., & Vagenas, D. (2013). Is there a bidirectional relationship between maternal well-being and child behavior problems in autism spectrum disorders? Longitudinal analysis of a population-defined sample of young children. *Autism Research, 6*(3), 201–211. https://doi.org/10.1002/aur.1279

Totsika, V., Toogood, S., Hastings, R. P., & Lewis, S. (2008). Persistence of challenging behaviours in adults with intellectual disability over a period of 11 years. *Journal of Intellectual Disability Research, 52*(5), 446–457. https://doi.org/10.1111/j.1365-2788.2008.01046.x

Tsiouris, J. A., Kim, S. Y., Brown, W. T., & Cohen, I. L. (2011). Association of aggressive behaviours with psychiatric disorders, age, sex and degree of intellectual disability: A large-scale survey. *Journal of Intellectual Disability Research, 55*(7), 636–649. https://doi.org/10.1111/j.1365-2788.2011.01418.x

Turygin, N. C., Matson, J. L., MacMillan, K., & Konst, M. (2013). The relationship between challenging behavior and symptoms of depression in intellectually disabled adults with and without autism spectrum disorders. *Journal of Developmental and Physical Disabilities, 25*(4), 475–484. https://doi.org/10.1007/s10882-012-9321-1

Woodman, A. C., Smith, L. E., Greenberg, J. S., & Mailick, M. R. (2016). Contextual factors predict patterns of change in functioning over 10 years among adolescents and adults with autism spectrum disorders. *Journal of Autism and Developmental Disorders, 46*(1), 176–189. https://doi.org/10.1007/s10803-015-2561-z

Zaidman-Zait, A., Mirenda, P., Duku, E., Szatmari, P., Georgiades, S., Volden, J., … Thompson, A. (2014). Examination of bidirectional relationships between parent stress and two types of problem behavior in children with autism spectrum disorder. *Journal of Autism and Developmental Disorders, 44*(8), 1908–1917. https://doi.org/10.1007/s10803-014-2064-3

Zeedyk, S. M., & Blacher, J. (2017). Longitudinal correlates of maternal depression among mothers of children with or without intellectual disability. *American Journal on Intellectual and Developmental Disabilities, 122*(5), 374–391. https://doi.org/10.1352/1944-7558-122.5.374

Zeedyk, S. M., & Blacher, J. (2015). Maternal depression and child behavior problems: Longitudinal considerations. *International Review of Research in Developmental Disabilities, 49*, 1–43. https://doi.org/10.1016/bs.irrdd.2015.06.005

Chapter 3
Neurobiology of Self-Injurious Behavior

3.1 Introduction

This chapter describes accumulating evidence from the neurobiology of genetic syndromes associated with self-injurious behavior (SIB), animal models of those syndromes, studies of the clinical efficacy of pharmacological and other treatments for those syndromes, and research into other repetitive behavior disorders, which suggests that the development of SIB is underpinned by abnormalities in multiple corticostriatal loops. The chapter further describes how environmental processes including psychosocial stressors and the social consequences of SIB drive a process in which SIB originating in difficulty in inhibiting aggressive and other self-directed responses initially acquires operant functions, but can then become a habitual response to environmental challenges and finally become compulsive in nature.

3.2 Genetic Syndromes Associated with Self-Injurious Behavior

3.2.1 Introduction

The rapid pace of development in techniques for genomic analysis and their increasing availability in clinical practice have in recent years led to the identification of numerous microdeletions, microduplications, single-gene mutations, and other genetic correlates, associated with neurodevelopmental conditions (NDCs) (Read & Donnai, 2015). The increasing number of conditions being identified, often in very small numbers of cases, raises difficult questions regarding the extent to which any aspect of a presumed behavioral phenotype is specific to a particular condition. Traditionally, this question would be addressed by comparing prevalences of the

F. Furniss, A. B. Biswas, *Self-Injurious Behavior in Individuals with Neurodevelopmental Conditions*, Autism and Child Psychopathology Series,
https://doi.org/10.1007/978-3-030-36016-0_3

feature concerned in people with the genetic condition and people with a comparable level of intellectual ability with no known NDC. This methodology has however been increasingly questioned, and direct comparisons of the prevalence of presumed aspects of the behavioral phenotype across known NDC groups are often now preferred (Arron, Oliver, Moss, Berg, & Burbidge, 2011). Nevertheless, in some conditions (e.g., Lesch-Nyhan syndrome and Smith-Magenis syndrome), SIB occurs in all or nearly all the people with the condition, while in others (e.g., Rett syndrome), SIB occurs sufficiently frequently as to be generally regarded as an aspect of the behavioral phenotype.

Consideration of genetic syndromes associated with SIB may be of help in understanding the development of SIB in others who do not have those syndromes (Devine & Symons, 2013). It is now clear that the genetic changes associated with NDCs for which SIB is considered part of the behavioral phenotype are diverse. It is possible therefore that self-injury is a heterogeneous disorder and that there is a unique developmental pathway for long-term SIB arising from the genetic condition associated with each NDC. Alternatively, there may be a common final causal pathway which may be reached from diverse starting points or a common central causal pathway which may be facilitated or inhibited by a range of factors. In the following section of this chapter, we therefore consider the genetics and physical and cognitive phenotypes of three syndromes associated with SIB: Lesch-Nyhan syndrome, Smith-Magenis syndrome, and Rett syndrome. The first two of these syndromes are almost always associated with SIB, while Rett syndrome is associated with a high prevalence of SIB but also with a very high prevalence of hand/arm stereotypies which may be related to SIB. For each of these syndromes, we then consider the phenomenology and behavioral context of SIB in the syndrome and then review key findings on the neurobiology and animal models of the syndrome, before examining research on response to a variety of treatments. We start with consideration of Lesch-Nyhan syndrome, because of the extremely high incidence of persistent SIB in the condition, because it has stimulated extensive research into the modelling of the condition, and because it arises from mutations of a single gene.

3.2.2 Lesch-Nyhan Syndrome

Lesch-Nyhan syndrome (LNS: OMIM#300322) is an extremely rare X-linked inherited disorder first described by Lesch and Nyhan (1964), affecting almost exclusively boys. Self-injurious behavior, which usually first takes the form of self-biting, often emerges as soon as the infant's teeth break through, and boys with LNS are usually engaging in SIB by the age of 3 years. The study of LNS has had a major influence on our understanding of the development of SIB for three reasons. Firstly, the characteristic development and relatively invariant initial topography of SIB seen in LNS first led Nyhan (1972) to propose the concept of a behavioral phenotype. Secondly, the cause of the condition was identified, only 3 years after it was first described, as a deficiency in hypoxanthine-guanine phosphoribosyltransferase

(HGPRT), an enzyme involved in recycling of the purine bases hypoxanthine and guanine in most cells throughout the body (Jinnah, 2009). Thirdly, although individuals with the typical condition have extremely low levels of HGPRT, with enzyme activity levels less than 1.6% of normal, over 600 mutations in the *HPRT1* gene responsible for the condition have now been identified, with varying influence on levels of HGPRT enzyme function and severity of the clinical syndrome (Fu et al., 2014). Some individuals, generally referred to as "variant" cases of LNS, have higher although still impaired HGPRT function, and these individuals are much less likely to engage in SIB, although they still experience to some degree many of the other features of the condition (Jinnah et al., 2010). Given this direct association between SIB and the level of activity of the enzyme activity caused by the mutated allele responsible for the syndrome, LNS appears to offer an extremely promising opportunity for understanding the etiology and development of SIB.

The prenatal and neonatal development of individuals with LNS is normal, but hypotonia and delayed motor development are apparent by 3–6 months of age, followed by the development of involuntary movements between 6 and 24 months of age, leaving children with LNS with a severe motor disability characterized by ongoing hypotonia and severe action dystonia, together with dysarthric speech (Harris, 2018; Jinnah et al., 2006). Some people with LNS experience other difficulties, such as severe gastroesophageal reflux or recurrent emesis (Jinnah, 2009).

3.2.2.1 Cognitive Phenotype of Lesch-Nyhan Syndrome

Comprehensive neurocognitive assessment of 15 children and adults with "typical" LNS together with 9 "variant" cases diagnosed with partial HGPRT deficiency and 13 typically developing control participants (Schretlen, Harris, Park, Jinnah, & Del Pozo, 2001) yielded intelligence quotient (IQ) estimates for 13 of the typical cases, ranging between 39 and 81 (mean 59), and for 9 variant cases ranging from 49 to 96 (mean 72). Comparison of profiles of performance across different tests showed that both typical and variant cases showed wide-ranging cognitive deficits when compared with control participants. Participants with partial HGPRT deficiency generally achieved mean test scores intermediate between those of control participants and those with typical LNS, but their scores usually did not differ significantly from those of participants with typical LNS. On measures of auditory divided attention and free recall word list learning however, both typical and variant cases experienced significant impairment by comparison with control participants, but participants with partial HGPRT deficiency performed significantly better than those with typical LNS. Matthews, Solan, and Barabas (1995) and Matthews, Solan, Barabas, and Robey (1999) used subtests from a standard IQ test to assess four areas of cognitive functioning of seven people with typical LNS, with ages ranging from 10 to 22 years, and retested the six who were still alive 4 years later. At initial testing, the six participants who were tested at both times had mean standard scores of 67.8 for verbal reasoning, 74 for abstract/visual reasoning, 59.3 for quantitative, and 64.7 for short-term memory. At retesting, the corresponding mean scores were 64.3, 62.3,

59.3, and 55.2, reflecting significant reductions for the abstract/visual reasoning and short-term memory scores. Matthews et al. (1999) observed that these changes in standard scores did not reflect actual loss of skills, but rather a failure to maintain the progress which would be expected in typically developing peers.

3.2.2.2 Phenomenology and Behavioral Context of Self-Injurious Behavior in Lesch-Nyhan Syndrome

The phenomenology and evolution of SIB in LNS, together with the broader behavioral phenotype, have been explored in several studies using parent or carer reports. Anderson and Ernst (1994) studied 40 males with LNS aged between 2 and 32 years. All were reported to engage in SIB (three additional participants who were reported as not engaging in SIB were excluded from the study as probably having been misdiagnosed). Thirty-nine of the 40 were reported to engage in multiple forms of SIB, with biting some part of the body the most common topography, but headbanging and extending some part of the body to strike against a doorframe while passing through it also commonly reported. Finger biting was however frequently, but not exclusively, reported to have been the form in which SIB first emerged. Anderson and Ernst (1994) also observed that SIB was reported to be experienced as painful and as increasing, rather than reducing, arousal levels. Most people with LNS were also reported by carers to be aware of when they were likely to be about to engage in SIB and to request, or cooperate with, use of restraints at these times. Robey, Reck, Giacomini, Barabas, and Eddey (2003) found that 58 (91%) of their participants were reported to engage in SIB and that for 53% of those who did so, SIB appeared first in the form of biting of lips and/or fingers. These two topographies were however also frequently reported to have disappeared from people's repertoires of SIB after having been exhibited in the past. Case reports have described emergence of apparently new topographies of SIB in school-aged children when established self-biting was prevented by total dental extraction (Gisbert de la Cuadra, Torres, Beltrán, Sánchez, & Puig, 2016). Anderson and Ernst (1994) noted that a high proportion of their participants also engaged in aggression toward other people, and other research has also indicated a broader behavioral and mental health phenotype. Schretlen et al. (2005) compared 22 people with typical LNS (aged 12–38 years), 11 people with variant LNS (aged 12–65 years), and 11 healthy control participants (aged 12–31) years using two standardized and widely used measures of emotional and behavioral difficulties, the Child Behavior Checklist (CBCL; Achenbach, 1991) and the American Association on Mental Retardation Adaptive Behavior Scale: Residential and Community, 2nd edition (ABS-RC2; Nihira, Leland, & Lambert, 1993). On the CBCL, participants with typical LNS received higher ratings on anxiety and depression, social problems, thought problems, attention problems, and aggression, than control participants. In each of these areas, the participants with variant LNS received scores intermediate between those of the typical LNS and control participants; with regard to thought problems and aggression, they received significantly lower ratings than the typical LNS participants, while for attention problems, they were rated as having significantly greater difficulties than control participants, with ratings not significantly different from those of participants with typical LNS. On the ABS-RC2, participants with typical LNS received higher ratings (indicating greater behavioral disturbance) than control participants in the areas of social behavior, trustworthiness, stereotyped and hyperactive behavior, self-abusive behavior, social behavior (primarily reflecting aggression toward others), and disturbing interpersonal behavior. Participants with variant LNS did not differ significantly from the control group on any ABS-RC2 measure, but were rated as having significantly lower levels of difficulty than participants with typical LNS in the areas of social behavior, self-abusive behavior, and disturbing interpersonal behavior.

3.2.2.3 Neurobiology of Lesch-Nyhan Syndrome

Recent research has confirmed that recycling of both hypoxanthine and guanine are impaired in both typical and variant cases of LNS (Fu et al., 2015), but has also suggested that only guanine recycling activity differentiates "typical" from "variant" groups in LNS, a finding potentially important given the role of guanine nucleotides in neuronal development and function (Schretlen et al., 2016). Nevertheless, the pathway from gene allele to behavioral phenotype in LNS is still far from clear. The motor difficulties associated in varying degrees of severity with both the typical and variant forms of LNS led to an initial focus on possible abnormalities of the basal ganglia and associated circuits in persons with LNS (Visser, Bär, & Jinnah, 2000). Recent neuroimaging studies have however found a broader pattern of differences between individuals with typical LNS, those with the variant syndrome, and healthy control participants. Schretlen et al. (2013) used voxel-based morphometry to analyze patterns of difference in gray matter volumes between age-matched groups of 21 people with typical LNS, 17 with the variant syndrome, and 33 healthy control participants. Initial analyses found that compared with healthy controls, people with typical LNS had a mean total intracranial volume reduction of 20%, while those with variant LNS had a reduction of 14%. People with typical LNS had larger reductions in white matter than in gray matter volumes (26% vs. 17%), while those with variant disease had similar reductions in white and gray matter volume. After adjustment for differences in total brain size, spatially distinct regional gray matter volume differences between groups were identified. Reductions in gray matter volumes were found for both typical and variant LNS groups in the caudate, thalamus, and anterior putamen, but also in multiple limbic, temporal, and frontal regions, while no significant differences were found in the occipital and parietal lobes, and only one region of difference in gray matter volume was noted in the cerebellum. Regions in which only the typical LNS group (not those with the variant syndrome) differed from healthy controls comprised the right dorsolateral prefrontal cortex, left and right orbital frontal cortex, right and left hippocampus and amygdala, left insula, and cingulate gyrus. Subsequent between-group comparisons showed that compared with patients with variant LNS, those with typical LNS showed reduced gray matter volumes in ventral striatum, parietal operculum, and prefrontal areas. Subsequent examination of white matter volumes (Schretlen et al., 2015) showed that by comparison with the control participants, both LNS groups also showed reduced white matter volumes in medial inferior white matter regions and that by comparison with the variant LNS group, the typical LNS group showed larger reductions in inferior frontal white matter adjoining limbic and temporal regions and the motor cortex.

With regard to neurotransmitter function, two autopsy studies of the brains of people with LNS found low concentrations of the neurotransmitter dopamine, its main metabolite homovanillic acid (HVA), and a key enzyme in its synthesis, tyrosine hydroxylase, in basal ganglia structures including the caudate nucleus, putamen, and nucleus accumbens, but normal levels of dopamine in the dopamine-producing cells of the substantia nigra (Lloyd et al., 1981; Saito et al., 1999). These findings of reduced striatal dopamine levels in LNS were corroborated by in vivo positron emission tomography (PET) studies using a marker binding to dopamine transporters (Wong et al., 1996) or a tracer analogue of a dopamine precursor assessing DOPA decarboxylase activity and dopamine storage processes (Ernst et al., 1996), which found reduced dopaminergic activity in the caudate and putamen but also in the ventral tegmental complex. Wong et al. (1996) also found a 30% reduction in caudate volume in participants with LNS compared with healthy controls. Overall, this pattern of results suggests either reduced numbers of dopaminergic neurons in LNS or reduced dendritic branching of those neurons.

3.2.2.4 Animal Models of Lesch-Nyhan Syndrome

Two groups of animal models of LNS have been developed. Genetically engineered HGPRT-deficient mice (Doetschman et al., 1987; Hooper, Hardy, Handyside, Hunter, & Monk, 1987; Kuehn, Bradley, Robertson, & Evans, 1987), and more recently rats (Meek et al., 2016), demonstrate a range of metabolic and other abnormalities also seen in human LNS, including depleted levels of brain dopamine and in some cases serotonin (Jinnah, 2009; Meek et al., 2016). Together with tissue culture studies, these animal models have contributed substantially to understanding of the complex cascade of metabolic consequences which can result from mutations in a single gene (Jinnah, 2009). The animals concerned do not however develop overt self-biting, nor the excessive self-grooming which is sometimes taken to be related to SIB in rodent models, nor any other salient features of the neurobehavioral phenotype of LNS, and so to date have not directly contributed to understanding of SIB in the syndrome.

A second, serendipitously developed model in which self-biting is observed, often of sufficient severity to break the skin, is generated by injecting the dopaminergic neurotoxin 6-hydroxydopamine (6-OHDA) intracisternally into the brains of neonatal rats (Breese et al., 1984a). As adults, these rats engage in SIB if given the dopamine precursor levodopa (L-DOPA) or the dopamine agonist apomorphine.

Dopamine levels are substantially reduced in the striatum, including the nucleus accumbens, and olfactory tubercles. The proportion of rats responding with SIB to administration of L-DOPA is dose-dependent, and the response can be observed from the age of 22 days onward (Breese et al., 1984b). Rats neonatally lesioned with 6-OHDA also showed elevated striatal serotonin levels, but a variety of other observations suggested that this effect was not responsible for the emergence of SIB (Breese et al., 1984b). Administration of haloperidol at 1 mg/kg was reported to reduce the incidence of tissue-damaging SIB but not of self-biting under L-DOPA challenge, whereas *cis*-flupentixol completely blocked all severities of self-biting induced by L-DOPA, suggesting that these behaviors in neonatal 6-OHDA treated rats are more associated with D_1 than D_2 receptor subtype functioning (Breese et al., 1984b). Breese et al. (1984b) also remarked that neonatally 6-OHDA-lesioned rats should be regarded as a model for vulnerability to induction of SIB rather than as a complete model of its causation, i.e., that activation of dopamine receptors need not be the mechanism by which SIB is induced in LNS. Subsequent research with 6-OHDA-lesioned rats (Breese et al., 2005) and a related model involving monkeys with unilateral ventral tegmental lesions which exhibited self-biting when given mixed D_1/D_2 agonists (Goldstein et al., 1986) have yielded numerous findings with implications for the relevance of these models to the human LNS phenotype, for tracing the multiple downstream effects of the dopaminergic depletion observed in these models, and for understanding of possible mechanisms underlying SIB in people with LNS. The relevance of the 6-OHDA-lesioned rat as a model for SIB in LNS has been strengthened by findings that in addition to their SIB, lesioned rats have impairments of learning and memory together with impaired habituation and alterations in startle responses and sensory gating (Breese et al., 2005). Further, these rats show hyperactivity between 21 and 45 days of age and learning and memory deficiencies. Administration of central nervous system stimulants such as amphetamine and methylphenidate produces dose-dependent reduction of this hyperactivity, together with amelioration of the cognitive difficulties, leading to neonatally 6-OHDA-lesioned rats being considered also as a model for attention deficit hyperactivity disorder (ADHD; Breese et al., 2005). As described in Chap. 2, recent research has identified attentional difficulties and overactivity/impulsivity as possible risk factors for SIB, and as described earlier in this chapter, people with LNS experience difficulties in these areas. Parents and carers of people with LNS describe exacerbation of their SIB during periods of stress, and "priming" experiences with stress (electric footshock) and apomorphine also potentiate the ability of apomorphine to induce SIB in neonatally lesioned rats. A combination of stress and apomorphine priming more than doubles the proportion of rats engaging in SIB during subsequent acute cumulative apomorphine dosing compared with priming by footshock or apomorphine alone, and combined priming has also been found to result in increased neostriatal concentrations of dopamine, its metabolites, and norepinephrine (Stodgell, Loupe, Schroeder, & Tessel, 1998). The 6-OHDA-lesioned rat thus appears to be a potential model not only of the striatal dopamine depletion seen in LNS but also of the role of personal and environmental factors in evoking

SIB. Its value in tracing the complex effects of the dopamine depletion has been demonstrated by a series of studies showing that neonatal 6-OHDA lesions result in hyper-innervation of striatal serotonergic (5-HT) neurons in adult rats, with accompanying increases in 5-HT_{1B} and 5-HT_2 receptor binding, and supersensitivity to 5-HT receptor agonists, together with increases in striatal met-enkephalin and substance P (Devine, 2012). The value of the model in understanding the specific processes leading to SIB and possible therapeutic agents can be seen in the results of studies using dopamine antagonist agents selective for D_1 or D_2 receptors, which find unchanged or increased binding to the D_2 receptors in the striatum and unchanged or decreased binding to D_1 receptors. However, it appears that despite their reduced density, it is the D_1 receptors which are implicated in SIB in this rodent model. Self-injurious behavior can be induced by administration of D_1 agonists, and the SIB-inducing effects of such agonists and L-DOPA are blocked by selective D_1 receptor antagonists but not by D_2 antagonists (Devine, 2012). It has been suggested therefore than the chronic dopamine deficiency caused by 6-OHDA lesioning results in supersensitivity of dopamine receptors in the remaining cells.

3.2.2.5 Psychopharmacological Therapies for Lesch-Nyhan Syndrome

Attempts to directly boost dopamine levels in people with LNS by provision of L-DOPA have produced effects on SIB (and aggression) ranging from slight improvement to significant worsening, but have also frequently been reported to worsen dystonia and hyperactivity (Bell, Kolobova, Crapper, & Ernst, 2016; Visser, Schretlen, Bloem, & Jinnah, 2011). Trials of fluphenazine, a D_1 and D_2 receptor antagonist, reported positive effects on SIB in people with LNS, but also serious negative motor side effects (Bell et al., 2016). Various antipsychotic drugs, which primarily target D_2 receptors but have some affinity for D_1 receptors, have been reported to improve SIB for some people with LNS but not others (Bell et al., 2016). Khasnavis, Reiner, et al. (2016) and Khasnavis, Torres, et al. (2016) reported a safety/tolerability study and a planned placebo-controlled crossover trial of ecopipam, a selective D_1 receptor antagonist not approved for general clinical use but with "orphan drug" designation. The trial was however discontinued owing to a high frequency of negative side effects, and results for the four participants who completed at least one ecopipam and one placebo period were mixed, including improvement for some participants during placebo periods and apparent improvement of SIB with ecopipam vs. placebo, in widely varying degrees, according to structured rating scales, but with parents' global impressions of change conflicting with the structured ratings in two out of three cases.

To date, all other medications trialled in LNS have produced mixed results. In a study of nine people with LNS, an attempt to boost serotonin levels by administering its metabolic precursor 5-hydroxytryptophan (5-HTP), together with carbidopa (to inhibit peripheral conversion of 5-HTP to serotonin, hence increasing the availability of 5-HTP in the central nervous system), and imipramine (a serotonin reuptake inhibitor), initially resulted in dramatic improvements in SIB which, however, were not maintained (Nyhan, 2000; Nyhan, Johnson, Kaufman, & Jones, 1980). S-Adenosylmethionine (SAMe) is found in human liver and brain and acts as a cofactor providing a methyl group to facilitate multiple metabolic pathways. Its administration increases brain serotonin levels in rats (Young & Shalchi, 2005), and it has been suggested that it may play a role in replenishing available purines (Lauber, Plecko, Pfiffner, Nuoffer, & Häberle, 2016). Case reports, open-label trials, and a single-subject double-blind placebo-controlled trial of its use with people with LNS have found substantial and durable reductions of SIB (and aggression to others) for some people, but worsening of symptoms in others (Bell et al., 2016).

3.2.2.6 Other Therapies for Lesch-Nyhan Syndrome

Several case reports have reported substantial and durable improvements in SIB (and, for some, aggression to others) for people with LNS treated with deep brain stimulation with electrodes inserted bilaterally into the globus pallidus internus (GPi). Behavioral improvements are reversed when stimulation is stopped, and the intervention appears to produce a strong GPi inhibition (Bell et al., 2016; Harris, 2018).

Several experimental case studies using behavioral interventions, primarily extinction and differential reinforcement of other or incompatible behaviors, together with relaxation and systematic desensitization to removal of restraints, have also demonstrated substantial reductions in SIB in people with LNS (Olson & Houlihan, 2000; Tunnicliffe & Oliver, 2011). Both successes and failures of generalization of treatment effects across behaviors, settings, and carers have been reported, together with variability in long-term outcomes (Olson & Houlihan, 2000). Cases in which reduction of one topography of SIB by behavioral treatment was accompanied by emergence, or increased frequency, of other topographies of SIB have also been noted. A "paradoxical" effect of attempts to use electric shock punishment of SIB, which has been reported to increase SIB in all cases where it was used, has also been reported for people with LNS. Although behavioral treatment continues to be regarded as an important component in supporting people with LNS to manage their SIB (Harris, 2018), research into behavioral treatments appears to have decreased markedly since the turn of the century. This may be because of difficulties in maintaining interventions (Olson & Houlihan, 2000) or a perception that behaviors constituting a behavioral phenotype will not respond to environmental interventions. Alternatively, the current tendency in behavioral research to insist that intervention must be tailored to the function of the behavior as determined by an experimental functional analysis (EFA: see Chap. 5) may have inhibited such research, since such analysis (Bergen, Holborn, & Scott-Huyghebaert, 2002) has found that the SIB of a man with LNS, although varying in response to changes to his social environment, did not do so in ways usually predicted by operant theory.

3.2.3 Smith-Magenis Syndrome

Smith-Magenis syndrome (SMS; OMIM#182290) is a neurodevelopmental condition characterized also by a complex of multiple congenital physical abnormalities. Most (90%) cases of SMS are caused by microdeletions in chromosomal region 17p11.2 (Greenberg et al., 1996; Smith, Dykens, & Greenberg, 1998). The remainder (10% of cases or under) are caused by a variety of mutations in the gene retinoic acid induced 1 (*RAI1*), located in the 17p11.2 region (Slager, Newton, Vlangos, Finucane, & Elsea, 2003). Although most of the microdeletion-related cases involve a deletion of approximately 4 mega base pairs (Mb), deletions can range in size from under 1.5 Mb to approximately 9 Mb with relatively little impact on the phenotype observed (Edelman et al., 2007; Vlangos, Yim, & Elsea, 2003). A variety of sources of evidence strongly suggest that most of the phenotypic features associated with SMS are a result of haploinsufficiency of *RAI1*. The gene encodes a chromatin-binding protein that appears to play a role in promoting expression of many different genes, including genes involved in neurodevelopment (Huang et al., 2016). Infants with SMS may have mild facial dysmorphisms and developmental delays, together with hypotonia, but are sociable, content, and apparently good sleepers, also happy to nap during daytime, although objective measures suggest that sleep is disturbed from as young as 6 months (Gropman, Duncan, & Smith, 2006). Infants and children with SMS show delayed motor development, oral motor dysfunction often leading to eating difficulties, and speech delays. As children develop, external features of the physical phenotype, including relatively minor craniofacial anomalies and brachydactyly, together with slowing of growth, become more apparent. The extended physical phenotype is multifaceted and variable. In a study of 27 children with SMS, Greenberg et al. (1996) found otolaryngologic abnormalities in 94%, eye abnormalities in 85%, hearing impairment in 68% (approximately 65% conductive and 35% sensorineural), scoliosis in 65%, and brain abnormalities (predominantly ventriculomegaly) in 52%. Cardiac, renal, thyroid, and immune system abnormalities were found in lower but substantial proportions of children. Almost 75% of the children in Greenberg et al.'s (1996) study had clinical symptoms or signs associated with peripheral neuropathy such as decreased deep tendon reflexes, decreased sensitivity to pain or temperature, or pes cavus or planus. Sleep disturbance, comprising fragmented and shortened total sleep cycles, frequent and prolonged nighttime awakenings, and daytime sleepiness, is evident throughout childhood and adolescence. An extensive behavioral phenotype is also associated with SMS, with difficulties including impulsivity, hyperactivity, attentional difficulties, and aggression toward property and/or other people all shown by over 80% of children with the syndrome (Dykens & Smith, 1998). Clinical observations have described older children, teenagers, and adults with SMS as exhibiting hyperacusis to certain frequencies of sound, thinking obsessively about specific topics, engaging in repetitive behaviors, and showing flight responses without any obvious precipitating event (Gropman et al., 2006; Osório, Garayzábal-Heinze, Villaverde, & Sampaio, 2013). A substantial proportion are described as having a heightened tendency to adhere to rigid routines, with distress if these are disrupted (Osório et al., 2013).

3.2.3.1 Cognitive Phenotype of Smith-Magenis Syndrome

Most children and adults with SMS experience moderate or severe intellectual disability (ID) (Osório et al., 2012; Udwin & Horn, 2001), although a small number have IQs within the normal range. Long-term memory and verbal comprehension have been reported as areas of relative strength, and working memory has been reported as an area of relative difficulty, for both children and adults (Osório et al., 2012; Udwin & Horn, 2001).

3.2.3.2 Phenomenology and Behavioral Context of Self-Injurious Behavior in Smith-Magenis Syndrome

Between 90 and 100% of children with SMS are reported to engage in SIB (Dykens & Smith, 1998; Finucane, Dirrigl, & Simon, 2001; Martin, Wolters, & Smith, 2006). Martin et al. (2006) found no association between children's cognitive abilities and levels of problem behavior. Finucane et al. (2001) however examined the prevalence and severity of 11 specific types of SIB in 29 children and adults with SMS and found that overall prevalence of SIB, and the number of different SIB topographies, increased with age and that the number of topographies engaged in was directly correlated with level of intellectual functioning. Finucane et al. (2001) concluded that with increasing age and ability levels, people with SMS add to their repertoire of SIB from among a small number of specific behaviors.

Children with SMS begin to engage in SIB from the age of approximately 18 months (Gropman et al., 2006). Pulling out of finger- and toenails and insertion of objects into bodily orifices are often mentioned as being apparently specific to SMS, but these behaviors are rather uncommon, and in children with SMS, insertion of objects is often confined to the ears and nose (Finucane et al., 2001). The forms of SIB most common in people with IDs of all etiologies (self-biting, self-hitting, and hitting the body against hard surfaces) appear to be the most common topographies at all ages in SMS (Dykens & Smith, 1998; Finucane et al., 2001). Some children with SMS are reported to engage in headbanging or rocking behaviors while falling asleep (Smith et al., 1998). Children with SMS also show high rates of stereotypy (especially mouthing of their hands or objects), aggression to others, overactivity, and impulsivity, together with the sleep difficulties mentioned above (Dykens & Smith, 1998). Although children with SMS show an overall level of communication skills consistent with their intellectual ability (Martin et al., 2006), it is likely that for many children with SMS, expressive language development is further hindered by oral-motor difficulties and hearing problems (Wolters et al., 2009); indeed, verbal dyspraxia is so severe in some children with SMS that they never acquire speech, despite having comparatively good understanding of language (Finucane & Haas-Givler, 2009).

In young children with SMS, standardized assessments of social skills suggest that these are age-appropriate and significantly higher than daily living, communication, and motor abilities, which are below expectation for typically developing children (Wolters et al., 2009). Studies including older children find that social skills are impaired by comparison with those of typically developing children, but also find that the social skills of children with SMS are stronger than their communication and self-help skills, and also that their social skills are better than would be expected on the basis of their overall intellectual ability (Martin et al., 2006). Taylor and Oliver (2008), in an observational study of five children with SMS, have shown that for three children episodes of SIB were preceded by (relatively) low levels of adult interaction and followed by increased levels of such interaction, consistent with the pattern which would be expected if the children's behavior were being reinforced by adult attention. Wilde, Silva, and Oliver (2013) further found that children with SMS preferentially directed attention to adults versus peers by comparison with children with Down syndrome (DS) and also showed more preferential looking directed toward adults than children with DS. Wilde, Mitchell, and Oliver (2016) observed children with SMS and DS in social situations in which the familiarity to the children of the adults present and levels of attention were manipulated. One of two adults (the child's mother or an unfamiliar adult) played actively with the child or left the room, while the second adult remained present throughout but ignored the child, responding to any approaches by indicating that they were busy and telling the child to play alone. In a complex pattern of results, children with both syndromes oriented to and/or approached adults less frequently in the low attention (adult ignoring) condition than in the high attention (adult playing) conditions, but the reduction in approaches was less for the children with SMS, a difference attributable primarily to the interactions between SMS children and their mothers rather than to those involving unfamiliar adults. Multiple sources of evidence thus suggest that motivation to interact with caregiving adults may be specifically high in children with SMS and that one function of problem behaviors in children with SMS may be accessing such attention (Oliver et al., 2013). Two studies using indirect (parent-informed) measures of the functions of problem behaviors in SMS have however concluded that although accessing attention may be one function of problem behavior, including SIB, for children with SMS, it is not more salient a function for these children than for children with IDs of nonspecific origin (Langthorne & McGill, 2012), and neither is it a specifically salient function of SIB in children with SMS (Sloneem, Oliver, Udwin, & Woodcock, 2011).

3.2.3.3 Neurobiology of Smith-Magenis Syndrome

Early studies using computerized tomography (CT) scanning found no obvious brain abnormalities in many people with SMS and only ventricular enlargement in many others. Greenberg et al. (1996) reported results from CT scans of 25 people with SMS; 9 showed ventriculomegaly, 2 showed enlarged cisterna magna, 1 enlarged foramen magnum, 1 showed partial absence of the cerebellar vermis together with prominent cerebrospinal fluid spaces, and 1 had dystrophic calcification of the right frontal lobe. Hypoplasia of the vermis was also described by Natacci et al. (2000) in a woman with SMS associated with an unusually large 17p11.2 deletion. Using magnetic resonance imaging (MRI) and positron emission tomography (PET), Boddaert et al. (2004) found reductions in gray matter in the insula and lenticular nucleus in five boys with SMS by comparison with both typically developing children and a control group of children with IDs of unknown cause. Significant hypoperfusion was found in the same regions in SMS as compared with children with IDs of unknown cause. Maya et al. (2014) described results from MRI of two females (one aged 3, one aged 24) who were subsequently diagnosed with SMS. The child's MRI revealed marked dilation of the lateral and third ventricles and a thin corpus callosum stretched over the enlarged ventricles, together with a thin brain stem and small vermis. The adult's scan showed bilateral periventricular subependymal nodules consistent with gray matter heterotopia. Capra et al. (2014) similarly found bilateral periventricular subependymal nodules on MRI of two children with SMS. Periventricular heterotopias, which have been found in people with several distinct microdeletion syndromes including 22q11.2 deletion syndrome and Williams syndrome, are collections of nerve cells in abnormal locations secondary to arrest of neuronal migration and have been suggested to represent a relatively nonspecific consequence of disrupted neuronal migration during development (Van Kogelenberg et al., 2010).

3.2.3.4 Animal Models of Smith-Magenis Syndrome

Mouse chromosome 11qB1.3-B2 is syntenic with human chromosome 17p11.2, with numbers and orders of genes highly conserved, and Walz et al. (2003) used chromosome engineering to create mice heterozygous for a deletion corresponding to the SMS "critical region" in humans, i.e., the region of overlap of deletions in humans with differing deletion sizes associated with SMS. These *Df(11)17/+* mice showed craniofacial abnormalities, and marked obesity, and over 20% experienced seizures. Walz et al. (2003) also created mice heterozygous for the corresponding microduplication, which in humans is associated with Potocki-Lupski syndrome, and by crossing these mice with those with the deletion obtained mice with a deletion on one chromosome but with the corresponding region duplicated on the other. These mice experienced none of the abnormalities found in the *Df(11)17/+* animals, implying a gene-dosage effect. Subsequent exploration of the behavioral phenotype of *Df(11)17/+* mice (Walz et al., 2004) showed that by comparison with "wild-type" mice, those with the deletion showed differences in circadian rhythm length and males with the deletion were hypoactive. Tests of anxiety, Pavlovian fear conditioning, and pain sensitivity however showed no differences between *Df(11)17/+* and wild-type mice, and mice with the deletion showed no signs of engaging in SIB. Subsequent research (Ricard et al., 2010) has however found behavior indicative of reduced levels of anxiety, and subtle changes in social behavior, in *Df(11)17/+* compared to wild-type mice.

Following the ascertainment of individuals with SMS who did not have typical deletions in 17p11.2, but did have mutations in *RAI1* (Slager et al., 2003), genotype-phenotype correlation studies identified a primary role for haploinsufficiency of *RAI1* in the development of many key features of the phenotype including ID, disturbance of the circadian rhythm, SIB, disturbance in social behaviors, and craniofacial features. Deletions in 17p11.2 however were implicated in the development of cardiac anomalies, speech and motor delay, hypotonia, short stature, and hearing loss (Bi et al., 2004; Girirajan et al., 2006). Mice haploinsufficient for *Rai1* showed obesity, craniofacial abnormalities, and proneness to seizures similar to those found in *Df(11)17/+* mice (Bi et al., 2005, 2007). Bi et al. (2007) showed that in the brains of these *Rai1+/−* mice, the *Rai1* gene was expressed predominantly in the hippocampus and cerebellum, with other sites of strong expression being the striatum, including the nucleus accumbens, and neurons in the cerebral cortex. Nonetheless, as for *Df(11)17/+* mice, *Rai1+/−* mice showed no differences from wild-type mice in anxiety, Pavlovian fear conditioning, or SIB. Most mice with both copies of *Rai1* inactivated (*Rai1−/−*) died early in development. Surviving *Rai1−/−* mice however displayed more severe neurobehavioral abnormalities including hindlimb clasping, overt seizures, motor impairment, and impaired conditioning of fear both to the general environment and to specific conditional stimuli. Intriguingly, mice with a deletion of an approximately 590 kb interval surrounding *Rai1* showed increased startle responses and impaired fear conditioning compared to wild-type mice, suggesting that the impact of *Rai1* on neurodevelopment is modified by other genes located relatively close to it. The relevance of both the *Df(11)17/+* and *Rai1+/−* mouse models to human SMS has been emphasized by findings that both types of mouse show behaviors indicative of circadian rhythm abnormalities (Lacaria, Gu, & Lupski, 2013).

Further insights into the role of *Rai1* have been provided by studies of *Dp(11)17/+* heterozygous microduplication mice, which show increased anxiety-related behaviors and changes in social behavior (Molina et al., 2008), and mice engineered to overexpress *Rai1*, which also show increased anxiety-related behaviors. The latter mice also show normal brain serotonin levels but reduced levels of the serotonin metabolite 5-hydroxyindoleacetic acid, suggesting abnormality of serotonin metabolism or reduced serotonin release and/or enhanced reuptake in presynaptic neurons (Girirajan et al., 2008; Girirajan & Elsea, 2009). These findings have stimulated attempts to delineate neurochemical pathways linking *Rai1* haploinsufficiency to aspects of the behavioral phenotype. Huang et al. (2016) demonstrated that RAI1 preferentially occupies DNA regions near active promoters and appears to play a general role in positively regulating steady-state gene expression. Using a conditional *Rai1* knockout mouse model, Huang et al. (2016) showed that in the cortex and striatum, RAI1 regulates genes involved in cell adhesion, axon guidance, and neuronal morphogenesis, suggesting that it may be involved in the development of neural circuits. RAI1 also enhances the expression of genes that function in interneuronal excitatory and inhibitory communication. In preparation for its release into the synaptic cleft, the excitatory neurotransmitter glutamate is accumulated within vesicles in the terminal of the presynaptic neuron through the action of vesicular glutamate transporters (VGLUTs) 1–3. VGLUT 1 is primarily expressed in cortical neurons, and VGLUT 2 is primarily expressed in subcortical neurons (Vigneault et al., 2015). Huang et al. (2016) found that in mouse cortex, RAI1 was expressed in 75% of excitatory neurons expressing *Vglut1* (encoding VGLUT1) as well as being expressed in 57% of inhibitory neurons expressing *Gad1* and/or *Gad2*, which encode glutamate decarboxylase 1 (GAD1; also known as GAD67) and glutamate decarboxylase 2 (GAD2; also known as GAD65), enzymes involved in the production of γ-aminobutyric acid (GABA). Selective deletion of *Rai1* from particular cell populations implicated *Rai1* deletion in subcortical VGLUT2-positive excitatory neurons in the motor function deficits shown by the knockout mice, while *Rai1* deletion in both GAD2-positive inhibitory and VGLUT2-positive subcortical excitatory neurons contributed to deficits in Pavlovian fear conditioning (Huang et al., 2016).

Mouse models of SMS have therefore been rather more successful than those created for LNS in replicating some features of the behavioral phenotype, including subtle disturbances in social behavior. The value of these models has been further emphasized by a demonstration that a social interaction deficit demonstrated by mice with one copy of *Rai1* inactivated could be reversed by normalizing the RAI1 level 3–4 weeks after birth, but not at a later stage in development (Huang et al., 2018). As has been the case with LNS mouse models, however, neither overt SIB nor excessive grooming resulting in lesions has been shown in these models.

3.2.3.5 Psychopharmacological Therapies for Smith-Magenis Syndrome

A phase shift in the circadian rhythm of melatonin secretion underlies the sleep difficulties of children with SMS, and administration of a β_1-adrenergic antagonist in the morning to reduce melatonin production, combined with administration of melatonin in the evening, has been reported to improve both sleeping patterns and behavioral disturbance (De Leersnyder, 2006; De Leersnyder et al., 2003). Laje, Bernert, Morse, Pao, and Smith (2010) asked parents or other caregivers of 62 individuals with SMS for retrospective information on use of psychotropic and other behavior-related medication. Caregivers of 16 people with SMS reported that they had never used psychotropic medication, but the mean age of the children concerned was only 4.5 years. Sleep aides, stimulants, and antidepressants were being or had been used by over one-third of the group, with α_2-adrenoceptor agonists, antipsychotics, and mood stabilizers all used by substantial numbers of people with SMS. For each broad class of medication considered, mean caregiver global ratings of its effect on the difficulties of the person with SMS were within the range "slightly worse" to "slightly better," with the exception of benzodiazepines, which were taken by only four people and were on average reported as making their difficulties "worse."

3.2.3.6 Other Therapies for Smith-Magenis Syndrome

Bass and Speak (2005) carried out a functional assessment of one form of SIB (inserting objects into a pre-existing wound) engaged in by a woman with SMS and a mild ID and concluded that the reinforcer that was most active in maintaining her SIB was the positive social attention, provided in settings outside the unit on which she was living, which followed episodes of SIB. A treatment program based on differential reinforcement of other behavior (providing such interaction following periods in which she refrained from SIB), minimizing the attention provided when she did engage in SIB, and asking her to self-monitor her SIB, reduced episodes of SIB from a mean of just over eight episodes per month in the 9 months prior to the intervention to under one a month in the first 9 months of the intervention period. The lowest monthly frequency of SIB during baseline (4 episodes per month, for a single month) equalled the highest monthly rate seen during intervention (also for only a single month). Episodes of aggression to others (which were not targeted by the intervention) also reduced in frequency during the intervention, whereas another form of SIB (pulling out nails), also not targeted by the intervention, showed no change.

3.2.4 Rett Syndrome

Rett syndrome (RTT, OMIM312750) is a severe neurodevelopmental condition in which apparently normal development up to the age of approximately 6–18 months is followed by deceleration in the rate of head growth and deterioration in motor skills, communication, and (it has generally been thought) intellectual functioning, together with the development of stereotyped hand movements (Bahi-Buisson, 2013). Although children with RTT meet early developmental milestones appropriately, parents and experienced professionals report subtle signs of difficulty from birth onward, often in motor development including unusual hand postures and feeding difficulties (Burford, 2005; Leonard et al., 2005; Leonard & Bower, 1998). RTT is almost entirely a condition affecting females, a fact explained when Amir et al. (1999) discovered that it was caused by mutation of an X-linked gene (*MECP2*) encoding methyl-CpG-binding protein 2 (MeCP2). Most affected individuals are female heterozygotes who, owing to X chromosome inactivation, have somatic mosaicism, with some cells with normal, and some with mutated, *MECP2*; in rare cases, males can inherit the mutation from their mother, but usually die young (Katz et al., 2016). Approximately 95% of individuals with an RTT diagnosis have a confirmed mutation in *MECP2* with eight hotspot mutations accounting for more than 60% of all cases (Katz et al., 2016). However, certain "atypical" forms of RTT have also been recognized, including an "early seizure" variant and a "congenital" variant (in which the apparently normal period of early development is not seen), which are usually, respectively, associated with mutations of *CDKL5* and *FOXG1* (Bahi-Buisson, 2013).

The slowing of head growth which is one of the earliest clear signs of RTT is followed by general growth retardation, hypotonia, and development of stereotyped hand movements, sometimes including hand-mouthing, and accompanied by loss of functional hand use (Bahi-Buisson, 2013). The condition progresses with loss of language and social skills, hypersensitivity to sound, and development of SIB, accompanied by loss of motor coordination and the development of ataxia and gait apraxia (Bahi-Buisson, 2013). Girls with RTT experience respiratory problems including hyperventilation, breath-holding, and abnormal cardiorespiratory coupling, and other autonomic difficulties include gastrointestinal dysfunction and cardiac electrical problems (Katz et al., 2016). A large-scale study found that 68.1% of people with RTT had epilepsy, with a mean age of onset of 4.68 years, which was poorly controlled in 32.6% of those with epilepsy (Nissenkorn et al., 2015). Seizures however tend to decrease in severity after the teenage years and beyond (Bahi-Buisson, 2013). Social interest and interaction recover to some extent in mid-childhood, but with further aging motor deterioration, generalized rigidity, dystonia, and progressively worsening scoliosis become serious issues (Bahi-Buisson, 2013).

3.2.4.1 Cognitive Phenotype of Rett Syndrome

Owing to the severity of their difficulties with motor control and expressive language, formal testing of the cognitive abilities of girls and women with RTT is very challenging. A widespread assumption has been that their intellectual development will have been arrested at the age at which motor deterioration commenced (Loffler & Gordon, 2018). Many parents of people with RTT have however always challenged this view, and recent research using eye-tracking technology to enable people with RTT to respond to formal testing have suggested that the receptive vocabulary of at least some people with RTT is mildly impaired or within the normal range (Ahonniska-Assa et al., 2018; Loffler & Gordon, 2018). The development of eye-tracking technology (Djukic & Valicenti McDermott, 2012; Djukic, Valicenti McDermott, Mavrommatis, & Martins, 2012) has also stimulated work into more specific aspects of cognition in RTT. Girls and women with RTT appear to have difficulties in recognition of facial emotional expressions (Djukic, Rose, Jankowski, & Feldman, 2014), anticipatory shifting of attention (Rose, Djukic, Jankowski, Feldman, & Rimler, 2016), sustaining attention (Rose, Wass, Jankowski, Feldman, & Djukic, 2017), and visual search (Rose, Wass, Jankowski, Feldman, & Djukic, 2019). Since people with RTT also have atypical cortical responses to visual stimuli (LeBlanc et al., 2015; Stauder, Smeets, van Mil, & Curfs, 2006), it is likely that these difficulties are associated with changes in cortical excitatory/inhibitory balance (LeBlanc et al., 2015).

3.2.4.2 Phenomenology and Behavioral Context of Self-Injurious Behavior in Rett Syndrome

The emergence of SIB in children with RTT is typically described as dating to the period of loss of early developmental skills and emergence of hand stereotypies (Bahi-Buisson, 2013), although there has been little systematic study of its early development. Early studies estimated that just under 50% of people with RTT engaged in SIB (Coleman, Brubaker, Hunter, & Smith, 1988; Sansom, Krishnan, Corbett, & Kerr, 1993). Cass et al. (2003) recorded an overall prevalence of 73.8% in a clinical case series of children and adults, despite considering only one topography of SIB (self-scratching). They observed this behavior in 55% of children under 5 and between 78.6% and 85.7% of older children, teenagers, and young adults. Cianfaglione et al. (2015) however found a much lower prevalence of SIB (28.2% overall) in a British national sample of girls and women with RTT, despite considering a broader range of topographies. Rubbing/scratching themselves was the most common topography engaged in by those who did self-injure (45.8% of cases), but self-hitting and self-biting were both engaged in by one-third of those who self-injured, with smaller numbers pulling at their own hair and/or skin and hitting themselves against surfaces. Cianfaglione et al. (2015) also observed that engaging in SIB was associated with the degree of overactivity and impulsivity and also with milder severity of overall signs and symptoms of RTT. Buchanan et al. (2019) reported data from a large (over 800 participants) study of females with RTT aged 3 years and over. A clinical rating scale recorded "self-mutilation," defined as pulling at one's own hair or ears, or self-scratching, while headbanging was included with throwing objects, spitting, etc. as "aggressive behavior," and "biting self and others" was again recorded separately. Each of these groups of behaviors was recorded as never occurring for over 80% of study participants. Aggressive behavior and biting self and others reduced with age, while self-mutilation showed no change. "Self-abuse," recorded in clinical records separately from the structured rating scale, was noted in 35.4% of the sample. Buchanan et al. (2019) confirmed Cianfaglione et al.'s (2015) finding that engaging in SIB was associated with milder severity of overall signs and symptoms of RTT and also noted overall a high prevalence of night waking (41%), daytime napping (37%), constipation (82%), and gastroesophageal reflux (44%) among their participants.

It appears therefore that although the prevalence of SIB in RTT is higher than those reported for children and adults with IDs of mixed or unknown origin, it is comparable with the prevalence of SIB in people with autism spectrum conditions (ASCs: see Chap. 2). Self-rubbing and scratching do however appear to be forms of SIB which are more common in RTT compared with other NDCs (Cianfaglione et al., 2015). In an observational study of ten girls and women, with less severe forms of typical or atypical RTT, Cianfaglione et al. (2016) found that while at home, eight of the ten engaged in hand stereotypies for over 30% of the time. Six engaged in SIB, including biting of the fingers, arm, and hand and hitting the head and mouth. Engagement in hand stereotypy was found to be unrelated to patterns of social interaction. The same was true for SIB for two participants, but for the remaining four, engagement in SIB was related to patterns of interaction with carers consistent with SIB being socially reinforced (Cianfaglione et al., 2016).

Over 80% of the parents of females with RTT surveyed by Coleman et al. (1988) described insensitivity to pain in their daughters, and almost as many reported that their daughter showed inappropriate levels of fear in unfamiliar situations. The parental survey of Sansom et al. (1993) reported that relatively brief episodes of low mood and anxiety were common in girls and women with RTT, with the latter in particular being associated with SIB and apparently related to environmental events including sudden noises, changes of routine, and unfamiliar people or places. Many case descriptions of females with RTT have also described difficulties with social interaction skills (Mount, Hastings, Reilly, Cass, & Charman, 2001). Later surveys using structured assessments to compare the profiles of females with RTT to those of females with severe or profound ID of mixed etiologies have confirmed that mood fluctuations and episodes of fear and anxiety, and difficulties in social relationship skills, are more common in those with RTT (Mount, Charman, Hastings, Reilly, & Cass, 2003; Mount, Charman, Hastings, Reilly, & Cass, 2002; Mount, Hastings, Reilly, Cass, & Charman, 2003). Compared with typically developing age-matched girls, girls with RTT show higher levels of urinary cortisol excretion (relative to lean body mass), indicative of possible differences in stress responses (Motil, Schultz, Abrams, Ellis, & Glaze, 2006).

3.2.4.3 Neurobiology of Rett Syndrome

Early postmortem and imaging studies with people with clinically diagnosed RTT revealed reduced brain and cerebral volumes, with reductions proportionally greater in prefrontal, posterior frontal, and anterior temporal regions and more limited in posterior temporal and posterior occipital regions. Widespread reduction in the size of individual neurons, with less dendritic arborization and spines than those observed in typically developing individuals, was also reported (Armstrong, 2005). Reduction in size of the caudate nucleus was also noted (Reiss et al., 1993). Subsequent studies of cortical regions suggested generalized reductions in white matter throughout the cortex, with gray matter reductions more pronounced in prefrontal, posterior frontal, and anterior temporal regions and less marked in the posterior occipital region (Carter et al., 2008). Subsequent research with girls with confirmed *MECP2* mutations replicated previous findings of absolute reductions throughout the brain, including cortex, with diffuse reductions in white matter, but suggested that relative decreases in gray matter were consistently seen only in the parietal lobe, particularly in dorsal parietum (Carter et al., 2008). Carter et al. (2008) did however find relative reductions in anterior frontal lobe volumes in girls with more severe overall presentation of RTT. Further, in a comparison of two monozygotic but clinically discordant twins with differing patterns of X-inactivation which resulted in one showing clear signs of RTT while the other had only minor language difficulties, Carter et al. found that both had occipital gray matter volumes comparable to those of typically developing girls, while only the clinically affected twin showed reduced volumes, particularly with respect to gray matter, in the whole brain and frontal, parietal, and temporal lobes.

Early studies of the neurochemistry of RTT found decreased cholinergic markers in basal forebrain structures, hippocampus, thalamus, and basal ganglia, variable findings with respect to dopaminergic and serotonergic activity, and increased β-endorphin levels in the thalamus (Wenk, 1997). Subsequent research has confirmed lower than normal levels of metabolites of both dopamine and serotonin in people with RTT and found that people with an *MECP2* mutation associated with more severe symptomatology had greater reductions in metabolite levels than those with a mutation associated with a milder phenotype (Samaco et al., 2009). Subsequent research, informed by the development of mouse models of RTT, suggests that MeCP2 deficiency affects multiple neural pathways and neurotransmitter systems and that it has impacts on both neuronal development and differentiation in the developing brain and ongoing processes of neuronal and synaptic homeostasis (Kaufmann, Stallworth, Everman, & Skinner, 2016). In human brain development, expression of the MeCP2 protein is first seen in brainstem structures and in the Cajal-Retzius cells which contribute to the organization of cortical development; then is seen in the thalamus, striatum, and hippocampus; and then progresses widely throughout the cortex (Shahbazian, Antalffy, Armstrong, & Zoghbi, 2002). Although the number of neurons expressing MeCP2 increases rapidly during gestation, the proportion of cortical neurons expressing MeCP2 continues to increase throughout early and middle childhood (Shahbazian et al., 2002), and it is likely therefore that dysfunction in various structures and neurotransmitter systems will become salient at different developmental stages (Kaufmann et al., 2016). For example, in early childhood, *N*-methyl-D-aspartate (NMDA) glutamate receptor densities were found to be higher in the cortical superior frontal gyrus of girls with RTT than in neurologically unimpaired girls, but by age 10 this pattern had reversed (Blue, Naidu, & Johnston, 1999a). A similar developmental pattern has been observed in the putamen (Blue, Naidu, & Johnston, 1999b), and elevated levels of glutamate reported in childhood (Horská et al., 2009). The potential effectiveness of pharmacological interventions may therefore vary across the various stages of the progression of RTT.

3.2.4.4 Animal Models of Rett Syndrome

Models of RTT have been developed in mice, rats, monkeys, and other species (Ip, Mellios, & Sur, 2018) and have led to considerable advances in understanding the processes involved in the development of RTT and identification and testing of potential therapeutic strategies (Ip et al., 2018; Katz et al., 2016; Kaufmann et al., 2016). The utility of mouse models in particular has been aided by the fact that some salient and specific features of RTT, such as the problems controlling breathing, can be assessed more directly and reliably in mice than more complex behavioral features of the condition (Katz et al., 2016). Male mice with a single inactivated copy of the *Mecp2* gene, or female mice with the gene inactivated on both X chromosomes, develop motor problems at 3–8 weeks of age, and most later develop breathing irregularities and unusual clasping of hindlimbs seemingly analogous to the hand/arm stereotypies seen in people with RTT; mice with the gene selectively deleted in brain rather than somatic tissues show essentially the same phenotype (Guy, Hendrich, Holmes, Martin, & Bird, 2001). Mice with *Mecp2* deletions or mutations have reduced volumes in many cortical areas (Allemang-Grand et al., 2017). Mouse models of specific deletions causing RTT in humans, and conditional knockout models enabling the effect of region-specific *Mecp2* inactivation to be examined, have further clarified the effects of loss of MeCP2 in human RTT. Male mice with a mutation similar to common RTT causing alleles show subtle abnormalities of social behavior and social memory, spatial memory, and diurnal activity patterns, together with impaired contextual fear conditioning (Moretti et al., 2006; Moretti, Bouwknecht, Teague, Paylor, & Zoghbi, 2005). These mice also show elevated anxiety and an abnormal stress response to being restrained, as evidenced by elevated serum corticosterone levels, mediated by increased corticotropin-releasing hormone gene expression in the paraventricular nucleus of the hypothalamus, the central amygdala, and the bed nucleus of the stria terminalis (McGill et al., 2006). Mice with reduced MeCP2 levels in forebrain regions (prefrontal cortex, striatum, nucleus accumbens, hippocampus, and amygdala) show hindlimb clasping, impaired motor coordination, heightened anxiety, abnormalities in social behavior, and impaired cue-dependent but unimpaired context-dependent fear conditioning (Gemelli et al., 2006). Viral-mediated specific deletion of *Mecp2* in the basolateral amygdala of mice (Adachi, Autry, Covington III, & Monteggia, 2009) replicated the increased anxiety and impaired cue-dependent but unimpaired context-dependent fear conditioning, but without the social interaction deficit. Mice with selective deletion of *Mecp2* from hypothalamic neurons, by contrast, show unimpaired cue- and context-dependent fear conditioning and only limited signs of increased anxiety, but show an exaggerated cortisol response to restraint stress together with aggression toward unfamiliar mice placed in their home cage after a period of single housing (Fyffe et al., 2008). Deleting *Mecp2* from dopaminergic and noradrenergic neurons reduces whole-brain levels of dopamine and norepinephrine and causes motor coordination problems, while deleting *Mecp2* from serotonergic neurons reduces serotonin levels and increases aggression, in mice so engineered (Samaco et al., 2009). Finally, loss of MeCP2 in GABAergic inhibitory neurons throughout the brain causes mice to develop many features related to the human RTT phenotype. These behaviors include forelimb and other stereotypies, excessive grooming leading to epidermal lesions (with unimpaired nociception), motor dysfunction, abnormalities in social behavior, reduced acoustic startle together with increased prepulse inhibition, and normal spatial learning on a maze task but impairment of spatial memory as reflected in performance on a post-training probe trial (Chao et al., 2010). Loss of MeCP2 from a subset of forebrain GABAergic neurons only also resulted in stereotypies, motor dysfunction, and abnormalities in social behavior, startle response, and prepulse inhibition, but without SIB (Chao et al., 2010). GABAergic neurons almost exclusively serve as interneurons, with functions including synchronization of circuit activity, providing context-dependent modulation of dynamic changes in excitation so as to maintain circuit functionality (Hattori,

Kuchibhotla, Froemke, & Komiyama, 2017; Rudy, Fishell, Lee, & Hjerling-Leffler, 2011). Three major subclasses, identified by their expression of parvalbumin (PV), somatostatin (SOM), and vasoactive intestinal polypeptide (VIP), constitute the majority of such neurons, and are believed to exercise different functions in circuit regulation, including modulation of experience-dependent plasticity of excitatory circuits, and to be dynamically involved in regulating and integrating diverse components of complex behaviors, providing context-dependent modulation (Ito-Ishida, Ure, Chen, Swann, & Zoghbi, 2015). Ito-Ishida et al. (2015) selectively deleted *Mecp2* from PV-positive and SOM-positive neurons in mice and demonstrated that removal of MeCP2 from PV-positive neurons led to motor, sensory, fear conditioning, and social deficits, while mice lacking MeCP2 in SOM-positive neurons developed seizures and stereotyped behaviors.

The importance of GABAergic processes in RTT has been further demonstrated by Banerjee et al. (2016), who found that male mice with a single inactivated copy of the *Mecp2* gene showed reduced visually driven excitatory and inhibitory conductances in primary visual cortex pyramidal neurons, together with alterations in their relative timing, thus reducing response reliability and selectivity. These changes were associated with reduced responses in PV-positive interneurons and were replicated in mice with MeCP2 removed from PV-positive inhibitory neurons only, supporting a significant role for abnormality of GABAergic processes in disrupting cortical processing in RTT. The potential relevance of GABAergic processes in the RTT phenotype, and their complex interplay with social processes, is provided by a study of the effect of MeCP2 deficiency on the behavior of female mice heterozygous for the *Mecp2* deletion in a naturalistic observational learning situation (Krishnan, Lau, Ewall, Huang, & Shea, 2017). Wild-type female mice with no previous maternal experience can learn to respond to distress calls from mouse pups if they are co-housed with first-time mothers and their pups. Mice heterozygous for the *Mecp2* deletion are impaired in this learning. Krishnan et al. (2017) found that expression of GAD1 (GAD67), a key enzyme in synthesis of GABA, was significantly increased in the auditory cortex 5 days after the initiation of maternal experience, and returned to baseline levels by the time pups were weaned, in both wild-type and *Mecp2* heterozygous mice. However, during the corresponding period, the *Mecp2* heterozygous mice showed transient increases in highly PV-expressing interneurons, and high-intensity perineuronal nets associated with them, not seen in wild-type mice. Loss of or impairment of MeCP2, in addition to its structural effects on brain development, thus apparently continues to dynamically impair or deform neuronal plasticity in response to learning opportunities, reducing or distorting learning outcomes.

Animal, and particularly knockout mouse, models of RTT have contributed substantially to understanding of the processes involved in RTT at the tissue, cell, and increasingly molecular level (Ip et al., 2018). This research also has potential implications for understanding several other NDCs where *MECP2* mutations have been reported in individual cases (Samaco et al., 2008). Some caution must however be exercised in extrapolating findings from these animal models to women with RTT. Much of the research has been conducted with male mice, with their single copy of *Mecp2* deleted or mutated, in order to avoid the phenotypic variability associated with X-chromosome silencing if female mice heterozygous for the deletion are used. Such female mice do show a phenotype similar in many respects to those of males with the gene deleted on their X-chromosome, but there are some differences potentially relevant to the cognitive/emotional phenotype in particular. For example, female mice heterozygous for the deletion show complex abnormalities in social behavior, and impaired context-dependent but unimpaired cue-dependent fear conditioning, but also show reduced signs of anxiety, normal baseline corticosterone levels, and a normal or attenuated corticosterone response to stress depending on their wider genotype (Philippe et al., 2018; Samaco et al., 2013).

3.2.4.5 Psychopharmacological Therapies for Rett Syndrome

The understanding of the consequences of MeCP2 deficiency gained from animal models and from studies using human cells (Ip et al., 2018) has led to identification of a wide range of possible therapeutic targets, including the *MECP2* gene and its protein product, but also a variety of mechanisms downstream of *MECP2* including neurotransmitter signalling pathways, growth factor signalling pathways, metabolic pathways, and ion channels (Katz et al., 2016; see Fig. 3.1). A correspondingly wide range of interventions have been proposed and/or tested in animals, including gene therapy, targeted re-activation of X-silenced copies of *MECP2*, and use of nerve growth factors including brain-derived neurotrophic factor and insulin-like growth factor 1, and treatments designed to boost growth factor levels. The latter class of interventions has already been translated to clinical trials with humans, to date with mixed outcomes (Katz et al., 2016: O'Leary et al., 2018). Although disturbances in neurotransmitter systems are in principle possible treatment targets, the variability in findings with regard to many neurotransmitters, which may result from real variability in their status in different phases of the development of RTT, raises challenges in selecting appropriate interventions for specific individuals (Kaufmann et al., 2016; Roux & Villard, 2010). Nevertheless, there have been several clinical studies of the effects of neurotransmitter modulators in RTT. Bromocriptine is a potent dopamine D_2 receptor agonist which also agonizes multiple other subtypes of dopaminergic, serotonergic, and adrenergic receptors. Zappella (Zappella, 1990; Zappella, Genazzani, Facchinetti, & Hayek, 1990) conducted an open-label and then a double-blind placebo-controlled half-crossover trial of bromocriptine with 13 and 10 girls with RTT, respectively. In the open trial, parents were also given guidance on interacting with their children, stimulating them with stories and music, and encouraging mobility. Bromocriptine was given for 6 months, withdrawn for 2 months, and resumed for 2 months. Eight of the 13 girls improved on more than one aspect of a comprehensive clinical evaluation (not however including SIB), but in many cases improvements were lost when treatment was withdrawn, and not always recovered with reinstatement of bromocriptine. In the double-blind trial, three out of ten girls showed some improvement with bromocriptine.

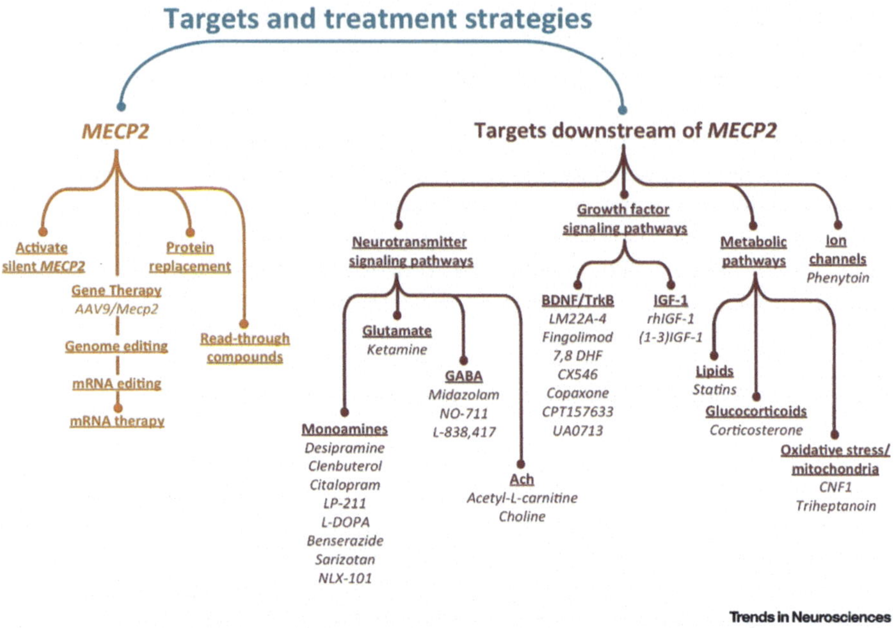

Fig. 3.1 Therapeutic targets and potential pharmacological strategies currently being explored in animal models for the treatment of RTT. Underlined headings indicate therapeutic targets; compounds that have been reported in the literature to be effective in improving behavioral outcome measures or physiological function in vivo are shown in italics. (Reproduced with permission of Elsevier Ltd. from Katz, D. M., Bird, A., Coenraads, M., Gray, S. J., Menon, D. U., Philpot, B. D., & Tarquinio, D. C. (2016). Rett syndrome: Crossing the threshold to clinical translation. *Trends in Neurosciences, 39*(2), 100–113. © 2016 Published by Elsevier Ltd)

Dextromethorphan, an NMDA receptor antagonist, has been reported in a preliminary trial to have a dose-dependent positive effect on receptive language, but no effect on clinically rated global severity (Smith-Hicks et al., 2017). A randomized, double-blind, placebo-controlled trial of desipramine, an inhibitor of norepinephrine and serotonin reuptake, was focused on possible effects of blocking norepinephrine reuptake on breathing difficulties in girls with RTT. Desipramine did not significantly improve breathing irregularities, and no incidental positive effects on the girls' emotional or behavioral difficulties were reported (Mancini et al., 2018). In a rare report of a treatment targeting neurotransmitter levels specifically impacting on SIB in a person with RTT, Temudo et al. (2009) noted that in one of two very young girls with RTT who had low levels of 5-hydroxyindoleacetic acid, indicating low levels of serotonin, treatment with the selective serotonin reuptake inhibitor fluoxetine decreased self-injurious stereotypies after 1 month. Overall, therefore, there is to date little evidence of positive effects of treatment with neurotransmitter modulators in RTT and even less of any effect on SIB. However, further trials with NMDA receptor antagonists are ongoing, and the limited effects seen with drugs targeting the dopamine and serotonin systems to date may be due to the variable involvement of these systems at different stages of the development of RTT.

3.2.4.6 Other Therapies for Rett Syndrome

Experimental functional analyses (EFAs) have been reported for stereotyped hand movements in a total of ten people with RTT (Roane, Piazza, Sgro, Volkert, & Anderson, 2001; Wales, Charman, & Mount, 2004) and of self-injurious hand-mouthing in three others (Iwata, Pace, & Willis, 1986; Oliver, Murphy, Crayton, & Corbett, 1993). In only one of these cases (reported by Oliver et al., 1993) was a possible social function of the behavior identified. Nevertheless, behavioral interventions, primarily involving physical interruption or blocking of stereotyped or self-injurious behaviors together with prompting and reinforcement of more adaptive hand behaviors, have been reported to reduce stereotyped or self-injurious behaviors in all five cases in which their use has been reported (Iwata et al., 1986; Paisey, Whitney, & Wainczak, 1993; Roane et al., 2001). Evans and Meyer (1999) however reported that interrupting hand stereotypies led to an increase in other problematic responses and found that reducing educational demands and increasing playful interactions with a teacher were the most effective methods of reducing the hand stereotypies of a girl with RTT. The use of new communication technologies (Simacek, Reichle, & McComas, 2016) and computer-supported systems for detecting and reinforcing constructive hand movements (Stasolla et al., 2015) may offer new possibilities for delivering behavioral interventions.

Research using female mice heterozygous for the *Mecp2* deletion has shown that post-weaning environmental enrichment (EE) and voluntary exercise normalize the reduced levels of anxiety shown in these mice and reduce their elevated basal serum corticosterone levels (Kondo et al., 2016). An intervention comprising 2–3 h of motor learning and exercise together with social, cognitive, and sensory experiences for 6 days per week over a 6-month period has been shown to improve gross motor skills in young (1 year 6 months to 5 years 2 months) girls with RTT (Downs et al., 2018). Participation in the intervention was accompanied by increases in blood levels of brain-derived neurotrophic factor, which Kondo et al. (2016) had found to be increased in the hippocampus of mice heterozygous for the *Mecp2* deletion given EE and exercise, but no effects were seen on the girls' mood (Downs et al., 2018).

Deep brain stimulation of the fimbria-fornix, which regulates hippocampal activity, has been shown to improve contextual but not cue-dependent fear conditioning in female mice heterozygous for the *Mecp2* deletion (Hao et al., 2015). This effect probably results from modulation of activity in both excitatory and inhibitory neurons (Lu et al., 2016) and has been suggested as a possible future therapy in RTT (Ip et al., 2018). Low doses of ketamine, an antagonist of NMDA receptors, have been shown to normalize cortical activity in mice lacking *Mecp2* (Patrizi et al., 2016) and are believed to act by inhibiting GABAergic inhibitory neurons (Katz et al., 2016). Ketamine may also stimulate long-term synaptic repair processes and thus may have multiple effects in RTT (Katz et al., 2016), and clinical trials are ongoing.

3.2.5 Three Genetic Syndromes Associated with Self-Injurious Behavior: Summary

The first conclusion which can clearly be drawn from considering the neurobiology of LNS, SMS, and RTT is that in each case mutations in a single gene affect a complex cascade of developmental processes resulting in changes in multiple brain regions and neurotransmitter systems. With regard to the overall phenotype associated with these syndromes, Table 3.1 presents a selective summary of the phenotypes associated with these conditions and their principal animal models.

In making cross-condition and cross-model comparisons, it should be remembered that mouse models in particular can show marked phenotypic differences dependent on the specific deletions or mutations involved, the broader genetic background, and gender. Further, some recent findings from mouse models require replication. Nevertheless, comparison of these genetic conditions identifies some commonalities of potential relevance to a broader understanding of the development of SIB. Perhaps the most striking point concerns the cognitive phenotype. Although research involving people with IDs has typically found a strong inverse association between ability and SIB, both LNS and SMS are typically associated with moderate levels of ID. Further, although people with RTT were formerly assumed to have severe levels of ID, recent research results are challenging this view. It seems possible therefore that none of these three syndromes in which SIB is a key element of the behavioral phenotype are characterized by very severe ID. All three conditions are however associated with hypotonia and other problems of motor coordination, and these contribute to speech difficulties, resulting in impairments in expressive language skills in the context of relatively stronger receptive skills. In all three conditions, complex difficulties in social interaction have been noted. In the case of individuals with SMS, this appears to take the form of increased motivation to interact with caregiving adults, while in the *Df(11)17/+* mouse model of SMS, it appears as an enhancement of the normal tendency of "wild-type" mice to spend more time in proximity to a stranger mouse most recently placed into a cage with them than to a previously introduced stranger. Mice with reduced levels of MeCP2, modelling RTT, by contrast appear to show lower interest in interacting with newly introduced mice. Gastrointestinal problems are common in people with LNS and RTT, and sleep difficulties and peripheral neuropathy and/or reduced pain sensation are reported in SMS and RTT. Aggression toward others, attentional difficulties, and stereotypy are reported as common in all three conditions, with impulsivity and/or hyperactivity noted in people with LNS and SMS and anxiety and/or inappropriate fears reported as commonly experienced by people with LNS and RTT. Reduced volumes in diverse cortical areas are reported for all three conditions, and reduced volumes in one or more of the basal ganglia structures have been reported for all three.

Table 3.1 Key features of the phenotypes of Lesch-Nyhan, Smith-Magenis, and Rett syndromes and their principal animal models. *N/A* not applicable, *ID* intellectual disability, *DA* dopamine, *5-HT* serotonin, *Ne* norepinephrine, *GABA* gamma-aminobutyric acid

Table 3.1 Key features of the phenotypes of Lesch-Nyhan, Smith-Magenis, and Rett syndromes and their principal animal models

Condition OR animal model of condition	Typical initial SIB topography	SIB increased by	Motor development	Language difficulties	Social interaction	Common health and related conditions	Cognitive phenotype	Behavioral and emotional phenotype	Brain anatomy	NT abnormalities
Lesch-Nyhan syndrome	Self-biting	Stress	Delayed, with hypotonia and severe action dystonia	Dysarthria	Impaired	Gastro-oesophageal reflux, emesis	I.Q. 39-81, impaired auditory divided attention and short-term memory	Aggression, anxiety, depression, attention difficulties, stereotypy, hyperactivity.	Reduced GM in frontal cortex, hippocampus, amygdala, left insula, cingulate gyrus, ventral striatum	Reduced DA levels in striatum
6-OHDA Neonatally lesioned rat	Self-biting	Stress		N/A		Reduced caloric intake	Impairments of learning and memory	Hyperactivity, impaired habituation, altered startle response and sensory gating		Reduced DA, increased 5-HT levels in striatum
Smith-Magenis syndrome	Self-biting, self-hitting, hitting self against surfaces		Delayed, with hypotonia and oral motor dysfunction	Verbal dyspraxia	Increased motivation for interaction with adults	Otolaryngolic problems, hearing impairment, sleep disturbance and peripheral neuropathy	Moderate ID to normal I.Q., impaired short-term memory	Aggression, attention difficulties, obsessive thinking, stereotypy, impulsivity, hyperactivity,	Reduced GM volumes in insula, putamen and globus pallidus, grey matter heteropia	
Df(11)17/+ mouse	None	N/A		N/A	Subtly impaired	Seizures, changes in circadian rhythm	Unimpaired fear conditioning	Hypoactivity (in males), reduced anxiety		

(continued)

Table 3.1 (continued)

Condition OR animal model of condition	Typical initial SIB topography	SIB increased by	Motor development	Language difficulties	Social interaction	Common health and related conditions	Cognitive phenotype	Behavioral and emotional phenotype	Brain anatomy	NT abnormalities
Rett syndrome	Self-rubbing or scratching		Deteriorates after normal early development with hypotonia, ataxia, gait apraxia and hand stereotypies	Expressive language lost after normal early development	Social skills deteriorate after normal early development; difficulty in recognising facial emotional expressions	Breathing difficulties, cardiac problems, gastro-intestinal problems, sleep disturbance, seizures, pain insensitivity	General ability uncertain but may range from severe ID to normal I.Q.	Aggression, inappropriate fear in unfamiliar situations, episodes of low mood and anxiety, attention difficulties, stereotypy	Reduced GM volumes in anterior frontal and parietal cortex; reduced volume of caudate, diffuse reductions in white matter	Changes in multiple neurotransmitter systems as condition progresses
Mecp2 deleted or mutated mouse	Excessive grooming leading to lesions		Impaired motor coordination, forelimb motor stereotypies	N/A	Subtle abnormalities of social behavior and memory	Seizures	Subtle abnormalities of spatial learning; impaired contextual fear conditioning	Aggression, anxiety, abnormal stress response, reduced startle response	Reduced volumes in many cortical areas	Reduced DA, 5-HT, Ne and GABA in neurons without *Mecp2*

N/A not applicable, *ID* intellectual disability, *DA* dopamine, *5-HT* serotonin, *Ne* norepinephrine, *GABA* gamma-aminobutyric acid

3.3 Other Animal Models of Self-Injurious Behavior

In the last decade, a large number of knockout mouse models with potential relevance to human NDCs, especially ASCs, have been generated. Many of these have targeted genes with products expected to exert pervasive effects on neurodevelopment, such as the SHANK proteins, which are believed to play an important role in the functioning of glutamatergic synapses (Eltokhi, Rappold, & Sprengel, 2018). Mice with knockout of the gene coding for the SHANK3 protein show excessive self-grooming leading to lesions which typically appear first on the face or back of the neck (Peça et al., 2011). Use of conditional knockout mice to investigate the effects of reduced *Shank3* expression in different brain areas of such mice shows that reduction of SHANK3 in the striatum is associated with repetitive behaviors but that excessive self-grooming leading to lesions is associated with SHANK3 deficiency in the cortex and hippocampus, albeit at a trend level lower than that seen in mice with brain-wide knockout of *Shank3* (Bey et al., 2018).

A second approach to modelling SIB in animals, rather than starting by reproducing in a nonhuman animal the genetic alteration associated with SIB in humans, begins by modelling neurotransmitter abnormalities observed in human conditions associated with SIB and/or genetic knockout models. One such model, the neonatally 6-OHDA-lesioned rat, was described above. In a second rat model, the administration of the long-acting psychostimulant pemoline, either in a single 300mg/kg dose or by several daily treatments with doses of 80–200 mg, results in stereotyped self-biting (Devine, 2012, 2014). Animals given lower doses (100mg/kg/day) mainly bite their tails, while higher doses (200 or 300 mg/kg/day) result in biting of the forepaws and ventrum (Kies & Devine, 2004). The pemoline model has a number of features which immediately increase its appeal as a model of human SIB. Firstly, when rats are treated with the repeated lower doses of pemoline, only some show SIB, suggesting that the pemoline treatment produces a model of vulnerability to, rather than complete causation of, SIB (Devine, 2014). The pemoline model thus offers the possibility to examine other factors which may interact with the pemoline-induced vulnerability to cause (or protect against) development of SIB. Among the factors which increase the probability of SIB developing and/or exacerbate its severity are cortical damage (Cromwell, Levine, & King, 1999), being raised in social isolation, especially if that is combined with an impoverished physical environment (Devine, 2014), social stress (Muehlmann et al., 2012), and innate responsivity to stress (Muehlmann, Wilkinson, & Devine, 2011). Repeated pemoline injections reduce striatal dopamine to less than 70% of baseline levels, while measures of neuronal metabolic activity after a course of pemoline show downregulation in a number of regions associated with limbic and basal ganglia function, including the striatum, ventral pallidum, and hippocampal subfields (Devine, 2014). The involvement of the basal ganglia is supported by the fact that pemoline-induced SIB is reduced by administration of a variety of D_1 and D_2 receptor antagonists and exacerbated by the selective serotonin reuptake inhibitor paroxetine, suggesting involvement of a dopaminergic mechanism with possible modulation by striatal serotonergic activity (Devine, 2014). Limbic system involvement is suggested by a therapeutic effect of sodium valproate on pemoline-induced SIB (Devine, 2014). Of further interest in this model of SIB is that pemoline treatment is first associated with increased levels of activity and stereotyped behaviors (STBs), with the latter replaced by self-biting as pemoline administrations continue (Devine, 2014; Kies & Devine, 2004).

As noted earlier, despite their helpfulness in tracing causal pathways of other features of the syndromes involved, many mouse models of syndromes associated with high prevalences of SIB either show no SIB at all or limited SIB produced by excessive self-grooming. Administration of the L-type calcium channel activator Bay K 8644, especially early in post-weaning development, induces dystonia together with active self-biting in mice (Devine, 2012). In a series of studies of these mice, Kasim and colleagues (Kasim, Egami, & Jinnah, 2002; Kasim & Jinnah, 2003) showed that Bay K 8644-induced SIB was increased by administration of the indirect dopamine agonists amphetamine and GBR 12909 or by a monoamine oxidase inhibitor, but also by the selective serotonin reuptake inhibitor (SSRI) fluoxetine. SIB was conversely reduced by drugs which deplete vesicular stores of dopamine or deplete serotonin, again implicating both dopaminergic and serotonergic systems in causation of SIB in these mice. In a further series of experiments using dopamine receptor subtype selective antagonists or selective knockouts, Kasim et al. (2006) demonstrated that Bay K 8644-induced SIB was associated with dopamine receptor functioning rather than increased presynaptic release of dopamine and further implicated D_1, D_3 and/or D_5, but not D_2 and D_4, receptors in the mediation of this effect.

One final influential animal model of SIB concerns the behaviors engaged in by primates who have been raised in isolation and/or in physically impoverished environments. As adults these primates (rhesus macaque monkeys being the species most extensively studied) show extensive and severe behavioral dysfunctions including impaired performance on tests of cognition, impulsivity, overeating and drinking, STBs (including body-directed STBs such as self-mouthing), exaggerated responses to minor changes in routine, and SIB including self-biting, headbanging, and eye-gouging (Schroeder, Loupe, & Tessel, 2008). Studies of the effects of variation in the amount of time spent in social isolation and the age at which isolation commences suggest that early deprivation of social experience is the major factor influencing later behavioral difficulties (Devine, 2014). The identification of a model of SIB comprising multiple self-injurious topographies resembling those seen in humans, and observed in a primate species, immediately suggests the relevance of the model to SIB in humans. The relevance of the model is further increased by the fact that even without severe early social isolation, some macaques housed singly or in groups in laboratory conditions develop SIB, with reported prevalence between 5 and 14% (Stanwicks, Hamel, & Novak, 2017). Further, macaques who engage in SIB show higher levels of STBs, impairments in social interaction, and sleep disturbance, than those who do not, mirroring several of the correlates of SIB in humans (Devine, 2014; Stanwicks et al., 2017). Isolation-reared macaques show abnormalities in basal ganglia functioning involving dopaminergic and peptidergic neurons, and also in the function of the limbic-hypothalamic-pituitary-adrenal axis (Devine, 2014), although whether the latter is implicated in causation of SIB or rather is a consequence of chronic engagement in SIB remains uncertain (Novak, El-Mallah, & Menard, 2014).

Although some studies of animal models of SIB have examined the interactions between biological vulnerability and subsequent social factors such as stress, there have been few attempts to examine interactions with the processes of social operant conditioning which are regarded as key factors in the causation of SIB within the operant model. Schaefer (1970) used shaping (a process in which reinforcement is delivered contingent on behaviors with a criterion for reinforcement which is progressively adjusted toward the desired behavioral topography) to train two laboratory-housed rhesus monkeys to hit their own heads with a forepaw with sufficient force to eventually produce lesions. Schaefer (1970) showed that the SIB could be brought under stimulus control (see Box 3.1) and that it was abolished when the monkeys were given free access to the food reinforcers which were used to shape the SIB. An attempt to subsequently shape one of the monkeys to bang his head against a wall however resulted in failure, which Schaefer attributed to the inadequacy of his shaping program. Layng, Andronis, and Goldiamond (1999) similarly shaped headbanging in two pigeons. Following shaping, the schedule on which the behavior was reinforced was gradually shifted from one reinforcer for every response to one reinforcer after completion of 40 responses. As is typical for such schedules, the birds responded rapidly and with considerable force, such that they periodically fell over. A pattern of responding emerged in which periods of high rate and vigorous responding alternated with periods in which the birds stopped headbanging for periods of up to 20 min after they had fallen over. Layng et al. (1999) subsequently brought the behavior under stimulus control, showing that the birds headbanged steadily when the discriminative stimulus for reinforcement was present and almost never when it was absent. The most interesting aspect of this study from a clinical perspective however were two further experiments in which headbanging in two additional pigeons was shaped, reinforced on a variable-interval schedule (see Box 3.1), extinguished, and then monitored while an alternative behavior (key-pecking) was shaped and then maintained under various reinforcement contingencies. When headbanging was placed on extinction, a typical "extinction burst" was seen, followed by a rapid decline in the behavior. As reinforcement for key-pecking was thinned and placed on interval schedules, however, episodes of headbanging recurred, particularly when schedules of reinforcement for headbanging were changed. Finally, continuing these conditions while very occasionally reinforcing headbanging led to a recurrence of high rates of headbanging. This animal model suggests therefore that if headbanging is developed by operant processes, the behavior will continue to occur sporadically, even if it is not being reinforced, if schedules of reinforcement for alternative behaviors thin and change, and that under these conditions even very occasional reinforcement of headbanging will maintain the behavior at stable levels.

Box 3.1 Operant Conditioning: Basic Concepts

An **operant** is a class of responses which have a common relationship with a reinforcing consequence. **Reinforcement** is a process in which a consequence which follows any member of the operant class strengthens the class. In basic research the strengthening of the operant is usually measured by an increase in the frequency with which the person or animal performs the response. However, strengthening of the operant may also be reflected in an increase in the vigor with which the response is performed and is typically also accompanied by increased resistance to extinction (see below). **Positive reinforcement** occurs when an operant is strengthened by an event which occurs contingent on the performance of a member of the operant class. **Negative reinforcement** occurs when an operant is strengthened by an event which ceases temporarily contingent on the performance of a member of the operant class. **Extinction** occurs when the contingency between the performance of responses which are members of the operant class and the presentation of a positive reinforcer or the removal of a negative reinforcer is discontinued. Extinction is normally seen as a progressive decrease in the frequency with which responses which are members of the operant class are performed.

Events which function as positive or negative reinforcers will not always have the same effects when presented contingent on a behavior. Their effectiveness as reinforcers varies. **Motivating operations** increase or decrease their reinforcing effects. Food deprivation, for example, will usually increase the reinforcement value of food, while satiation will usually decrease its reinforcing value. Motivating operations which increase the value of a reinforcer are often termed **establishing operations**, while those which decrease the value of a reinforcer are sometimes referred to as **abolishing operations**. Establishing operations, in addition to causing variation in the reinforcing power of contingent stimuli, also have an evocative action, increasing the probability of responses which have previously led to relevant reinforcement.

Stimuli which are present only when reinforcement occurs may come to exert control over the behavior so that responding occurs during the presence of those stimuli but occurs at low or zero rate in their absence. Such stimuli are termed **discriminative stimuli** and are often represented by the notation S^D. Other discriminative stimuli, present only when reinforcement does not occur, may also exert control over behavior so that relevant responses are rarely produced when the stimuli are present. Such negative discriminative stimuli are sometimes represented by the notation S^Δ. In operant theory, although discriminative stimuli control responding, they are not viewed as causes of the behavior concerned. The behavior is caused by the reinforcement contingency, and the control exerted by discriminative stimuli depends entirely on that contingency. When extinction occurs, a discriminative stimulus will cease to control the behavior; a discriminative stimulus has no power to elicit behavior independent of the reinforcement contingency.

In **continuous reinforcement** (**CRF**), a reinforcer follows every response. In a **fixed-ratio** (**FR**) schedule, reinforcement follows every Nth response. FR schedules typically result in a steady, high rate of responding. In a **variable-ratio** (**VR**) schedule, the number of responses required to produce a reinforcer varies randomly (sometimes within set limits) around a mean value. VR schedules typically produce very high and stable rates of responding. In a **fixed-interval** (**FI**) schedule, reinforcement occurs following the first response which the person or animal makes after a fixed time period has elapsed. FI schedules usually result in so-called scalloping in which there is a pause in responding immediately after each reinforcement followed by an accelerating trend in responding as time passes. In a **variable-interval** (**VI**) schedule, reinforcement follows the first response following a certain interval of time, but that interval varies randomly around a mean value. VI schedules typically result in steady responding at a lower rate than those found under variable-ratio schedules. Finally, a **fixed-time** (**FT**) schedule is one in which reinforcement is provided after a fixed interval of time irrespective of behavior, and a **variable-time** (**VT**) schedule is the corresponding variable schedule.

Demonstrations that behaviors resembling SIB in humans can be established by operant processes in animals do not of course necessarily imply that such processes are involved in the natural development of SIB. Further evidence does exist however that reinforcement processes can play a role in the SIB engaged in by captive primates. An experimental functional analysis (EFA; see Chap. 5) carried out by Dorey, Rosales-Ruiz, Smith, and Lovelace (2009) on the SIB (self-biting) of a zoo-housed olive baboon suggested that her SIB was maintained by contingent (human) social interaction, and Dorey et al. (2009) showed that an intervention involving providing attention contingent on an alternative behavior (lip-smacking), while not responding to SIB, reduced the rate of SIB. The effect reported by Layng et al. (1999) in which changes in reinforcement of another behavior exacerbate SIB has also been reported for the SIB engaged in by partial isolate-reared rhesus macaques, which show bursts of SIB when an alternative response is moved from continuous reinforcement to extinction (Gluck & Sackett, 1974).

Evidence from a variety of animal models (6-OHDA-lesioned rats, pemoline-treated rats, Bay K 8644-treated mice, and isolation-reared monkeys) thus implicates striatal dopaminergic dysfunction, and particularly dysfunction of D_1, D_3, and/or D_5 receptors, in the causation of SIB, possibly as a result of development of supersensitivity in these receptors. However, there is also evidence from SHANK3 knockout mice and pemoline-treated rats of serotonergic modulation of these processes, and from BAY K 8644 treated mice, pemoline-treated rats, and isolation-reared monkeys, of cortical and limbic system involvement.

3.4 Neural Circuits Associated with Prominent Risk Markers for Self-Injurious Behavior

3.4.1 Stereotyped Behaviors

With each of these candidates for a neurobiological substrate for SIB, the question arises as to whether the dysfunction observed is specific to SIB or general to broader behavioral phenotypes, including those which appear to be risk factors for development of chronic SIB. As noted in Chap. 2, two of the most frequently reported risk markers are engagement in STBs and overactivity/impulsivity. Partly because of their salience within the NDCs (e.g., in ASCs and ADHD), the neurobiology of these characteristics has received substantial attention.

With regard to STBs, abnormalities in the basal ganglia appear to play a key role in disrupting neural circuits involving also the cortex and cerebellum, with changes in the basal ganglia being the most commonly reported finding from neuroimaging studies of people with conditions associated with STBs and of animal models of those syndromes (Wilkes & Lewis, 2018). The strongest evidence is for involvement of the cortico-striato-thalamo-cortical motor loop (Muehlmann & Lewis, 2012) (see Fig. 3.2).

The striatum receives projections from the intralaminar nuclei of the thalamus, from the pars compacta of the substantia nigra, and (to the nucleus accumbens) from the ventral tegmentum (not shown in Fig. 3.2), but also inputs from many cortical regions. While fibers from "association" regions of the cortex project mainly to the caudate nucleus within the striatal complex, glutamatergic neurons originating in motor areas of the frontal lobe exert an excitatory effect directed primarily at the putamen. The outputs from the striatum are provided by "medium spiny neurons" (MSNs) which direct GABAergic inhibitory projections to the lateral (external) and medial (internal) sections of the globus pallidus and to the pars reticulata of the substantia nigra.

Approximately half of the striatal MSNs express D_1 dopamine receptors and A_1 adenosine receptors and have their activity modulated by excitatory dopaminergic input from the pars compacta of the substantia nigra, use the neuropeptides dynorphin and substance P as cotransmitters with GABA, and project directly to the internal globus pallidus and to the pars reticulata of the substantia nigra, from where further inhibitory GABAergic fibers connect to nuclei within the thalamus. The remainder of the striatal MSNs express D_2 dopamine receptors and A_2 adenosine receptors and have their activity modulated by inhibitory dopaminergic input from the pars compacta of the substantia nigra, use the neuropeptide enkephalin as a cotransmitter with GABA, and are connected to the thalamus via an indirect pathway. These indirect pathway neurons project to the external globus pallidus, from where a further inhibitory GABAergic projection runs to the subthalamic nucleus, from where excitatory glutamatergic projections to the internal globus pallidus and to the pars reticulata of the substantia nigra rejoin the "direct" pathway (Crossman & Neary, 2019; Muehlmann & Lewis, 2012). Activation of the direct pathway thus

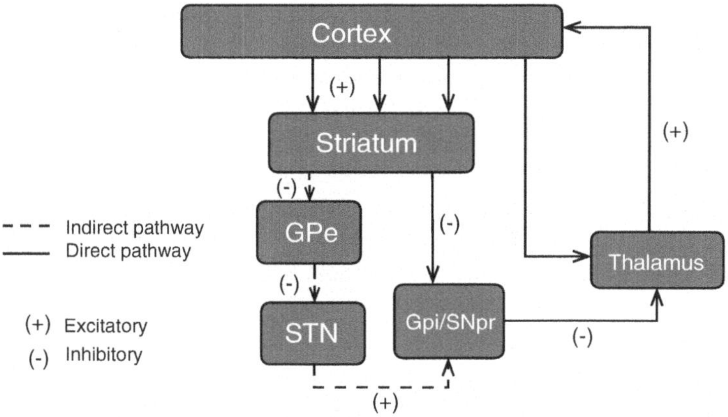

Fig. 3.2 Cortical basal ganglia circuitry. GPe, external segment of globus pallidus; GPi, internal segment of the globus pallidus; SNpr, substantia nigra pars reticulata; STN, subthalamic nucleus. (Reproduced with permission of Blackwell Publishing Ltd. from Muehlmann, A. M., & Lewis, M. H. (2012). Abnormal repetitive behaviours: Shared phenomenology and pathophysiology. *Journal of Intellectual Disability Research, 56*(5), 427–440. © 2012 The Authors. Journal of Intellectual Disability Research © 2012 Blackwell Publishing Ltd)

increases activity of the excitatory glutamatergic connections from the thalamic nuclei to frontal motor cortex which complete the cortico-striato-thalamo-cortical motor loop, while activation of the indirect pathway reduces such activity. The traditional view of these pathways is that once a motor action is initiated, the direct pathway supports the ongoing performance of that action, whereas the indirect pathway suppresses potentially interfering competitive or incompatible motor actions (Crossman & Neary, 2019). In addition to the wealth of evidence suggesting involvement of basal ganglia dysfunction in STB, several studies have focused specifically on the roles of the direct and indirect striatal-thalamic pathways. Working with deer mice, which develop STBs if reared in standard laboratory conditions, Presti and Lewis (2005) showed that STB was associated with reduced met-enkephalin levels and increased dynorphin/enkephalin content ratios in the dorsolateral striatum, suggesting that STB resulted from a hyperactivation of the direct cortico-striato-thalamo-cortical pathway which itself was caused by hypoactivation of the indirect pathway. Further evidence for this possibility comes from the finding that reduced levels of a marker of neuronal activity in the subthalamic nucleus were associated with STB (Tanimura, Vaziri, & Lewis, 2010). However, administration of a selective adenosine A_2 receptor agonist attenuated STB only when a selective A_1 agonist was co-administered, suggesting a dynamic interaction between the direct and indirect pathways possibly related to an inhibitory effect of A_1 receptor stimulation on dopamine release from presynaptic dopaminergic terminals (Tanimura et al., 2010). A recent study using optogenetic techniques (Yizhar, Fenno, Davidson, Mogri, & Deisseroth, 2011) to target stimulation at D_1 MSNs projecting to the substantia nigra pars reticulata (Bouchekioua et al., 2018) has suggested that activation of the direct pathway is sufficient to induce motor stereotypies in mice. Given the existence of multiple mechanisms for coordinated control of, and interactions between, the direct and indirect pathways (Benarroch, 2016), and the complexities of determining neuronal activation patterns following photoactivation in vivo (Bepari et al., 2012; Kravitz, Owen, & Kreitzer, 2013), further research will be necessary to confirm whether the direct pathway alone is involved in this effect. Given the likely involvement of D_1 receptors in the 6-OHDA model of SIB however, evidence of a role for the direct cortico-striato-thalamo-cortical pathway in induction of stereotypy, even if the indirect pathway is also involved, would strengthen the case for overlap in neural circuits underpinning SIB and STBs.

3.4.2 Attention Deficit Hyperactivity Disorder

Many recent studies have reported associations between attentional difficulties and impulsivity/overactivity with SIB (see Chap. 2), and people with LNS, SMS, and RTT all experience difficulties with attention. Research from murine models of these disorders also suggests presence of attentional problems impacting on learning performance, most notably in the findings of puzzling discrepancies between performance on contextual and cue-dependent aversive conditioning. Unsurprisingly given the established clinical differentiation of inattentive, impulsive-hyperactive, and combined subtypes of ADHD, research has identified a number of abnormalities in distinct neural circuits related to different aspects of the condition. Since the turn of the present century, Sonuga-Barke and colleagues (Sonuga-Barke, 2002, 2003; Sonuga-Barke, Bitsakou, & Thompson, 2010; Sonuga-Barke, Cortese, Fairchild, & Stringaris, 2016; Sonuga-Barke, Dalen, & Remington, 2003) have proposed and elaborated a multi-pathway model of ADHD. Sonuga-Barke (2002, 2003) originally proposed a dual-pathway model in which the symptoms of ADHD were suggested to result from a combination of deficits in "executive function" involving a prefrontal cortex-striato-thalamo-cortical pathway, essentially parallel to the motor pathway described above apart from the cortical regions involved, together with fundamental changes in reinforcement processes. In general, the operant approach predicts that the reinforcing effect of a stimulus varies according to its quality, size, and the immediacy with which it is delivered following a behavior. The "dual-pathway" model of ADHD proposed that in children with ADHD, the parameters of these effects are shifted so that immediacy of reinforcement exerts greater effect than quality and size, such that children with ADHD, compared to those without, are more likely to choose to obtain smaller reinforcers delivered rapidly following a behavior rather than larger reinforcers delivered with a delay. This increased discounting of delayed reinforcement is argued to lead to a general aversion to delay of reinforcement, which appears behaviorally as impulsivity in choice situations and as inattention and self-stimulatory (or self-distracting) overactivity in non-choice situations. Sonuga-Barke (2002, 2003) again proposed that changes in a cortico-striato-thalamo-cortical loop underpinned these difficulties. This comprised the orbito-frontal cortex and anterior cingulate cortex and the nucleus accumbens, with feedback to the cortex again via the globus pallidus, substantia nigra pars reticulata, and subthalamic nucleus. In this case however, functional connections between the amygdala and the cortical areas involved, thalamus, and nucleus accumbens were hypothesized to link the cortico-striato-thalamo-cortical loop with the limbic system.

With advances in functional MRI methods, in particular resting-state functional MRI (R-fMRI) techniques in which imaging is conducted without the participant engaging in a specific task, the extent and complexity of neural networks have become better understood, and the number of candidate networks potentially involved in ADHD has increased (Castellanos & Aoki, 2016; Castellanos & Proal, 2012). Current conceptualizations of ADHD stress the involvement of the "default mode network," an extensive system involved in self-referential brain activity including self-monitoring, which is believed to be dysregulated in many psychiatric conditions (Menon, 2011). The involvement of an "executive control circuit" including the dorsolateral prefrontal cortex, anterior prefrontal cortex, anterior cingulate cortex, anterior insula, and inferior parietal lobe, together with the caudate and cerebellum, has however been supported by R-fMRI studies and by fMRI using a variety of tasks (Castellanos & Proal, 2012), as has the involvement of the reward circuit involving the orbitofrontal cortex, nucleus accumbens, and amygdala (Castellanos & Aoki, 2016; Van Dessel et al., 2018).

3.5 Toward an Integration of Neurobiological and Operant Models of Self-Injurious Behavior

The neural systems research described above strongly supports the involvement of disruptions in multiple cortico-striatal-thalamo-cortical loops in vulnerability for, or causation of, SIB. As noted in Sect. 3.2 of this chapter however, it is also the case that specific impairments in learning are also seen in syndromes specifically associated with SIB and/or animal models of those syndromes and that behavioral interventions have shown potential to reduce levels of SIB in individuals with these syndromes. However, there have been relatively few attempts to develop models of the interaction between biological and social learning processes in the development of SIB. Among the most sophisticated of these are the models presented by Oliver et al. (2013) of the causation of SIB in Cornelia de Lange syndrome and SMS. Even these models however assume no fundamental dysfunction in learning processes in the development of SIB and even more strikingly make no assumptions regarding the long-term effects of operant processes on the neural networks involved in causation of SIB.

The development of integrated biobehavioral models of SIB in people with NDCs has probably been inhibited by the insistence of many working within the operant framework on strictly operational definitions of operant learning processes. In other fields however, alternative models of goal-directed learning have led to more fruitful conceptualizations of interactions between neural and social processes in the development of clinical conditions. Central to these has been the assumption that the process of operant reinforcement, in which a behavior performed within a context of antecedent stimuli is strengthened by a reinforcer delivered contingent on that response, actually involves two separate processes. The first is a strengthening of the association between the response and the reinforcer, enhancing goal-directed control of the behavior; the second is a strengthening of the association between the antecedent stimuli and the behavior, increasing habitual performance of the behavior in response to antecedent stimuli. Additionally, the process of operant reinforcement provides the individual with information regarding the current value of the reinforcing stimulus. Dissociation between habitual and goal-directed control of the behavior can be demonstrated by breaking the link between the response and reinforcer delivery (i.e., operant extinction) or by devaluing the reinforcer (e.g., by satiation), which will reduce goal-directed but not habitual control of the behavior. Pavlovian conditioning during operant learning processes introduces further dimensions to the learning which takes place. The complex of contextual antecedent stimuli present during operant learning, through association with the reinforcer, may acquire secondary reinforcing properties and the ability to energize performance of the behavior which led to the reinforcer via Pavlovian-instrumental transfer (Cartoni, Balleine, & Baldassarre, 2016). This multiple-process model of operant learning, which evolved from basic research into instrumental learning (Dickinson, 1985), has facilitated dialogue between behavioral and neural systems research and proven fruitful in understanding a number of conditions characterized by engagement in behaviors which are costly or even harmful to the person engaging in them, such as overeating, OCD, and drug dependence (Balleine, 2005; Everitt, 2014; Everitt & Robbins, 2016; Gillan, Robbins, Sahakian, van den Heuvel, & van Wingen, 2016; Vaghi et al., 2019).

The neural system supporting action-outcome learning must necessarily respond dynamically to changes in both reinforcer value and response-reinforcement contingencies involving multiple response options. Research involving rats, humans, and other primates suggests that this is achieved by a complex system including the basolateral amygdala (BLA) and insular cortex (Balleine, Killcross, & Dickinson, 2003; Parkes & Balleine, 2013; Parkes, Ferreira, & Coutureau, 2016), the medial prefrontal/medial orbital cortex in humans (the prelimbic region of the medial prefrontal cortex in rats) (Corbit & Balleine, 2003; Coutureau, Marchand, & Di Scala, 2009; Killcross & Coutureau, 2003; Naneix, Marchand, Di Scala, Pape, & Coutureau, 2009; Ostlund & Balleine, 2005), the mediodorsal thalamus (Corbit, Muir, & Balleine, 2003), and the posterior dorsomedial striatum (caudate and nucleus accumbens in humans) (Balleine & O'Doherty, 2010; Parkes, Bradfield, & Balleine, 2015; Shiflett, Brown, & Balleine, 2010; Yin, Ostlund, Knowlton, & Balleine, 2005). Habit learning by contrast appears to depend on areas within the anterior dorsolateral striatum (putamen in humans) and sensorimotor cortical areas (Balleine & O'Doherty, 2010).

Under normal circumstances, the goal-directed (action-outcome learning) and habit (stimulus-response learning) systems are believed to interact dynamically to enable the individual to optimize outcomes with minimal necessary effort. In contexts where reinforcer values are stable and response-reinforcer contingencies are unchanging, the activity of the habit system will be predominant; where reinforcer values and/or response-reinforcer contingencies are changing, the goal-directed system will become engaged. Under certain conditions however, the habit system may become so dominant that changes in reinforcer value and response-reinforcer contingencies no longer affect the behavior, which will become a habitual response to the stimulus contexts in which the behavior has been learned (Yin & Knowlton, 2006). Dickinson (1985), reporting experiments in which rats were trained to press a lever to obtain sucrose pellets, showed that the habit system became predominant with "overtraining," i.e., when reinforcement of the response continued well after the rats were already responding at a high rate. Dickinson argued however that the effect was not due to overtraining per se, but to the fact that during overtraining, unlike in early acquisition of the response, the animals were responding at such a high rate that they no longer experienced any correlation between their rate of responding and the rate of reinforcement. Consistent with this proposition, relatively brief training with a variable-interval schedule, in which the animal also experiences a relatively low correlation between its rate of responding and the rate of reinforcement, also resulted in the resistance to extinction suggestive of dominance of habitual responding (Dickinson, 1985).

The shift from goal-directed to stimulus-response control of behavior can be facilitated by chronic stress and involves predominance of the corticostriatal system involving the putamen and sensorimotor cortex over that involving the caudate and nucleus accumbens and medial prefrontal/medial orbital cortex (Everitt & Robbins, 2016; Yin, Knowlton, & Balleine, 2004). Stimuli associated with reinforcement by Pavlovian learning may initially serve to increase instrumental responding through Pavlovian-instrumental transfer, but may also facilitate the shift toward habitual control by acquiring conditional reinforcing properties, resulting in the behavior effectively being continually reinforced even if delivery of the primary reinforcer is intermittent (Hogarth, Balleine, Corbit, & Killcross, 2013; Hogarth, Dickinson, & Duka, 2010). Importantly, major impediments to the shift toward habitual control of responding are situations where multiple responses lead to multiple reinforcers (Yin & Knowlton, 2006). The ability for a person to use a communication system to request reinforcers, therefore, should provide some protection against SIB coming under the control of the habit system, in addition to its potential to compete directly with SIB as a means of obtaining reinforcement.

The shift from goal-directed to habitual control of a behavior, aided by Pavlovian processes, is sufficient to produce a pattern of responding in which a behavior appears to be elicited by antecedent stimuli or events, is highly resistant to extinction, and may suddenly reappear in response to antecedent stimuli after a long period in which it has not occurred (i.e., relapse). A very substantial body of evidence now implicates these processes in other clinical conditions which are often costly to the person engaging in them and have typically been regarded as highly resistant to treatment, including substance abuse (Everitt, 2014; Everitt & Robbins, 2016) and OCD (Gillan et al., 2016). The transition from habitual control of behavior to compulsivity, in the sense that a person persists in a behavior even though it is causing them direct harm, appears however to involve additional processes. Approximately 20% of humans who take addictive drugs, and about 20% of rats responding for cocaine in rodent models of drug abuse, become compulsive users.

Research using a rodent model suggests that the development of compulsivity is not simply a continuation of the strengthening of antecedent control implicate in habit formation, but results from extended self-administration of cocaine (Jonkman, Pelloux, & Everitt, 2012b). Further research has shown that compulsive responding for cocaine in rats depends on a specific region within the dorsolateral striatum (Jonkman, Pelloux, & Everitt, 2012a), is associated with reduced serotonin turnover in prefrontal cortical areas and striatum, is associated with reduced dopamine turnover in dorsal striatum but not prefrontal areas, and can be reduced in a dose-dependent manner by the SSRI citalopram (Pelloux, Dilleen, Economidou, Theobald, & Everitt, 2012). Additionally, research with the cocaine-seeking rat model of substance abuse has suggested that rats which experience impulsivity (including increased discounting of delayed reinforcement), anxiety, and novelty-seeking may be at increased risk of developing compulsivity in stimulant seeking (Everitt & Robbins, 2016).

Although we have rather neglected the obviously important role of cortical influences in the above account, the research described above strongly suggests that exposure to particular reinforcement contingencies can have effects more complex than simply increasing the probability of a person engaging in SIB in a particular stimulus context. In particular, extended exposure to reinforcement during high rates of responding, or exposure to reinforcement schedules such as variable-interval schedules which can result in relatively low correlations between rates of responding and rates of reinforcement, drives a process in which antecedent stimulus control of responding through a habit loop involving the putamen and sensorimotor cortex will predominate over outcome-directed responding mediated by a neural circuit involving the caudate and nucleus accumbens and medial prefrontal/medial orbital cortex. The long-term effects of this shift will be manifested as decreased sensitivity to degradation of the response-reinforcer contingency (e.g., operant extinction) and the value of the reinforcer (e.g., by presentation of the reinforcer on a time-based schedule or so-called noncontingent reinforcement). On a day-to-day basis, carers supporting the person who engages in SIB will face situations in which a particular environmental event (e.g., a vehicle in which a person is travelling stopping at a red light) clearly and obviously elicits a burst of SIB which however does not stop when the condition which provoked it has ended. The engagement of Pavlovian processes may further exacerbate and broaden stimulus control of the SIB, so that on the following day, the person may start to engage in SIB as the vehicle approaches the traffic signal even though it does not have to stop.

Studies of the processes leading to this shift toward habitual, stimulus-response control of behavior have identified stress as a further factor promoting the shift, and environments offering multiple response, multiple-reinforcer contingencies as a powerful barrier to it. However, extended exposure to reinforcement, specifically under conditions characterized by relatively low correlations between rates of responding and rates of reinforcement, will be expected to lead to compulsive behavior in some individuals. Although compromised cortical control is probably important in the development of compulsive behavior, impulsivity, anxiety, and novelty-seeking may also increase vulnerability to its development.

3.6 Development of Self-Injurious Behavior: A General Biobehavioral Model

The perspective on instrumental learning outlined above suggests that social-environmental processes play a key role in the development of SIB, not just in causing short-term changes in the probability of a person engaging in SIB but also resulting in changes in the neural circuits controlling SIB.

Figure 3.3 outlines the key processes which we propose to be involved. A major problem for any model of the development of SIB is to explain the initial emergence of self-injurious behavioral topographies. The operant theory of the shaping of SIB from non-injurious STBs is an elegant and persuasive account of how such topographies might evolve. Such evolution has however been observed in only very few cases, and the fact that SIB and STB typically emerge at comparable (very young) ages suggests that this process is probably not involved in the initial emergence of SIB in all cases (Furniss & Biswas, 2012). One alternative possibility for the initial emergence of SIB is indicated by the often-reported fact that people who engage in SIB are also highly likely to engage in aggression toward other people. Such aggression can be unconditionally elicited by aversive stimulation (e.g., pain) or by operant extinction or shifts in reinforcement schedules (i.e., "frustration") (Azrin, Hutchinson, & Hake, 1966, 1967; Azrin, Rubin, & Hutchinson, 1968; Hutchinson, Azrin, & Hunt, 1968; Kelly & Hake, 1970). This aggression may be directed to a variety of targets (Macurik, Kohn, & Kavanaugh, 1978), including previously neutral stimuli associated with the aversive experience (Lyon & Ozolins, 1970; Romanczyk & Matthews, 1998; Schroeder, Reese, Hellings, Loupe, & Tessel, 1999). In the model presented in Fig. 3.3, we hypothesize that SIB emerges when such elicited aggression is directed against the person's own body, either because developmental immaturity and motor difficulties make other targets inaccessible or because motor difficulties lead to the person accidentally making contact with themselves (Langthorne & McGill, 2008). In either case, the model predicts that motor difficulties underpinned by functional disturbance in the motor cortex-striato-thalamo-cortical motor loop will be a risk factor for emergence of SIB. Impaired motor control may also cause or exacerbate a discrepancy between expressive and receptive language abilities which may increase frustration in the face of two of the most commonly reported early antecedents of SIB, frustration of a desire and rapid situational transitions (Berkson, 2002). The aversiveness of these events however will also be increased if the person experiences impulsivity with delay intolerance and/or "insistence on sameness," both characteristics also involving striatal connections, with the orbitofrontal cortex-nucleus accumbens-amygdala reward circuit mediating delay intolerance and the caudate nucleus, possibly together with connected prefrontal regions including the inferior frontal gyrus, specifically implicated in "insistence on sameness" (Langen et al., 2009, 2014; Traynor et al., 2018).

After the initial emergence of SIB, the model posits potentially rapid increases both in the rate and intensity of SIB, mediated by operant reinforcement and Pavlovian-instrumental transfer, and in the range of stimuli which elicit SIB, mediated by Pavlovian associations between originally eliciting stimuli and others.

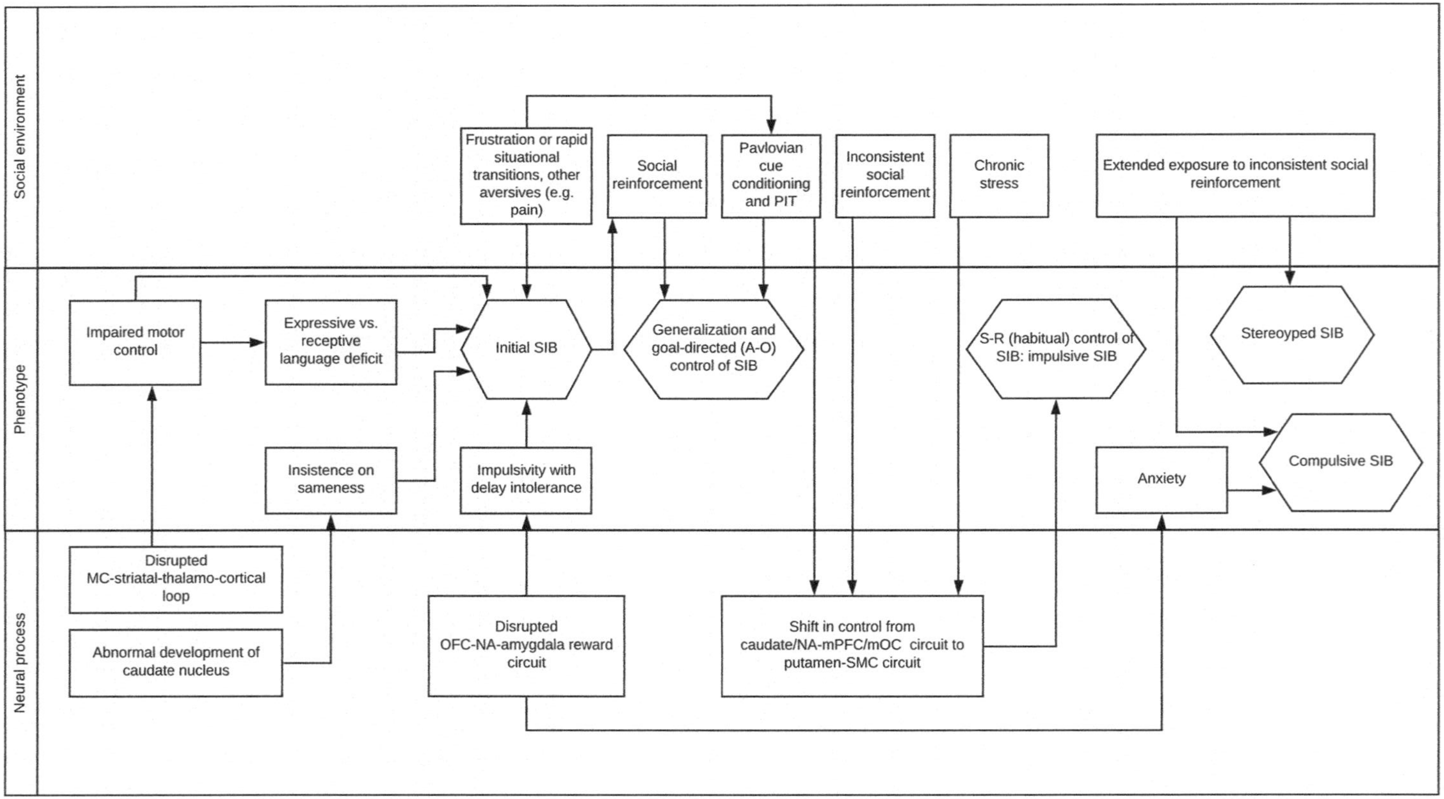

Fig. 3.3 Hypothesized processes in the emergence and development of SIB. *MC* motor cortex, *OFC* orbitofrontal cortex, *NA* nucleus accumbens, *PIT* Pavlovian-instrumental transfer, *A-O* action-outcome, *mPFC* medial prefrontal cortex, *mOC* medial orbitofrontal cortex, *SMC* sensorimotor cortex, *S-R* stimulus-response

The model assumes however (as does the operant model of the shaping of SIB from STB) that as carers become accustomed to the person engaging in SIB, their responses to SIB will become more variable. In the case of the present model however, it is hypothesized that the primary effect of this change (which we somewhat imprecisely label "inconsistent social reinforcement") is to reduce the correlation between change in the rate of SIB and the rate of reinforcement, engaging the transition in control of the behavior from the posterior dorsostriatal-medial prefrontal/medial orbitofrontal cortex action-outcome circuit to the anterior dorsostriatal-motor cortex stimulus-response circuit. Chronic stress (if experienced by the person engaging in SIB) will facilitate this transition. In terms of the phenomenology of SIB, the transition will be experienced as a change from "communicative" to impulsive SIB. In certain situations, the person will immediately begin to engage in SIB, even if the reinforcer previously motivating the behavior is freely available. The model then assumes that for some people, with extended exposure to inconsistent social reinforcement and ongoing Pavlovian conditioning of additional eliciting stimuli, two final outcomes are possible. For some people, hyperactivation of the direct cortico-striato-thalamo-cortical motor circuit and/or hypoactivation of the indirect circuit may result in SIB becoming stereotypical, with the person engaging in SIB more or less continuously over extended periods of time. For others however, especially those experiencing anxiety related to dysfunction of the amygdala, SIB may become compulsive, with the person engaging in the behavior only in certain stimulus contexts but then appearing to be driven to do so irrespective of the consequences.

This model may account for some of the inconsistencies in findings regarding risk factors for development and maintenance of SIB. Higher intellectual ability may, for example, be a risk factor for the initial development of SIB simply because it will be associated with more rapid learning of operant and Pavlovian contingencies or perhaps because more able infants with language and/or independence skills compromised by motor difficulties may experience more frustration than others. Higher ability will also however facilitate learning of other action-outcome contingencies, thus reducing the risk of transition to S-R control of SIB. Lower ability, if it results in a very impoverished behavioral repertoire, will by contrast increase the risk of transition from goal-directed to habitual SIB. The model also posits specific and differential roles for characteristics associated with ASCs at different points in the evolution of SIB. Insistence on sameness is hypothesized to play a role in the initial emergence of SIB by increasing the range of environmental changes and transitions which will be experienced as aversive, while the neural mechanisms mediating motor stereotypy and anxiety are hypothesized to facilitate the final evolution of SIB into stereotypical or compulsive forms, respectively.

The proposed model also accounts for the steady decrease in remission rates of SIB with increasing age and posits a dual role for impulsivity and specifically of discounting of delayed reinforcement, which is hypothesized to be involved both in the initial emergence of SIB and, for some people, in the transition to compulsivity. In other regards however, the model is probably incomplete. People with syndromes highly associated with SIB experience attentional difficulties which may well disrupt learning processes and be involved in the development of SIB. Those with SMS and RTT may well have reduced pain sensitivity, and the proposed model neglects not only the possible role which such insensitivity may play in the development and maintenance of SIB but also the possibility that hyperalgesia may be associated with SIB in other individuals (Symons et al., 2015).

The model however provides a unified account of the development of what have previously been described as "subtypes" of SIB and generally concurs with phenomenological classifications (e.g., Mace & Mauk, 1995) in suggesting that "operant," impulsive, stereotypic, and compulsive presentations of SIB will be seen at various stages in its evolution. Unlike classifications which distinguish between "operant" and "biological" subtypes of SIB, however, the model proposes that both environmental contingencies and neurobiological risk factors are involved at all stages in the development of SIB. Further, unlike the models of SIB in SMS and Cornelia de Lange syndrome proposed by Oliver et al. (2013), in which environmental contingencies modify only the behavioral phenotype, this model proposes that such contingencies are key drivers of changes in neural circuitry mediating the transitions from goal-directed to habitual/impulsive and then stereotypical or compulsive SIB. Further, the model proposes that while pharmacological interventions may have a role when SIB becomes predominantly habitual/impulsive or compulsive in nature, behavioral interventions will continue to be of potential benefit at all stages in the development of SIB.

Figure 3.4 summarizes the key stages in the development of SIB and behavioral interventions which may reduce SIB at each stage in its progression and/or disrupt

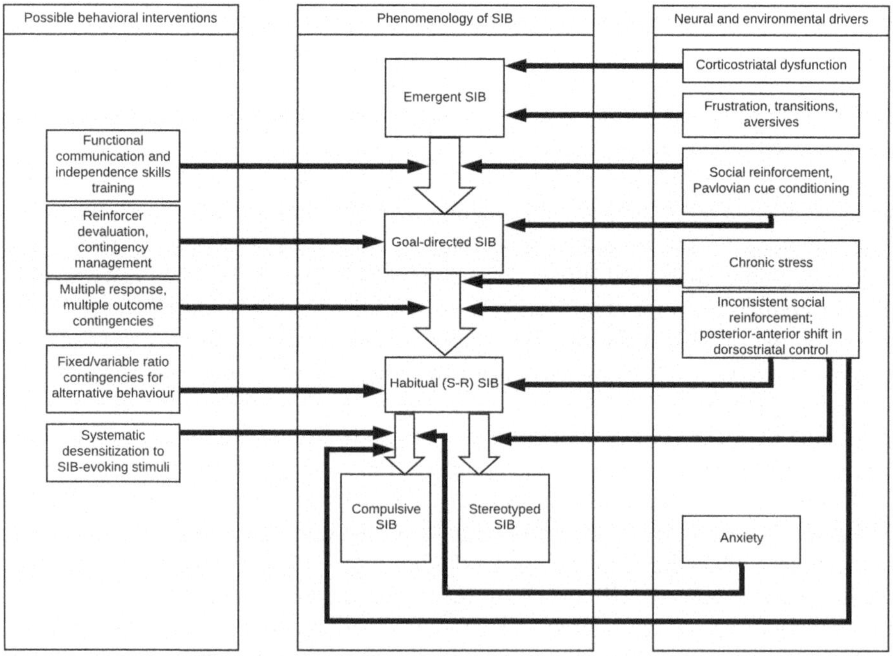

Fig. 3.4 Neural and environmental drivers of the development of SIB, with options for behavioral interventions to reduce SIB and block or reverse its progression

the progression of the behavior. The model has clear implications for stratification of both behavioral and pharmacological interventions, and in Chaps. 5 and 6, we will consider how the clinician can assess the presentation of SIB and tailor intervention to the individual stage of progression of SIB being experienced by a person.

References

Achenbach, T. M. (1991). *Manual for the Child Behavior Checklist/4–18 and 1991 Profile*. Burlington, VT: Department of Psychiatry, University of Vermont.

Adachi, M., Autry, A. E., Covington, H. E., III, & Monteggia, L. M. (2009). MeCP2-mediated transcription repression in the basolateral amygdala may underlie heightened anxiety in a mouse model of Rett syndrome. *Journal of Neuroscience, 29*(13), 4218–4227. https://doi.org/10.1523/JNEUROSCI.4225-08.2009

Ahonniska-Assa, J., Polack, O., Saraf, E., Wine, J., Silberg, T., Nissenkorn, A., & Ben-Zeev, B. (2018). Assessing cognitive functioning in females with Rett syndrome by eye-tracking methodology. *European Journal of Paediatric Neurology, 22*(1), 39–45. https://doi.org/10.1016/j.ejpn.2017.09.010

Allemang-Grand, R., Ellegood, J., Spencer Noakes, L., Ruston, J., Justice, M., Nieman, B. J., & Lerch, J. P. (2017). Neuroanatomy in mouse models of Rett syndrome is related to the severity of Mecp2 mutation and behavioral phenotypes. *Molecular Autism, 8*(1). https://doi.org/10.1186/s13229-017-0138-8

Amir, R. E., Van Den Veyver, I. B., Wan, M., Tran, C. Q., Francke, U., & Zoghbi, H. Y. (1999). Rett syndrome is caused by mutations in X-linked *MECP2*, encoding methyl- CpG-binding protein 2. *Nature Genetics, 23*(2), 185–188. https://doi.org/10.1038/13810

Anderson, L. T., & Ernst, M. (1994). Self-injury in Lesch-Nyhan disease. *Journal of Autism and Developmental Disorders, 24*(1), 67–81. https://doi.org/10.1007/BF02172213

Armstrong, D. D. (2005). Neuropathology of Rett syndrome. *Journal of Child Neurology, 20*(9), 747–753. https://doi.org/10.1177/08830738050200090901

Arron, K., Oliver, C., Moss, J., Berg, K., & Burbidge, C. (2011). The prevalence and phenomenology of self-injurious and aggressive behaviour in genetic syndromes. *Journal of Intellectual Disability Research, 55*(2), 109–120. https://doi.org/10.1111/j.1365-2788.2010.01337.x

Azrin, N. H., Hutchinson, R. R., & Hake, D. F. (1966). Extinction-induced aggression. *Journal of the Experimental Analysis of Behavior, 9*(3), 191–204. https://doi.org/10.1901/jeab.1966.9-191

Azrin, N. H., Hutchinson, R. R., & Hake, D. F. (1967). Attack, avoidance, and escape reactions to aversive shock. *Journal of the Experimental Analysis of Behavior, 10*(2), 131–148. https://doi.org/10.1901/jeab.1967.10-131

Azrin, N. H., Rubin, H. B., & Hutchinson, R. R. (1968). Biting attack by rats in response to aversive shock. *Journal of the Experimental Analysis of Behavior, 11*(5), 633–639. https://doi.org/10.1901/jeab.1968.11-633

Bahi-Buisson, N. (2013). Genetically determined encephalopathy: Rett syndrome. *Handbook of Clinical Neurology, 111*, 281–286. https://doi.org/10.1016/B978-0-444-52891-9.00031-2

Balleine, B. W. (2005). Neural bases of food-seeking: Affect, arousal and reward in corticostriatolimbic circuits. *Physiology and Behavior, 86*(5), 717–730. https://doi.org/10.1016/j.physbeh.2005.08.061

Balleine, B. W., Killcross, A. S., & Dickinson, A. (2003). The effect of lesions of the basolateral amygdala on instrumental conditioning. *Journal of Neuroscience, 23*(2), 666–675. https://doi.org/10.1523/JNEUROSCI.23-02-00666.2003

Balleine, B. W., & O'Doherty, J. P. (2010). Human and rodent homologies in action control: corticostriatal determinants of goal-directed and habitual action. *Neuropsychopharmacology, 35*(1), 48–69. https://doi.org/10.1038/npp.2009.131

Banerjee, A., Rikhye, R. V., Breton-Provencher, V., Tangb, X., Li, C., Li, K., … Sur, M. (2016). Jointly reduced inhibition and excitation underlies circuit-wide changes in cortical processing in Rett syndrome. *Proceedings of the National Academy of Sciences of the United States of America, 113*(46), E7287–E7296. https://doi.org/10.1073/pnas.1615330113

Bass, M. N., & Speak, B. L. (2005). A behavioural approach to the assessment and treatment of severe self-injury in a woman with Smith-Magenis syndrome: A single case study. *Behavioural and Cognitive Psychotherapy, 33*(3), 361–368. https://doi.org/10.1017/S1352465805002110

Bell, S., Kolobova, I., Crapper, L., & Ernst, C. (2016). Lesch-Nyhan syndrome: Models, theories, and therapies. *Molecular Syndromology, 7*(6), 302–311. https://doi.org/10.1159/000449296

Benarroch, E. E. (2016). Intrinsic circuits of the striatum. *Neurology, 86*(16), 1531–1542. https://doi.org/10.1212/WNL.0000000000002599

Bepari, A. K., Sano, H., Tamamaki, N., Nambu, A., Tanaka, K. F., & Takebayashi, H. (2012). Identification of optogenetically activated striatal medium spiny neurons by *Npas4* expression. *PLoS One, 7*(12). https://doi.org/10.1371/journal.pone.0052783

Bergen, A. E., Holborn, S. W., & Scott-Huyghebaert, V. C. (2002). Functional analysis of self-injurious behavior in an adult with Lesch-Nyhan syndrome. *Behavior Modification, 26*(2), 187–204. https://doi.org/10.1177/0145445502026002004

Berkson, G. (2002). Early development of stereotyped and self-injurious behaviors: II. age trends. *American Journal on Mental Retardation, 107*(6), 468–477+493. https://doi.org/10.1352/0895-8017(2002)107<0468:EDOSAS>2.0.CO;2

Bey, A. L., Wang, X., Yan, H., Kim, N., Passman, R. L., Yang, Y., … Jiang, Y. (2018). Brain region-specific disruption of *Shank3* in mice reveals a dissociation for cortical and striatal circuits in autism-related behaviors. *Translational Psychiatry, 8*(1):94. https://doi.org/10.1038/s41398-018-0142-6.

Bi, W., Ohyama, T., Nakamura, H., Yan, J., Visvanathan, J., Justice, M. J., & Lupski, J. R. (2005). Inactivation of *Rai1* in mice recapitulates phenotypes observed in chromosome engineered mouse models for Smith-Magenis syndrome. *Human Molecular Genetics, 14*(8), 983–995. https://doi.org/10.1093/hmg/ddi085

Bi, W., Saifi, G. M., Shaw, C. J., Walz, K., Fonseca, P., Wilson, M., … Lupski, J. R. (2004). Mutations of RAI1, a PHD-containing protein, in nondeletion patients with Smith-Magenis syndrome. *Human Genetics, 115*(6), 515–524. https://doi.org/10.1007/s00439-004-1187-6

Bi, W., Yan, J., Shi, X., Yuva-Paylor, L. A., Antalffy, B. A., Goldman, A., … Lupski, J. R. (2007). *Rai1* deficiency in mice causes learning impairment and motor dysfunction, whereas *Rai1* heterozygous mice display minimal behavioral phenotypes. *Human Molecular Genetics, 16*(15), 1802–1813. https://doi.org/10.1093/hmg/ddm128.

Blue, M. E., Naidu, S., & Johnston, M. V. (1999a). Altered development of glutamate and GABA receptors in the basal ganglia of girls with Rett syndrome. *Experimental Neurology, 156*(2), 345–352. https://doi.org/10.1006/exnr.1999.7030

Blue, M. E., Naidu, S., & Johnston, M. V. (1999b). Development of amino acid receptors in frontal cortex from girls with Rett syndrome. *Annals of Neurology, 45*(4), 541–545. https://doi.org/10.1002/1531-8249(199904)45:4<541::AID-ANA21>3.0.CO;2-2

Boddaert, N., De Leersnyder, H., Bourgeois, M., Munnich, A., Brunelle, F., & Zilbovicius, M. (2004). Anatomical and functional brain imaging evidence of lenticulo-insular anomalies in Smith Magenis syndrome. *NeuroImage, 21*(3), 1021–1025. https://doi.org/10.1016/j.neuroimage.2003.10.040

Bouchekioua, Y., Tsutsui-Kimura, I., Sano, H., Koizumi, M., Tanaka, K. F., Yoshida, K., … Mimura, M. (2018). Striatonigral direct pathway activation is sufficient to induce repetitive behaviors. *Neuroscience Research, 132*, 53–57. https://doi.org/10.1016/j.neures.2017.09.007

Breese, G. R., Baumeister, A. A., McCown, T. J., Emerick, S. G., Frye, G. D., & Mueller, R. A. (1984a). Neonatal-6-hydroxydopamine treatment: Model of susceptibility for self-mutilation in the Lesch-Nyhan syndrome. *Pharmacology Biochemistry and Behavior, 21*(3), 459–461. https://doi.org/10.1016/S0091-3057(84)80110-0

Breese, G. R., Baumeister, A. A., McCown, T. J., Emerick, S. G., Frye, G. D., Crotty, K., & Mueller, R. A. (1984b). Behavioral differences between neonatal and adult 6-hydroxydopamine-treated rats to dopamine agonists: Relevance to neurological symptoms in clinical syndromes with reduced brain dopamine. *Journal of Pharmacology and Experimental Therapeutics, 231*(2), 343–354. Retrieved from http://jpet.aspetjournals.org/content/231/2/343

Breese, G. R., Knapp, D. J., Criswell, H. E., Moy, S. S., Papadeas, S. T., & Blake, B. L. (2005). The neonate-6-hydroxydopamine-lesioned rat: A model for clinical neuroscience and neurobiological principles. *Brain Research Reviews, 48*(1), 57–73. https://doi.org/10.1016/j.brainresrev.2004.08.004

Buchanan, C. B., Stallworth, J. L., Scott, A. E., Glaze, D. G., Lane, J. B., Skinner, S. A., … Kaufmann, W. E. (2019). Behavioral profiles in Rett syndrome: Data from the natural history study. *Brain and Development, 41*(2), 123–134. https://doi.org/10.1016/j.braindev.2018.08.008

Burford, B. (2005). Perturbations in the development of infants with Rett disorder and the implications for early diagnosis. *Brain and Development, 27*(SUPPL. 1), S3–S7. https://doi.org/10.1016/j.braindev.2005.03.013

Capra, V., Biancheri, R., Morana, G., Striano, P., Novara, F., Ferrero, G. B., … Guerrini, R. (2014). Periventricular nodular heterotopia in Smith-Magenis syndrome. *American Journal of Medical Genetics, Part A, 164*(12), 3142–3147. https://doi.org/10.1002/ajmg.a.36742

Carter, J. C., Lanham, D. C., Pham, D., Bibat, G., Naidu, S., & Kaufmann, W. E. (2008). Selective cerebral volume reduction in Rett syndrome: A multiple-approach MR imaging study. *American Journal of Neuroradiology, 29*(3), 436–441. https://doi.org/10.3174/ajnr.A0857

Cartoni, E., Balleine, B., & Baldassarre, G. (2016). Appetitive Pavlovian-instrumental transfer: A review. *Neuroscience and Biobehavioral Reviews, 71*, 829–848. https://doi.org/10.1016/j.neubiorev.2016.09.020

Cass, H., Reilly, S., Owen, L., Wisbeach, A., Weekes, L., Slonims, V., … Charman, T. (2003). Findings from a multidisciplinary clinical case series of females with Rett syndrome. *Developmental Medicine and Child Neurology, 45*(5), 325–337. https://doi.org/10.1017/S0012162203000616

Castellanos, F. X., & Aoki, Y. (2016). Intrinsic functional connectivity in Attention-Deficit/Hyperactivity Disorder: A science in development. *Biological Psychiatry: Cognitive Neuroscience and Neuroimaging, 1*(3), 253–261. https://doi.org/10.1016/j.bpsc.2016.03.004

Castellanos, F. X., & Proal, E. (2012). Large-scale brain systems in ADHD: Beyond the prefrontal-striatal model. *Trends in Cognitive Sciences, 16*(1), 17–26. https://doi.org/10.1016/j.tics.2011.11.007

Chao, H., Chen, H., Samaco, R. C., Xue, M., Chahrour, M., Yoo, J., … Zoghbi, H. Y. (2010). Dysfunction in GABA signalling mediates autism-like stereotypies and Rett syndrome phenotypes. *Nature, 468*(7321), 263–269. https://doi.org/10.1038/nature09582

Cianfaglione, R., Clarke, A., Kerr, M., Hastings, R. P., Oliver, C., Moss, J., … Felce, D. (2015). A national survey of Rett syndrome: Behavioural characteristics. *Journal of Neurodevelopmental Disorders, 7*(1), 11. https://doi.org/10.1186/s11689-015-9104-y

Cianfaglione, R., Meek, A., Clarke, A., Kerr, M., Hastings, R. P., & Felce, D. (2016). Direct observation of the behaviour of females with Rett syndrome. *Journal of Developmental and Physical Disabilities, 28*(3), 425–441. https://doi.org/10.1007/s10882-016-9478-0

Coleman, M., Brubaker, J., Hunter, K., & Smith, G. (1988). Rett syndrome: A survey of North American patients. *Journal of Intellectual Disability Research, 32*(2), 117–124. https://doi.org/10.1111/j.1365-2788.1988.tb01397.x

Corbit, L. H., & Balleine, B. W. (2003). The role of prelimbic cortex in instrumental conditioning. *Behavioural Brain Research, 146*(1-2), 145–157. https://doi.org/10.1016/j.bbr.2003.09.023

Corbit, L. H., Muir, J. L., & Balleine, B. W. (2003). Lesions of mediodorsal thalamus and anterior thalamic nuclei produce dissociable effects on instrumental conditioning in rats. *European Journal of Neuroscience, 18*(5), 1286–1294. https://doi.org/10.1046/j.1460-9568.2003.02833.x

Coutureau, E., Marchand, A. R., & Di Scala, G. (2009). Goal-directed responding is sensitive to lesions to the prelimbic cortex or basolateral nucleus of the amygdala but not to their disconnection. *Behavioral Neuroscience, 123*(2), 443–448. https://doi.org/10.1037/a0014818

Cromwell, H. C., Levine, M. S., & King, B. H. (1999). Cortical damage enhances pemoline-induced self-injurious behavior in prepubertal rats. *Pharmacology Biochemistry and Behavior, 62*(2), 223–227. https://doi.org/10.1016/S0091-3057(98)00152-X

Crossman, A. R., & Neary, D. (2019). *Neuroanatomy: An illustrated colour text.* Amsterdam: Elsevier.

De Leersnyder, H. (2006). Inverted rhythm of melatonin secretion in Smith-Magenis syndrome: From symptoms to treatment. *Trends in Endocrinology and Metabolism, 17*(7), 291–298. https://doi.org/10.1016/j.tem.2006.07.007

De Leersnyder, H., De Blois, M., Munnich, A., Bresson, J. L., Mogenet, A., Salefranque, F., … Delhotal-Landes, B. (2003). β1-adrenergic antagonists and melatonin reset the clock and restore sleep in a circadian disorder, Smith-Magenis syndrome. *Journal of Medical Genetics, 40*(1), 74–78.

Devine, D. P. (2012). Animal models of self-injurious behaviour: An overview. *Methods in Molecular Biology, 829*, 65–84. https://doi.org/10.1007/978-1-61779-458-2_4

Devine, D. P. (2014). Self-injurious behaviour in autistic children: A neuro-developmental theory of social and environmental isolation. *Psychopharmacology, 231*(6), 979–997. https://doi.org/10.1007/s00213-013-3279-2

Devine, D. P., & Symons, F. J. (2013). Biological vulnerability and risk for self-injury in intellectual and developmental disabilities. *International Review of Research in Developmental Disabilities, 44*, 37–67. https://doi.org/10.1016/B978-0-12-401662-0.00002-6

Dickinson, A. (1985). Actions and habits: The development of behavioural autonomy. *Philosophical Transactions of the Royal Society of London B, 308*, 67–78.

Djukic, A., Rose, S. A., Jankowski, J. J., & Feldman, J. F. (2014). Rett syndrome: Recognition of facial expression and its relation to scanning patterns. *Pediatric Neurology, 51*(5), 650–656. https://doi.org/10.1016/j.pediatrneurol.2014.07.022

Djukic, A., & Valicenti McDermott, M. (2012). Social preferences in Rett syndrome. *Pediatric Neurology, 46*(4), 240–242. https://doi.org/10.1016/j.pediatrneurol.2012.01.011

Djukic, A., Valicenti McDermott, M., Mavrommatis, K., & Martins, C. L. (2012). Rett syndrome: Basic features of visual processing—A pilot study of eye-tracking. *Pediatric Neurology, 47*(1), 25–29. https://doi.org/10.1016/j.pediatrneurol.2012.04.009

Doetschman, T., Gregg, R. G., Maeda, N., Hooper, M. L., Melton, D. W., Thompson, S., & Smithies, O. (1987). Targetted correction of a mutant HPRT gene in mouse embryonic stem cells. *Nature, 330*(6148), 576–578. https://doi.org/10.1038/330576a0

Dorey, N. R., Rosales-Ruiz, J., Smith, R., & Lovelace, B. (2009). Functional analysis and treatment of self-injury in a captive olive baboon. *Journal of Applied Behavior Analysis, 42*(4), 785–794. https://doi.org/10.1901/jaba.2009.42-785

Downs, J., Rodger, J., Li, C., Tan, X., Hu, N., Wong, K., … Leonard, H. (2018). Environmental enrichment intervention for Rett syndrome: An individually randomised stepped wedge trial. *Orphanet Journal of Rare Diseases, 13*(1), 3. https://doi.org/10.1186/s13023-017-0752-8

Dykens, E. M., & Smith, A. C. M. (1998). Distinctiveness and correlates of maladaptive behaviour in children and adolescents with Smith-Magenis syndrome. *Journal of Intellectual Disability Research, 42*(6), 481–489. https://doi.org/10.1046/j.1365-2788.1998.4260481.x

Edelman, E. A., Girirajan, S., Finucane, B., Patel, P. I., Lupski, J. R., Smith, A. C. M., & Elsea, S. H. (2007). Gender, genotype, and phenotype differences in Smith-Magenis syndrome: A meta-analysis of 105 cases. *Clinical Genetics, 71*(6), 540–550. https://doi.org/10.1111/j.1399-0004.2007.00815.x

Eltokhi, A., Rappold, G., & Sprengel, R. (2018). Distinct phenotypes of *Shank2* mouse models reflect neuropsychiatric spectrum disorders of human patients with *SHANK2* variants. *Frontiers in Molecular Neuroscience, 11*, 240. https://doi.org/10.3389/fnmol.2018.00240

Ernst, M., Zametkin, A. J., Matochik, J. A., Pascualvaca, D., Jons, P. H., Hardy, K., … Cohen, R. M. (1996). Presynaptic dopaminergic deficits in Lesch-Nyhan disease. *New England Journal of Medicine, 334*(24), 1568–1572. https://doi.org/10.1056/NEJM199606133342403

Evans, I. M., & Meyer, L. H. (1999). Modifying adult interactional style as positive behavioural intervention for a child with Rett syndrome. *Journal of Intellectual and Developmental Disability, 24*(3), 191–205. https://doi.org/10.1080/13668259900033981

Everitt, B. J. (2014). Neural and psychological mechanisms underlying compulsive drug seeking habits and drug memories - indications for novel treatments of addiction. *European Journal of Neuroscience, 40*(1), 2163–2182. https://doi.org/10.1111/ejn.12644

Everitt, B. J., & Robbins, T. W. (2016). Drug addiction: Updating actions to habits to compulsions ten years on. *Annual Review of Psychology, 67*, 23–50. https://doi.org/10.1146/annurev-psych-122414-033457

Finucane, B., Dirrigl, K. H., & Simon, E. W. (2001). Characterization of self-injurious behaviors in children and adults with Smith-Magenis syndrome. *American Journal on Mental Retardation, 106*(1), 52–58. https://doi.org/10.1352/0895-8017(2001)106<0052:COSIBI>2.0.CO;2

Finucane, B., & Haas-Givler, B. (2009). Smith-Magenis syndrome: Genetic basis and clinical implications. *Journal of Mental Health Research in Intellectual Disabilities, 2*(2), 134–148. https://doi.org/10.1080/19315860802627619

Fu, R., Ceballos-Picot, L., Rosa, J., Larovere, L. E., Yamada, Y., Nguyen, K. V., … Jinnah, H. A. (2014). Genotype-phenotype correlations in neurogenetics: Lesch-Nyhan disease as a model disorder. *Brain, 137*(5), 1282–1303. https://doi.org/10.1093/brain/awt202

Fu, R., Sutcliffe, D., Zhao, H., Huang, X., Schretlen, D. J., Benkovic, S., & Jinnah, H. A. (2015). Clinical severity in Lesch-Nyhan disease: The role of residual enzyme and compensatory pathways. *Molecular Genetics and Metabolism, 114*(1), 55–61. https://doi.org/10.1016/j.ymgme.2014.11.001

Furniss, F., & Biswas, A. B. (2012). Recent research on aetiology, development and phenomenology of self-injurious behaviour in people with intellectual disabilities: A systematic review and implications for treatment. *Journal of Intellectual Disability Research, 56*(5), 453–475. https://doi.org/10.1111/j.1365-2788.2012.01534.x

Fyffe, S. L., Neul, J. L., Samaco, R. C., Chao, H., Ben-Shachar, S., Moretti, P., … Zoghbi, H. Y. (2008). Deletion of *Mecp2* in *Sim1*-expressing neurons reveals a critical role for MeCP2 in feeding behavior, aggression, and the response to stress. *Neuron, 59*(6), 947–958. https://doi.org/10.1016/j.neuron.2008.07.030

Gemelli, T., Berton, O., Nelson, E. D., Perrotti, L. I., Jaenisch, R., & Monteggia, L. M. (2006). Postnatal loss of methyl-CpG binding protein 2 in the forebrain is sufficient to mediate behavioral aspects of Rett syndrome in mice. *Biological Psychiatry, 59*(5), 468–476. https://doi.org/10.1016/j.biopsych.2005.07.025

Gillan, C. M., Robbins, T. W., Sahakian, B. J., van den Heuvel, O. A., & van Wingen, G. (2016). The role of habit in compulsivity. *European Neuropsychopharmacology, 26*(5), 828–840. https://doi.org/10.1016/j.euroneuro.2015.12.033

Girirajan, S., & Elsea, S. H. (2009). Distorted Mendelian transmission as a function of genetic background in *Rai1*-haploinsufficient mice. *European Journal of Medical Genetics, 52*(4), 224–228. https://doi.org/10.1016/j.ejmg.2008.12.002

Girirajan, S., Patel, N., Slager, R. E., Tokarz, M. E. M. E., Bucan, M., Wiley, J. L., & Elsea, S. H. (2008). How much is too much? phenotypic consequences of *Rai1* overexpression in mice. *European Journal of Human Genetics, 16*(8), 941–954. https://doi.org/10.1038/ejhg.2008.21

Girirajan, S., Vlangos, C. N., Szomju, B. B., Edelman, E., Trevors, C. D., Dupuis, L., … Elsea, S. H. (2006). Genotype-phenotype correlation in Smith-Magenis syndrome: Evidence that multiple genes in 17p11.2 contribute to the clinical spectrum. *Genetics in Medicine, 8*(7), 417–427. https://doi.org/10.1097/01.gim.0000228215.32110.89

Gisbert de la Cuadra, L., Torres, R. J., Beltrán, L. M., Sánchez, A., & Puig, J. G. (2016). Development of new forms of self-injurious behavior following total dental extraction in Lesch–Nyhan disease. *Nucleosides, Nucleotides and Nucleic Acids, 35*(10-12), 524–528. https://doi.org/10.1080/15257770.2016.1184276

Gluck, J. P., & Sackett, G. P. (1974). Frustration and self-aggression in social isolate rhesus monkeys. *Journal of Abnormal Psychology, 83*(3), 331–334. https://doi.org/10.1037/h0036584

Goldstein, M., Kuga, S., Kusano, N., Meller, E., Dancis, J., & Schwarcz, R. (1986). Dopamine agonist induced self-mutilative biting behavior in monkeys with unilateral ventromedial tegmental lesions of the brainstem: Possible pharmacological model for Lesch-Nyhan syndrome. *Brain Research, 367*(1-2), 114–120. https://doi.org/10.1016/0006-8993(86)91584-2

Greenberg, F., Lewis, R. A., Potocki, L., Glaze, D., Parke, J., Killian, J., … Lupski, J. R. (1996). Multi-disciplinary clinical study of Smith-Magenis syndrome (deletion 17p11.2). *American Journal of Medical Genetics, 62*(3), 247–254. https://doi.org/10.1002/(SICI)1096-8628(19960329)62:3<247::AID-AJMG9>3.0.CO;2-Q

Gropman, A. L., Duncan, W. C., & Smith, A. C. M. (2006). Neurologic and developmental features of the Smith-Magenis syndrome (del 17p11.2). *Pediatric Neurology, 34*(5), 337–350. https://doi.org/10.1016/j.pediatrneurol.2005.08.018

Guy, J., Hendrich, B., Holmes, M., Martin, J. E., & Bird, A. (2001). A mouse *Mecp2*-null mutation causes neurological symptoms that mimic Rett syndrome. *Nature Genetics, 27*(3), 322–326. https://doi.org/10.1038/85899

Hao, S., Tang, B., Wu, Z., Ure, K., Sun, Y., Tao, H., … Tang, J. (2015). Forniceal deep brain stimulation rescues hippocampal memory in Rett syndrome mice. *Nature, 526*(7573), 430–434. https://doi.org/10.1038/nature15694

Harris, J. C. (2018). Lesch-Nyhan syndrome and its variants: Examining the behavioral and neurocognitive phenotype. *Current Opinion in Psychiatry, 31*(2), 96–102. https://doi.org/10.1097/YCO.0000000000000388

Hattori, R., Kuchibhotla, K. V., Froemke, R. C., & Komiyama, T. (2017). Functions and dysfunctions of neocortical inhibitory neuron subtypes. *Nature Neuroscience, 20*(9), 1199–1208. https://doi.org/10.1038/nn.4619

Hogarth, L., Balleine, B. W., Corbit, L. H., & Killcross, S. (2013). Associative learning mechanisms underpinning the transition from recreational drug use to addiction. *Annals of the New York Academy of Sciences, 1282(1)*, 12–24. https://doi.org/10.1111/j.1749-6632.2012.06768.x

Hogarth, L., Dickinson, A., & Duka, T. (2010). The associative basis of cue-elicited drug taking in humans. *Psychopharmacology, 208*(3), 337–351. https://doi.org/10.1007/s00213-009-1735-9

Hooper, M., Hardy, K., Handyside, A., Hunter, S., & Monk, M. (1987). HPRT-deficient (Lesch-Nyhan) mouse embryos derived from germline colonization by cultured cells. *Nature, 326*(6110), 292–295. https://doi.org/10.1038/326292a0

Horská, A., Farage, L., Bibat, G., Nagae, L. M., Kaufmann, W. E., Barker, P. B., & Naidu, S. (2009). Brain metabolism in Rett syndrome: Age, clinical, and genotype correlations. *Annals of Neurology, 65*(1), 90–97. https://doi.org/10.1002/ana.21562

Huang, W., Guenthner, C. J., Xu, J., Nguyen, T., Schwarz, L. A., Wilkinson, A. W., … Luo, L. (2016). Molecular and neural functions of *Rai1*, the causal gene for Smith-Magenis syndrome. *Neuron, 92*(2), 392–406. https://doi.org/10.1016/j.neuron.2016.09.019

Huang, W., Wang, D. C., Allen, W. E., Klope, M., Hu, H., Shamloo, M., & Luo, L. (2018). Early adolescent *Rai1* reactivation reverses transcriptional and social interaction deficits in a mouse model of Smith-Magenis syndrome. *Proceedings of the National Academy of Sciences of the United States of America, 115*(42), 10744–10749. https://doi.org/10.1073/pnas.1806796115

Hutchinson, R. R., Azrin, N. H., & Hunt, G. M. (1968). Attack produced by intermittent reinforcement of a concurrent operant response. *Journal of the Experimental Analysis of Behavior, 11*(4), 489–495. https://doi.org/10.1901/jeab.1968.11-489

Ip, J. P. K., Mellios, N., & Sur, M. (2018). Rett syndrome: Insights into genetic, molecular and circuit mechanisms. *Nature Reviews Neuroscience, 19*(6), 368–382. https://doi.org/10.1038/s41583-018-0006-3

Ito-Ishida, A., Ure, K., Chen, H., Swann, J. W., & Zoghbi, H. Y. (2015). Loss of MeCP2 in parvalbumin-and somatostatin-expressing neurons in mice leads to distinct Rett syndrome-like phenotypes. *Neuron, 88*(4), 651–658. https://doi.org/10.1016/j.neuron.2015.10.029

Iwata, B. A., Pace, G. M., & Willis, K. D. (1986). Operant studies of self-injurious hand biting in the Rett syndrome. *American Journal of Medical Genetics, 24*(SUPPL. 1), 157–166. https://doi.org/10.1002/ajmg.1320250518

Jinnah, H. A. (2009). Lesch-Nyhan disease: From mechanism to model and back again. *DMM Disease Models and Mechanisms, 2*(3-4), 116–121. https://doi.org/10.1242/dmm.002543

Jinnah, H. A., Ceballos-Picot, I., Torres, R. J., Visser, J. E., Schretlen, D. J., Verdu, A., … Puig, J. G. (2010). Attenuated variants of Lesch-Nyhan disease. *Brain, 133*(3), 671–689. https://doi.org/10.1093/brain/awq013

Jinnah, H. A., Visser, J. E., Harris, J. C., Verdu, A., Larovere, L., Ceballos-Picot, I., … Reich, S. G. (2006). Delineation of the motor disorder of Lesch-Nyhan disease. *Brain, 129*(5), 1201–1217. https://doi.org/10.1093/brain/awl056

Jonkman, S., Pelloux, Y., & Everitt, B. J. (2012a). Differential roles of the dorsolateral and mid-lateral striatum in punished cocaine seeking. *Journal of Neuroscience, 32*(13), 4645–4650. https://doi.org/10.1523/JNEUROSCI.0348-12.2012

Jonkman, S., Pelloux, Y., & Everitt, B. J. (2012b). Drug intake is sufficient, but conditioning is not necessary for the emergence of compulsive cocaine seeking after extended self-administration. *Neuropsychopharmacology, 37*(7), 1612–1619. https://doi.org/10.1038/npp.2012.6

Kasim, S., Blake, B. L., Fan, X., Chartoff, E., Egami, K., Breese, G. R., … Jinnah, H. A. (2006). The role of dopamine receptors in the neurobehavioral syndrome provoked by activation of L-type calcium channels in rodents. *Developmental Neuroscience, 28*(6), 505–517. https://doi.org/10.1159/000095113

Kasim, S., Egami, K., & Jinnah, H. A. (2002). Self-biting induced by activation of L-type calcium channels in mice: Serotonergic influences. *Developmental Neuroscience, 24*(4), 322–327. https://doi.org/10.1159/000066747

Kasim, S., & Jinnah, H. A. (2003). Self-biting induced by activation of L-type calcium channels in mice: Dopaminergic influences. *Developmental Neuroscience, 25*(1), 20–25. https://doi.org/10.1159/000071464

Katz, D. M., Bird, A., Coenraads, M., Gray, S. J., Menon, D. U., Philpot, B. D., & Tarquinio, D. C. (2016). Rett syndrome: Crossing the threshold to clinical translation. *Trends in Neurosciences, 39*(2), 100–113. https://doi.org/10.1016/j.tins.2015.12.008

Kaufmann, W. E., Stallworth, J. L., Everman, D. B., & Skinner, S. A. (2016). Neurobiologically-based treatments in Rett syndrome: Opportunities and challenges. *Expert Opinion on Orphan Drugs, 4*(10), 1043–1055. https://doi.org/10.1080/21678707.2016.1229181

Kelly, J. F., & Hake, D. F. (1970). An extinction-induced increase in an aggressive response with humans. *Journal of the Experimental Analysis of Behavior, 14*(2), 153–164. https://doi.org/10.1901/jeab.1970.14-153

Khasnavis, T., Reiner, G., Sommerfeld, B., Nyhan, W. L., Chipkin, R., & Jinnah, H. A. (2016). A clinical trial of safety and tolerability for the selective dopamine D1 receptor antagonist ecopipam in patients with Lesch-Nyhan disease. *Molecular Genetics and Metabolism, 117*(4), 401–406. https://doi.org/10.1016/j.ymgme.2016.02.005

Khasnavis, T., Torres, R. J., Sommerfeld, B., Puig, J. G., Chipkin, R., & Jinnah, H. A. (2016). A double-blind, placebo-controlled, crossover trial of the selective dopamine D1 receptor antagonist ecopipam in patients with Lesch-Nyhan disease. *Molecular Genetics and Metabolism, 118*(3), 160–166. https://doi.org/10.1016/j.ymgme.2016.04.012

Kies, S. D., & Devine, D. P. (2004). Self-injurious behaviour: A comparison of caffeine and pemoline models in rats. *Pharmacology Biochemistry and Behavior, 79*(4), 587–598. https://doi.org/10.1016/j.pbb.2004.09.010

Killcross, S., & Coutureau, E. (2003). Coordination of actions and habits in the medial prefrontal cortex of rats. *Cerebral Cortex, 13*(4), 400–408. https://doi.org/10.1093/cercor/13.4.400

Kondo, M. A., Gray, L. J., Pelka, G. J., Leang, S., Christodoulou, J., Tam, P. P. L., & Hannan, A. J. (2016). Affective dysfunction in a mouse model of Rett syndrome: Therapeutic effects of environmental stimulation and physical activity. *Developmental Neurobiology, 76*(2), 209–224. https://doi.org/10.1002/dneu.22308

Kravitz, A. V., Owen, S. F., & Kreitzer, A. C. (2013). Optogenetic identification of striatal projection neuron subtypes during in vivo recordings. *Brain Research, 1511*, 21–32. https://doi.org/10.1016/j.brainres.2012.11.018

Krishnan, K., Lau, B. Y. B., Ewall, G., Huang, Z. J., & Shea, S. D. (2017). MECP2 regulates cortical plasticity underlying a learned behaviour in adult female mice. *Nature Communications, 8*, 14077. https://doi.org/10.1038/ncomms14077

Kuehn, M. R., Bradley, A., Robertson, E. J., & Evans, M. J. (1987). A potential animal model for Lesch-Nyhan syndrome through introduction of HPRT mutations into mice. *Nature, 326*(6110), 295–298. https://doi.org/10.1038/326295a0

Lacaria, M., Gu, W., & Lupski, J. R. (2013). Circadian abnormalities in mouse models of Smith-Magenis syndrome: Evidence for involvement of *RAI1*. *American Journal of Medical Genetics, Part A, 161*(7), 1561–1568. https://doi.org/10.1002/ajmg.a.35941

Laje, G., Bernert, R., Morse, R., Pao, M., & Smith, A. C. (2010). Pharmacological treatment of disruptive behavior in Smith-Magenis syndrome. *American Journal of Medical Genetics, Part C: Seminars in Medical Genetics, 154*(4), 463–468. https://doi.org/10.1002/ajmg.c.30282

Langen, M., Bos, D., Noordermeer, S. D. S., Nederveen, H., Van Engeland, H., & Durston, S. (2014). Changes in the development of striatum are involved in repetitive behavior in autism. *Biological Psychiatry, 76*(5), 405–411. https://doi.org/10.1016/j.biopsych.2013.08.013

Langen, M., Schnack, H. G., Nederveen, H., Bos, D., Lahuis, B. E., de Jonge, M. V., … Durston, S. (2009). Changes in the developmental trajectories of striatum in autism. *Biological Psychiatry, 66*(4), 327-333. doi:https://doi.org/10.1016/j.biopsych.2009.03.017

Langthorne, P., & McGill, P. (2008). Functional analysis of the early development of self-injurious behavior: Incorporating gene-environment interactions. *American Journal on Mental Retardation, 113*(5), 403–417+419. https://doi.org/10.1352/2008.113:403-417

Langthorne, P., & McGill, P. (2012). An indirect examination of the function of problem behavior associated with fragile x syndrome and Smith-Magenis syndrome. *Journal of Autism and Developmental Disorders, 42*(2), 201–209. https://doi.org/10.1007/s10803-011-1229-6

Lauber, M., Plecko, B., Pfiffner, M., Nuoffer, J. M., & Häberle, J. (2016). The effect of S-adenosylmethionine on self-mutilation in a patient with Lesch–Nyhan disease. In E. Morava, M. Baumgartner, M. Patterson, S. Rahman, J. Zschocke, & V. Peters (Eds.), *JIMD reports* (Vol. 32, pp. 51–57). Berlin: Springer. https://doi.org/10.1007/8904_2016_571

Layng, T. V. J., Andronis, P. T., & Goldiamond, I. (1999). Animal models of psychopathology: The establishment, maintenance, attenuation, and persistence of head-banging by pigeons. *Journal of Behavior Therapy and Experimental Psychiatry, 30*(1), 45–61. https://doi.org/10.1016/S0005-7916(99)00003-8

LeBlanc, J. J., DeGregorio, G., Centofante, E., Vogel-Farley, V. K., Barnes, K., Kaufmann, W. E., … Nelson, C. A. (2015). Visual evoked potentials detect cortical processing deficits in Rett syndrome. *Annals of Neurology, 78*(5), 775–786. https://doi.org/10.1002/ana.24513

Leonard, H., & Bower, C. (1998). Is the girl with Rett syndrome normal at birth? *Developmental Medicine and Child Neurology, 40*(2), 115–121. https://doi.org/10.1111/j.1469-8749.1998.tb15371.x

Leonard, H., Moore, H., Carey, M., Fyfe, S., Hall, S., Robertson, L., … De Klerk, N. (2005). Genotype and early development in Rett syndrome: The value of international data. *Brain and Development, 27*(SUPPL. 1), S59–S68. https://doi.org/10.1016/j.braindev.2005.03.023

Lesch, M., & Nyhan, W. L. (1964). A familial disorder of uric acid metabolism and central nervous system function. *The American Journal of Medicine, 36*(4), 561–570. https://doi.org/10.1016/0002-9343(64)90104-4

Lloyd, K. G., Hornykiewicz, O., Davidson, L., Shannak, K., Farley, I., Goldstein, M., … Fox, I. H. (1981). Biochemical evidence of dysfunction of brain neurotransmitters in the Lesch-Nyhan syndrome. *New England Journal of Medicine, 305*(19), 1106–1111. https://doi.org/10.1056/NEJM198111053051902

Loffler, G., & Gordon, G. E. (2018). Cognitive function in Rett syndrome: Profoundly impaired or near normal? *European Journal of Paediatric Neurology, 22*(1), 2–3. https://doi.org/10.1016/j.ejpn.2017.12.006

Lu, H., Ash, R. T., He, L., Kee, S. E., Wang, W., Yu, D., … Zoghbi, H. Y. (2016). Loss and gain of MeCP2 cause similar hippocampal circuit dysfunction that is rescued by deep brain stimulation in a Rett syndrome mouse model. *Neuron, 91*(4), 739–747. https://doi.org/10.1016/j.neuron.2016.07.018

Lyon, D. O., & Ozolins, D. (1970). Pavlovian conditioning of shock-elicited aggression: a discrimination procedure. *Journal of the Experimental Analysis of Behavior, 13*(3), 325–331. https://doi.org/10.1901/jeab.1970.13-325

Mace, F. C., & Mauk, J. E. (1995). Bio-behavioral diagnosis and treatment of self-injury. *Mental Retardation and Developmental Disabilities Research Reviews, 1*(2), 104–110. https://doi.org/10.1002/mrdd.1410010206

Macurik, K. M., Kohn, J. P., & Kavanaugh, E. (1978). An alternative target in the study of schedule-induced aggression in pigeons. *Journal of the Experimental Analysis of Behavior, 29*(2), 337–339. https://doi.org/10.1901/jeab.1978.29-337

Mancini, J., Dubus, J., Jouve, E., Roux, J., Franco, P., Lagrue, E., … Micallef, J. (2018). Effect of desipramine on patients with breathing disorders in Rett syndrome. *Annals of Clinical Translational Neurology, 5*(2), 118–127. https://doi.org/10.1002/acn3.468

Martin, S. C., Wolters, P. L., & Smith, A. C. M. (2006). Adaptive and maladaptive behavior in children with Smith-Magenis syndrome. *Journal of Autism and Developmental Disorders, 36*(4), 541–552. https://doi.org/10.1007/s10803-006-0093-2

Matthews, W. S., Solan, A., & Barabas, G. (1995). Cognitive functioning in Lesch-Nyhan syndrome. *Developmental Medicine and Child Neurology, 37*(8), 715–722. https://doi.org/10.1111/j.1469-8749.1995.tb15017.x

Matthews, W. S., Solan, A., Barabas, G., & Robey, K. (1999). Cognitive functioning in Lesch-Nyhan syndrome: A 4-year follow up study. *Developmental Medicine and Child Neurology, 41*(4), 260–262. https://doi.org/10.1017/S0012162299000547

Maya, I., Vinkler, C., Konen, O., Kornreich, L., Steinberg, T., Yeshaya, J., … Baris, H. N. (2014). Abnormal brain magnetic resonance imaging in two patients with Smith-Magenis syndrome. *American Journal of Medical Genetics, Part A, 164*(8), 1940–1946. https://doi.org/10.1002/ajmg.a.36583

McGill, B. E., Bundle, S. F., Yaylaoglu, M. B., Carson, J. P., Thaller, C., & Zoghbi, H. Y. (2006). Enhanced anxiety and stress-induced corticosterone release are associated with increased *Crh* expression in a mouse model of Rett syndrome. *Proceedings of the National Academy of Sciences of the United States of America, 103*(48), 18267–18272. https://doi.org/10.1073/pnas.0608702103

Meek, S., Thomson, A. J., Sutherland, L., Sharp, M. G. F., Thomson, J., Bishop, V., … Burdon, T. (2016). Reduced levels of dopamine and altered metabolism in brains of HPRT knock-out rats: A new rodent model of Lesch-Nyhan disease. *Scientific Reports, 6*, 25592. https://doi.org/10.1038/srep25592

Menon, V. (2011). Large-scale brain networks and psychopathology: A unifying triple network model. *Trends in Cognitive Sciences, 15*(10), 483–506. https://doi.org/10.1016/j.tics.2011.08.003

Molina, J., Carmona-Mora, P., Chrast, J., Krall, P. M., Canales, C. P., Lupski, J. R., … Walz, K. (2008). Abnormal social behaviors and altered gene expression rates in a mouse model for Potocki-Lupski syndrome. *Human Molecular Genetics, 17*(16), 2486–2495. https://doi.org/10.1093/hmg/ddn148

Moretti, P., Bouwknecht, J. A., Teague, R., Paylor, R., & Zoghbi, H. Y. (2005). Abnormalities of social interactions and home-cage behavior in a mouse model of Rett syndrome. *Human Molecular Genetics, 14*(2), 205–220. https://doi.org/10.1093/hmg/ddi016

Moretti, P., Levenson, J. M., Battaglia, F., Atkinson, R., Teague, R., Antalffy, B., … Zoghbi, H. Y. (2006). Learning and memory and synaptic plasticity are impaired in a mouse model of Rett syndrome. *Journal of Neuroscience, 26*(1), 319–327. https://doi.org/10.1523/JNEUROSCI.2623-05.2006

Motil, K. J., Schultz, R. J., Abrams, S., Ellis, K. J., & Glaze, D. G. (2006). Fractional calcium absorption is increased in girls with Rett syndrome. *Journal of Pediatric Gastroenterology and Nutrition, 42*(4), 419–426. https://doi.org/10.1097/01.mpg.0000189370.22288.0c

Mount, R. H., Charman, T., Hastings, R. P., Reilly, S., & Cass, H. (2003). Features of autism in Rett syndrome and severe mental retardation. *Journal of Autism and Developmental Disorders, 33*(4), 435–442. https://doi.org/10.1023/A:1025066913283

Mount, R. H., Charman, T., Hastings, R. P., Reilly, S., & Cass, H. (2002). The Rett syndrome behaviour questionnaire (RSBQ): Refining the behavioural phenotype of Rett syndrome. *Journal of Child Psychology and Psychiatry, and Allied Disciplines, 43*(8), 1099–1110. https://doi.org/10.1111/1469-7610.00236

Mount, R. H., Hastings, R. P., Reilly, S., Cass, H., & Charman, T. (2001). Behavioural and emotional features in Rett syndrome. *Disability and Rehabilitation, 23*(3-4), 129–138. https://doi.org/10.1080/09638280150504207

Mount, R. H., Hastings, R. P., Reilly, S., Cass, H., & Charman, T. (2003). Towards a behavioral phenotype for Rett syndrome. *American Journal on Mental Retardation, 108*(1), 1–12+69. https://doi.org/10.1352/0895-8017(2003)108<0001:TABPFR>2.0.CO;2

Muehlmann, A. M., Kies, S. D., Turner, C. A., Wolfman, S., Lewis, M. H., & Devine, D. P. (2012). Self-injurious behaviour: Limbic dysregulation and stress effects in an animal model. *Journal of Intellectual Disability Research, 56*(5), 490–500. https://doi.org/10.1111/j.1365-2788.2011.01485.x

Muehlmann, A. M., & Lewis, M. H. (2012). Abnormal repetitive behaviours: Shared phenomenology and pathophysiology. *Journal of Intellectual Disability Research, 56*(5), 427–440. https://doi.org/10.1111/j.1365-2788.2011.01519.x

Muehlmann, A. M., Wilkinson, J. A., & Devine, D. P. (2011). Individual differences in vulnerability for self-injurious behavior: Studies using an animal model. *Behavioural Brain Research, 217*(1), 148–154. https://doi.org/10.1016/j.bbr.2010.10.012

Naneix, F., Marchand, A. R., Di Scala, G. D., Pape, J., & Coutureau, E. (2009). A role for medial prefrontal dopaminergic innervation in instrumental conditioning. *Journal of Neuroscience, 29*(20), 6599–6606. https://doi.org/10.1523/JNEUROSCI.1234-09.2009

Natacci, F., Corrado, L., Pierri, M., Rossetti, M., Zuccarini, C., Riva, P., … Larizza, L. (2000). Patient with large 17p11.2 deletion presenting with Smith-Magenis syndrome and Joubert syndrome phenotype. *American Journal of Medical Genetics, 95*(5), 467–472. https://doi.org/10.1002/1096-8628(20001218)95:5<467::AID-AJMG11>3.0.CO;2-T

Nihira, K., Leland, H., & Lambert, N. (1993). *AAMR adaptive behavior scale—Residential and Community Examiner's Manual*. Austin, TX: Pro-ed.

Nissenkorn, A., Levy-Drummer, R. S., Bondi, O., Renieri, A., Villard, L., Mari, F., … Ben-Zeev, B. (2015). Epilepsy in Rett syndrome—Lessons from the Rett networked database. *Epilepsia, 56*(4), 569–576. https://doi.org/10.1111/epi.12941

Novak, M. A., El-Mallah, S. N., & Menard, M. T. (2014). Use of the cross-translational model to study self-injurious behavior in human and nonhuman primates. *ILAR Journal, 55*(2), 274–283. https://doi.org/10.1093/ilar/ilu001

Nyhan, W. L. (1972). Behavioral phenotypes in organic genetic disease: Presidential address to the Society for Pediatric Research, May 1, 1971. *Pediatric Research, 6*(1), 1–9. https://doi.org/10.1203/00006450-197201000-00001

Nyhan, W. L. (2000). Dopamine function in Lesch-Nyhan disease. *Environmental Health Perspectives, 108*(SUPPL. 3), 409–411. Retrieved from: http.//ehpnetl.niehs.nih.gov/docs/2000/suppl-3/4094/1/lnyhan/abstract.html.

Nyhan, W. L., Johnson, H. G., Kaufman, I. A., & Jones, K. L. (1980). Serotonergic approaches to the modification of behavior in the Lesch-Nyhan syndrome. *Applied Research in Mental Retardation, 1*(1-2), 25–40. https://doi.org/10.1016/0270-3092(80)90014-4

O'Leary, H. M., Kaufmann, W. E., Barnes, K. V., Rakesh, K., Kapur, K., Tarquinio, D. C., … Sahin, M. (2018). Placebo-controlled crossover assessment of mecasermin for the treatment of Rett syndrome. *Annals of Clinical Translational Neurology, 5*(3), 323–332. https://doi.org/10.1002/acn3.533

Oliver, C., Adams, D., Allen, D., Bull, L., Heald, M., Moss, J., … Woodcock, K. (2013). Causal models of clinically significant behaviors in Angelman, Cornelia de Lange, Prader-Willi and

Smith-Magenis syndromes. *International Review of Research in Developmental Disabilities, 44*, 167–211. https://doi.org/10.1016/B978-0-12-401662-0.00006-3

Oliver, C., Murphy, G., Crayton, L., & Corbett, J. (1993). Self-injurious behavior in Rett syndrome: Interactions between features of Rett syndrome and operant conditioning. *Journal of Autism and Developmental Disorders, 23*(1), 91–109. https://doi.org/10.1007/BF01066421

Olson, L., & Houlihan, D. (2000). A review of behavioral treatments used for Lesch-Nyhan syndrome. *Behavior Modification, 24*(2), 202–222. https://doi.org/10.1177/0145445500242003

Osório, A., Cruz, R., Sampaio, A., Garayzábal, E., Carracedo, T., & Fernández-Prieto, M. (2012). Cognitive functioning in children and adults with Smith-Magenis syndrome. *European Journal of Medical Genetics, 55*(6-7), 394–399. https://doi.org/10.1016/j.ejmg.2012.04.001

Osório, A., Garayzábal-Heinze, E., Villaverde, M. L., & Sampaio, A. (2013). Neurodevelopmental features of Smith-Magenis syndrome: Strengths and weaknesses. *International Journal of Developmental Disabilities, 59*(3), 156–165. https://doi.org/10.1179/2047387712Y.0000000011

Ostlund, S. B., & Balleine, B. W. (2005). Lesions of medial prefrontal cortex disrupt the acquisition but not the expression of goal-directed learning. *Journal of Neuroscience, 25*(34), 7763–7770. https://doi.org/10.1523/JNEUROSCI.1921-05.2005

Paisey, T. J. H., Whitney, R. B., & Wainczak, S. M. (1993). Case study: Noninvasive behavioral treatment of self-injurious hand stereotypy in a child with Rett syndrome. *Behavioral Interventions, 8*(2), 133–145. https://doi.org/10.1002/bin.2360080206

Parkes, S. L., & Balleine, B. W. (2013). Incentive memory: Evidence the basolateral amygdala encodes and the insular cortex retrieves outcome values to guide choice between goal-directed actions. *Journal of Neuroscience, 33*(20), 8753–8763. https://doi.org/10.1523/JNEUROSCI.5071-12.2013

Parkes, S. L., Bradfield, L. A., & Balleine, B. W. (2015). Interaction of insular cortex and ventral striatum mediates the effect of incentive memory on choice between goal-directed actions. *Journal of Neuroscience, 35*(16), 6464–6471. https://doi.org/10.1523/JNEUROSCI.4153-14.2015

Parkes, S. L., Ferreira, G., & Coutureau, E. (2016). Acquisition of specific response-outcome associations requires NMDA receptor activation in the basolateral amygdala but not in the insular cortex. *Neurobiology of Learning and Memory, 128*, 40–45. https://doi.org/10.1016/j.nlm.2015.12.005

Patrizi, A., Picard, N., Simon, A. J., Gunner, G., Centofante, E., Andrews, N. A., & Fagiolini, M. (2016). Chronic administration of the N-methyl-D-aspartate receptor antagonist ketamine improves Rett syndrome phenotype. *Biological Psychiatry, 79*(9), 755–764. https://doi.org/10.1016/j.biopsych.2015.08.018

Peça, J., Feliciano, C., Ting, J. T., Wang, W., Wells, M. F., Venkatraman, T. N., … Feng, G. (2011). *Shank3* mutant mice display autistic-like behaviours and striatal dysfunction. *Nature, 472*(7344), 437–442. https://doi.org/10.1038/nature09965

Pelloux, Y., Dilleen, R., Economidou, D., Theobald, D., & Everitt, B. J. (2012). Reduced forebrain serotonin transmission is causally involved in the development of compulsive cocaine seeking in rats. *Neuropsychopharmacology, 37*(11), 2505–2514. https://doi.org/10.1038/npp.2012.111

Philippe, T. J., Vahid-Ansari, F., Donaldson, Z. R., Le François, B., Zahrai, A., Turcotte-Cardin, V., … Albert, P. R. (2018). Loss of MeCP2 in adult 5-HT neurons induces 5-HT1A autoreceptors, with opposite sex-dependent anxiety and depression phenotypes. *Scientific Reports, 8*(1), 5788. https://doi.org/10.1038/s41598-018-24167-8

Presti, M. F., & Lewis, M. H. (2005). Striatal opioid peptide content in an animal model of spontaneous stereotypic behavior. *Behavioural Brain Research, 157*(2), 363–368. https://doi.org/10.1016/j.bbr.2004.08.003

Read, A., & Donnai, D. (2015). *New Clinical Genetics* (3rd. Edition). Banbury, Oxfordshire. Scion Publishing Ltd.

Reiss, A. L., Faruque, F., Naidu, S., Abrams, M., Beaty, T., Bryan, R. N., & Moser, H. (1993). Neuroanatomy of Rett syndrome: A volumetric imaging study. *Annals of Neurology, 34*(2), 227–234. https://doi.org/10.1002/ana.410340220

Ricard, G., Molina, J., Chrast, J., Gu, W., Gheldof, N., Pradervand, S., … Walz, K. (2010). Phenotypic consequences of copy number variation: Insights from Smith-Magenis and Potocki-Lupski syndrome mouse models. *PLoS Biology, 8*(11), e1000543. https://doi.org/10.1371/journal.pbio.1000543

Roane, H. S., Piazza, C. C., Sgro, G. M., Volkert, V. M., & Anderson, C. M. (2001). Analysis of aberrant behaviour associated with Rett syndrome. *Disability and Rehabilitation, 23*(3-4), 139–148. https://doi.org/10.1080/09638280150504216

Robey, K. L., Reck, J. F., Giacomini, K. D., Barabas, G., & Eddey, G. E. (2003). Modes and patterns of self-mutilation in persons with Lesch-Nyhan disease. *Developmental Medicine and Child Neurology, 45*(3), 167–171. https://doi.org/10.1017/S001216220300032X

Romanczyk, R. G., & Matthews, A. L. (1998). Physiological state as antecedent: utilization in functional analysis. In J.K. Luiselli & M.J. Cameron (Eds.), *Antecedent Control: Innovative Approaches to Behavioral Support* (pp.115–138). Baltimore, MD: Paul H. Brookes.

Rose, S. A., Djukic, A., Jankowski, J. J., Feldman, J. F., & Rimler, M. (2016). Aspects of attention in Rett syndrome. *Pediatric Neurology, 57*, 22–28. https://doi.org/10.1016/j.pediatrneurol.2016.01.015

Rose, S. A., Wass, S., Jankowski, J. J., Feldman, J. F., & Djukic, A. (2017). Sustained attention in the face of distractors: A study of children with Rett syndrome. *Neuropsychology, 31*(4), 403–410. https://doi.org/10.1037/neu0000369

Rose, S. A., Wass, S., Jankowski, J. J., Feldman, J. F., & Djukic, A. (2019). Impaired visual search in children with Rett syndrome. *Pediatric Neurology, 92*, 26–31. https://doi.org/10.1016/j.pediatrneurol.2018.10.002

Roux, J.-C., & Villard, L. (2010). Biogenic amines in Rett syndrome: The usual suspects. *Behavior Genetics, 40*(1), 59–75. https://doi.org/10.1007/s10519-009-9303-y

Rudy, B., Fishell, G., Lee, S., & Hjerling-Leffler, J. (2011). Three groups of interneurons account for nearly 100% of neocortical GABAergic neurons. *Developmental Neurobiology, 71*(1), 45–61. https://doi.org/10.1002/dneu.20853

Saito, Y., Ito, M., Hanaoka, S., Ohama, E., Akaboshi, S., & Takashima, S. (1999). Dopamine receptor upregulation in Lesch-Nyhan syndrome: A postmortem study. *Neuropediatrics, 30*(2), 66–71. https://doi.org/10.1055/s-2007-973462

Samaco, R. C., Fryer, J. D., Ren, J., Fyffe, S., Chao, H.-T., Sun,Y., Greer, J. J., Zoghbi, H. Y., & Neul, J. L. (2008). A partial loss of function allele of Methyl-CpG-binding protein 2 predicts a human neurodevelopmental syndrome. *Human Molecular Genetics 17* (12), 1718–1727. https://doi.org/10.1093/hmg/ddn062

Samaco, R. C., Mandel-Brehm, C., Chao, H., Ward, C. S., Fyffe-Maricich, S. L., Ren, J., … Neul, J. L. (2009). Loss of MeCP2 in aminergic neurons causes cell-autonomous defects in neurotransmitter synthesis and specific behavioral abnormalities. *Proceedings of the National Academy of Sciences of the United States of America, 106*(51), 21966–21971. https://doi.org/10.1073/pnas.0912257106

Samaco, R. C., Mcgraw, C. M., Ward, C. S., Sun, Y., Neul, J. L., & Zoghbi, H. Y. (2013). Female *Mecp2+/-* mice display robust behavioral deficits on two different genetic backgrounds providing a framework for pre-clinical studies. *Human Molecular Genetics, 22*(1), 96–109. https://doi.org/10.1093/hmg/dds406

Sansom, D., Krishnan, V. H. R., Corbett, J., & Kerr, A. (1993). Emotional and behavioural aspects of Rett syndrome. *Developmental Medicine and Child Neurology, 35*(4), 340–345. https://doi.org/10.1111/j.1469-8749.1993.tb11646.x

Schaefer, H. H. (1970). Self-injurious behavior: shaping "head-banging" in monkeys. *Journal of Applied Behavior Analysis, 3*(2), 111–116. https://doi.org/10.1901/jaba.1970.3-111

Schretlen, D. J., Callon, W., Ward, R. E., Fu, R., Ho, T., Gordon, B., … Jinnah, H. A. (2016). Do clinical features of Lesch-Nyhan disease correlate more closely with hypoxanthine or guanine recycling? *Journal of Inherited Metabolic Disease, 39*(1), 85–91. https://doi.org/10.1007/s10545-015-9869-x

Schretlen, D. J., Harris, J. C., Park, K. S., Jinnah, H. A., & Del Pozo, N. O. (2001). Neurocognitive functioning in Lesch-Nyhan disease and partial hypoxanthine-guanine phosphoribosyltransferase deficiency. *Journal of the International Neuropsychological Society, 7(7)*, 805–812. https://doi.org/10.1017/S135561770177703X

Schretlen, D. J., Varvaris, M., Ho, T. E., Vannorsdall, T. D., Gordon, B., Harris, J. C., & Jinnah, H. A. (2013). Regional brain volume abnormalities in Lesch-Nyhan disease and its variants: A cross-sectional study. *The Lancet Neurology, 12(12)*, 1151–1158. https://doi.org/10.1016/S1474-4422(13)70238-2

Schretlen, D. J., Varvaris, M., Vannorsdall, T. D., Gordon, B., Harris, J. C., & Jinnah, H. A. (2015). Brain white matter volume abnormalities in Lesch-Nyhan disease and its variants. *Neurology, 84*(2), 190–196. https://doi.org/10.1212/WNL.0000000000001128

Schretlen, D. J., Ward, J., Meyer, S. M., Yun, J., Puig, J. G., Nyhan, W. L., … Harris, J. C. (2005). Behavioral aspects of Lesch-Nyhan disease and its variants. *Developmental Medicine and Child Neurology, 47*(10), 673–677. https://doi.org/10.1017/S0012162205001374

Schroeder, S. R., Loupe, P. S., & Tessel, R. E. (2008). Animal Models of self-injurious behavior. Induction, prevention, and recovery. *International Review of Research in Mental Retardation, 36*, 195–231. https://doi.org/10.1016/S0074-7750(08)00006-2

Schroeder, S. R., Reese, R. M., Hellings, J., Loupe, P., & Tessel R. E. (1999). The causes of self-injurious behavior and their clinical applications. In N.A. Wieseler & R.H. Hanson (Eds.), *Challenging Behavior of Persons with Mental Health Disorders and Severe Developmental Disabilities* (pp. 65-87). Washington, D.C.: American Association on Mental Retardation.

Shahbazian, M. D., Antalffy, B., Armstrong, D. L., & Zoghbi, H. Y. (2002). Insight into Rett syndrome: MeCP2 levels display tissue- and cell-specific differences and correlate with neuronal maturation. *Human Molecular Genetics, 11*(2), 115–124. https://doi.org/10.1093/hmg/11.2.115

Shiflett, M. W., Brown, R. A., & Balleine, B. W. (2010). Acquisition and performance of goal-directed instrumental actions depends on ERK signaling in distinct regions of dorsal striatum in rats. *Journal of Neuroscience, 30*(8), 2951–2959. https://doi.org/10.1523/JNEUROSCI.1778-09.2010

Simacek, J., Reichle, J., & McComas, J. J. (2016). Communication intervention to teach requesting through aided AAC for two learners with Rett syndrome. *Journal of Developmental and Physical Disabilities, 28*(1), 59–81. https://doi.org/10.1007/s10882-015-9423-7

Slager, R. E., Newton, T. L., Vlangos, C. N., Finucane, B., & Elsea, S. H. (2003). Mutations in *RAI1* associated with Smith-Magenis syndrome. *Nature Genetics, 33*(4), 466–468. https://doi.org/10.1038/ng1126

Sloneem, J., Oliver, C., Udwin, O., & Woodcock, K. A. (2011). Prevalence, phenomenology, aetiology and predictors of challenging behaviour in Smith-Magenis syndrome. *Journal of Intellectual Disability Research, 55*(2), 138–151. https://doi.org/10.1111/j.1365-2788.2010.01371.x

Smith, A. C. M., Dykens, E., & Greenberg, F. (1998). Behavioral phenotype of Smith-Magenis syndrome (del 17p11.2). *American Journal of Medical Genetics - Neuropsychiatric Genetics, 81*(2), 179–185. https://doi.org/10.1002/(SICI)1096-8628(19980328)81:2<179::AID-AJMG10>3.0.CO;2-E

Smith-Hicks, C. L., Gupta, S., Ewen, J. B., Hong, M., Kratz, L., Kelley, R., … Naidu, S. (2017). Randomized open-label trial of dextromethorphan in Rett syndrome. *Neurology, 89*(16), 1684–1690. https://doi.org/10.1212/WNL.0000000000004515

Sonuga-Barke, E., Bitsakou, P., & Thompson, M. (2010). Beyond the dual pathway model: Evidence for the dissociation of timing, inhibitory, and delay-related impairments in Attention-Deficit/Hyperactivity Disorder. *Journal of the American Academy of Child and Adolescent Psychiatry, 49*(4), 345–355. https://doi.org/10.1097/00004583-201004000-00009

Sonuga-Barke, E. J. S. (2002). Psychological heterogeneity in AD/HD—A dual pathway model of behaviour and cognition. *Behavioural Brain Research, 130*(1-2), 29–36. https://doi.org/10.1016/S0166-4328(01)00432-6

Sonuga-Barke, E. J. S. (2003). The dual pathway model of AD/HD: An elaboration of neurodevelopmental characteristics. *Neuroscience and Biobehavioral Reviews, 27*(7), 593–604. https://doi.org/10.1016/j.neubiorev.2003.08.005

Sonuga-Barke, E. J. S., Cortese, S., Fairchild, G., & Stringaris, A. (2016). Annual research review: Transdiagnostic neuroscience of child and adolescent mental disorders - differentiating decision making in attention-deficit/hyperactivity disorder, conduct disorder, depression, and anxiety. *Journal of Child Psychology and Psychiatry, and Allied Disciplines, 57*(3), 321–349. https://doi.org/10.1111/jcpp.12496

Sonuga-Barke, E. J. S., Dalen, L., & Remington, B. (2003). Do executive deficits and delay aversion make independent contributions to preschool attention-deficit/hyperactivity disorder symptoms? *Journal of the American Academy of Child and Adolescent Psychiatry, 42*(11), 1335–1342. https://doi.org/10.1097/01.chi.0000087564.34977.21

Stanwicks, L. L., Hamel, A. F., & Novak, M. A. (2017). Rhesus macaques (Macaca mulatta) displaying self-injurious behavior show more sleep disruption than controls. *Applied Animal Behaviour Science, 197*, 62–67. https://doi.org/10.1016/j.applanim.2017.09.002

Stasolla, F., Perilli, V., Di Leone, A., Damiani, R., Albano, V., Stella, A., & Damato, C. (2015). Technological aids to support choice strategies by three girls with Rett syndrome. *Research in Developmental Disabilities, 36*, 36–44. https://doi.org/10.1016/j.ridd.2014.09.017

Stauder, J. E. A., Smeets, E. E. J., van Mil, S. G. M., & Curfs, L. G. M. (2006). The development of visual- and auditory processing in Rett syndrome: An ERP study. *Brain and Development, 28*(8), 487–494. https://doi.org/10.1016/j.braindev.2006.02.011

Stodgell, C. J., Loupe, P. S., Schroeder, S. R., & Tessel, R. E. (1998). Cross-sensitization between footshock stress and apomorphine on self- injurious behavior and neostriatal catecholamines in a rat model of Lesch- Nyhan syndrome. *Brain Research, 783*(1), 10–18. https://doi.org/10.1016/S0006-8993(97)01128-1

Symons, F. J., Tervo, R. C., Barney, C. C., Damerow, J., Selim, M., McAdams, B., … Kennedy, W. (2015). Peripheral innervation in children with global developmental delay. *Journal of Child Neurology, 30*(13), 1722–1727. https://doi.org/10.1177/0883073815579704

Tanimura, Y., Vaziri, S., & Lewis, M. H. (2010). Indirect basal ganglia pathway mediation of repetitive behavior: Attenuation by adenosine receptor agonists. *Behavioural Brain Research, 210*(1), 116–122. https://doi.org/10.1016/j.bbr.2010.02.030

Taylor, L., & Oliver, C. (2008). The behavioural phenotype of Smith-Magenis syndrome: Evidence for a gene-environment interaction. *Journal of Intellectual Disability Research, 52*(10), 830–841. https://doi.org/10.1111/j.1365-2788.2008.01066.x

Temudo, T., Rios, M., Prior, C., Carrilho, I., Santos, M., Maciel, P., … Artuch, R. (2009). Evaluation of CSF neurotransmitters and folate in 25 patients with Rett disorder and effects of treatment. *Brain and Development, 31*(1), 46–51. https://doi.org/10.1016/j.braindev.2008.05.003

Traynor, J. M., Doyle-Thomas, K. A. R., Hanford, L. C., Foster, N. E., Tryfon, A., Hyde, K. L., … Hall, G. B. C. (2018). Indices of repetitive behaviour are correlated with patterns of intrinsic functional connectivity in youth with autism spectrum disorder. *Brain Research, 1685*, 79–90. https://doi.org/10.1016/j.brainres.2018.02.009

Tunnicliffe, P., & Oliver, C. (2011). Phenotype-environment interactions in genetic syndromes associated with severe or profound intellectual disability. *Research in Developmental Disabilities, 32*(2), 404–418. https://doi.org/10.1016/j.ridd.2010.12.008

Udwin, O., & Horn, I. (2001). Abilities and attainment in Smith-Magenis syndrome. *Developmental Medicine and Child Neurology, 43*(12), 823–828. https://doi.org/10.1111/j.1469-8749.2001.tb00170.x

Vaghi, M. M., Cardinal, R. N., Apergis-Schoute, A. M., Fineberg, N. A., Sule, A., & Robbins, T. W. (2019). Action-outcome knowledge dissociates from behavior in obsessive-compulsive disorder following contingency degradation. *Biological Psychiatry: Cognitive Neuroscience and Neuroimaging, 4*(2), 200–209. https://doi.org/10.1016/j.bpsc.2018.09.014

Van Dessel, J., Sonuga-Barke, E., Mies, G., Lemiere, J., Van der Oord, S., Morsink, S., & Danckaerts, M. (2018). Delay aversion in attention deficit/hyperactivity disorder is mediated by amygdala and prefrontal cortex hyper-activation. *Journal of Child Psychology and Psychiatry, and Allied Disciplines, 59*(8), 888–899. https://doi.org/10.1111/jcpp.12868

Van Kogelenberg, M., Ghedia, S., McGillivray, G., Bruno, D., Leventer, R., MacDermot, K., … Robertson, S. (2010). Periventricular heterotopia in common microdeletion syndromes. *Molecular Syndromology, 1*(1), 35–41. https://doi.org/10.1159/000274491

Vigneault, É., Poirel, O., Riad, M., Prud'homme, J., Dumas, S., Turecki, G., … El Mestikawy, S. (2015). Distribution of vesicular glutamate transporters in the human brain. *Frontiers in Neuroanatomy, 9*(MAR), 23. https://doi.org/10.3389/fnana.2015.00023

Visser, J. E., Bär, P. R., & Jinnah, H. A. (2000). Lesch-Nyhan disease and the basal ganglia. *Brain Research Reviews, 32*(2-3), 449–475. https://doi.org/10.1016/S0165-0173(99)00094-6

Visser, J. E., Schretlen, D. J., Bloem, B. R., & Jinnah, H. A. (2011). Levodopa is not a useful treatment for Lesch-Nyhan disease. *Movement Disorders, 26*(4), 746–749. https://doi.org/10.1002/mds.23478

Vlangos, C. N., Yim, D. K. C., & Elsea, S. H. (2003). Refinement of the Smith-Magenis syndrome critical region to ~950 kb and assessment of 17p11.2 deletions. Are all deletions created equally? *Molecular Genetics and Metabolism, 79*(2), 134–141. https://doi.org/10.1016/S1096-7192(03)00048-9

Wales, L., Charman, T., & Mount, R. H. (2004). An analogue assessment of repetitive hand behaviours in girls and young women with Rett syndrome. *Journal of Intellectual Disability Research, 48*(7), 672–678. https://doi.org/10.1111/j.1365-2788.2003.00590.x

Walz, K., Caratini-Rivera, S., Bi, W., Fonseca, P., Mansouri, D. L., Lynch, J., … Lupski, J. R. (2003). Modeling del(17)(p11.2p11.2) and dup(17)(p11.2p11.2) contiguous gene syndromes by chromosome engineering in mice: Phenotypic consequences of gene dosage imbalance. *Molecular and Cellular Biology, 23*(10), 3646–3655. https://doi.org/10.1128/MCB.23.10.3646-3655.2003

Walz, K., Spencer, C., Kaasik, K., Lee, C. C., Lupski, J. R., & Paylor, R. (2004). Behavioral characterization of mouse models for Smith-Magenis syndrome and dup(17)(p11.2p11.2). *Human Molecular Genetics, 13*(4), 367–378. https://doi.org/10.1093/hmg/ddh044

Wenk, G. L. (1997). Rett syndrome: Neurobiological changes underlying specific symptoms. *Progress in Neurobiology, 51*(4), 383–391. https://doi.org/10.1016/S0301-0082(96)00059-7

Wilde, L., Mitchell, A., & Oliver, C. (2016). Differences in social motivation in children with Smith–Magenis syndrome and Down syndrome. *Journal of Autism and Developmental Disorders, 46*(6), 2148–2159. https://doi.org/10.1007/s10803-016-2743-3

Wilde, L., Silva, D., & Oliver, C. (2013). The nature of social preference and interactions in Smith-Magenis syndrome. *Research in Developmental Disabilities, 34*(12), 4355–4365. https://doi.org/10.1016/j.ridd.2013.09.014

Wilkes, B. J., & Lewis, M. H. (2018). The neural circuitry of restricted repetitive behavior: Magnetic resonance imaging in neurodevelopmental disorders and animal models. *Neuroscience and Biobehavioral Reviews, 92*, 152–171. https://doi.org/10.1016/j.neubiorev.2018.05.022

Wolters, P. L., Gropman, A. L., Martin, S. C., Smith, M. R., Hildenbrand, H. L., Brewer, C. C., & Smith, A. C. M. (2009). Neurodevelopment of children under 3 years of age with Smith-Magenis syndrome. *Pediatric Neurology, 41*(4), 250–258. https://doi.org/10.1016/j.pediatrneurol.2009.04.015

Wong, D. F., Harris, J. C., Naidu, S., Yokoi, F., Marenco, S., Dannals, R. F., … Breese, G. R. (1996). Dopamine transporters are markedly reduced in Lesch-Nyhan disease in vivo. *Proceedings of the National Academy of Sciences of the United States of America, 93*(11), 5539–5543. https://doi.org/10.1073/pnas.93.11.5539

Yin, H. H., & Knowlton, B. J. (2006). The role of the basal ganglia in habit formation. *Nature Reviews Neuroscience, 7*(6), 464–476. https://doi.org/10.1038/nrn1919

Yin, H. H., Knowlton, B. J., & Balleine, B. W. (2004). Lesions of dorsolateral striatum preserve outcome expectancy but disrupt habit formation in instrumental learning. *European Journal of Neuroscience, 19*(1), 181–189. https://doi.org/10.1111/j.1460-9568.2004.03095.x

Yin, H. H., Ostlund, S. B., Knowlton, B. J., & Balleine, B. W. (2005). The role of the dorsomedial striatum in instrumental conditioning. *European Journal of Neuroscience, 22*(2), 513–523. https://doi.org/10.1111/j.1460-9568.2005.04218.x

Yizhar, O., Fenno, L., Davidson, T., Mogri, M., & Deisseroth, K. (2011). Optogenetics in neural systems. *Neuron, 71*(1), 9–34. https://doi.org/10.1016/j.neuron.2011.06.004

Young, S. N., & Shalchi, M. (2005). The effect of methionine and S-adenosylmethionine on S-adenosylmethionine levels in the rat brain. *Journal of Psychiatry and Neuroscience, 30*(1), 44–48. Retrieved from https://jpn.ca/vol30-issue1/30-1-44/

Zappella, M. (1990). A double blind trial of bromocriptine in the Rett syndrome. *Brain and Development, 12*(1), 148–150. https://doi.org/10.1016/S0387-7604(12)80198-7

Zappella, M., Genazzani, A., Facchinetti, F., & Hayek, G. (1990). Bromocriptine in the Rett syndrome. *Brain and Development, 12*(2), 221–225. https://doi.org/10.1016/S0387-7604(12)80329-9

Chapter 4
Ethical and Practical Issues in Working with People Who Self-Injure

4.1 Ethical Issues in Responding to Self-Injurious Behavior

Some people who engage in self-injurious behavior (SIB) hit themselves so hard that the impact forces involved, relative to body weight, approximate the lower end of those experienced in combat sports (Newell, Challis, Boros, & Bodfish, 2002; Newell, Sprague, Pain, Deutsch, & Meinhold, 1999). People may repeatedly target the same body site, causing bruising, contusions, and other injuries (Symons & Thompson, 1997). People who bang their heads against hard surfaces may do so with such force that other people, seeing the behavior, fear that fractures of the skull may result. Head- or face-directed SIB may cause detached retinas, damaged teeth, fractured noses, or damaged ears. The research on age-related prevalence of SIB reviewed in Chap. 2 suggests that prolonged engagement in SIB may be associated with premature mortality, and the negative social consequences of such prolonged engagement can result in seriously diminished opportunities and quality of life.

Given these multiple negative outcomes of engaging in SIB, it is hardly surprising that there is little debate regarding the desirability of intervention to reduce SIB and its negative consequences. Although some concerns may be raised regarding the use of restraint and other restrictive methods to prevent people from engaging in SIB, and the use of assessment methods which may temporarily increase rates of SIB, there appears to be little debate regarding the ethics of intervention. Indeed, there is some concern that clinicians may require encouragement to avoid drifting into "therapeutic nihilism" regarding SIB (Cooper et al., 2009) and to instead adopt evidence-based methods of intervention (Oliver, Licence, & Richards, 2017). It is of interest that this position concerning approaches to SIB in people with neurodevelopmental conditions (NDCs), and especially those who have intellectual disabilities (IDs), contrasts somewhat with the situation regarding people without NDCs who engage in non-suicidal self-injury (NSSI). With regard to the latter group, there is vigorous debate regarding both the ethics and the likely therapeutic consequences

F. Furniss, A. B. Biswas, *Self-Injurious Behavior in Individuals with Neurodevelopmental Conditions*, Autism and Child Psychopathology Series,
https://doi.org/10.1007/978-3-030-36016-0_4

of attempting to prevent SIB versus managing the behavior safely while working therapeutically with the person concerned (Edwards & Hewitt, 2011; Gutridge, 2010; Pickard & Pearce, 2017; Sullivan, 2017).

Comparable ethical issues are rarely discussed in the context of SIB engaged in by people with NDCs, perhaps because contemporary behavioral approaches in particular assume that their methods reduce SIB specifically by enabling the person concerned to achieve by other means the outcomes previously achieved by SIB. Nevertheless, methods which attempt to prevent SIB or to reduce harm consequent upon SIB, without addressing the function of the behavior, continue to be widely used with people with NDCs. These methods include the use of protective appliances, padding of hard surfaces against which people bang their heads, and manual or mechanical physical restraint (Embregts et al., 2019; Harris, 1996; Hastings & Noone, 2005; Heyvaert, Saenen, Maes, & Onghena 2014, 2015; Jones, Allen, Moore, Phillips, & Lowe, 2007; Lefèvre-Utile et al., 2018; Wilkins, 2012). In addition to the ethical issues raised by the use of such methods, practical concerns include their safety and the possibility that their use may exacerbate SIB and/or lead to diversification in topographies of SIB (Jones et al., 2007).

Other ethical issues will however arise even in cases where obviously intrusive interventions such as restraint are not being considered. Antecedent interventions, particularly those which are focused on avoiding situations and stimulus contexts which elicit SIB, may be highly effective in reducing the behavior, but may also impact negatively on the person's social opportunities and quality of life. In some cases, the person engaging in SIB and/or their families or other carers will not regard the SIB as a high priority for intervention. This may be because they have experienced previous failed attempts to reduce the behavior and regard currently proposed interventions as unlikely to be effective. There will be other cases however where they consider that the SIB is being effectively managed and that assisting the person concerned in other areas of their life will bring greater benefits than focusing on SIB. More able people with NDCs may wish to reduce their SIB but may consider that they engage in the behavior as a way of coping with environmental stressors arising from the behavior of other people, and that the appropriate intervention would involve encouraging the people causing their stress to modify their own behaviors. In other cases, successful intervention with SIB may require high levels of supervision by carers which even if they do not involve any degree of physical intervention are highly social intrusive. In the remainder of this chapter, we consider some of the legal and ethical frameworks relevant to negotiating these complexities.

4.2 Consent and Capacity in Relation to Assessment and Intervention with Self-Injurious Behavior

The general principle that medical interventions (and, by extension, those of other health and social care professionals) should only be carried out with the informed consent of the person involved is regarded as a cornerstone of ethical practice.

The principle is however of relatively recent origin. For most of the history of medicine, patients were expected to trust in the doctor's judgment regarding the choice of treatment methods, with a choice only to accept or reject medical care. In the USA, it was not until the late 1950s that a court first awarded damages to a plaintiff's estate on the grounds that the risks involved in a medical procedure had not been adequately explained (Morse & Wilson, 2016). The establishment of the principle in law however raised the question of the extent of the information which must be available to the patient/client in order to enable her/him to provide or withhold such informed consent. There have been two main approaches to this question. The first defines the information required as being that which a reasonably competent and prudent doctor would provide to the patient. The second approach suggests that the patient should be aware of any "material risks" involved in the proposed intervention, where a material risk is any risk which a reasonable person, in what the doctor knows (or should know) to be the patient's position, would regard as significant in deciding whether or not to accept intervention (Morse & Wilson, 2016). The potential tensions between these two approaches, and judgments as to what constitutes a material risk, continue to evolve. A 2015 decision of the UK Supreme Court, for example, concluded that material risks comprised not only those which a reasonable person in the patient's position would regard as significant but also those which the doctor is (or should be) reasonably aware would be significant to the individual patient (Dunn, Fulford, Herring, & Handa, 2018).

Given these complexities in deciding whether consent is truly informed when given by adults where there are no concerns about their overall capacity to give such consent, further challenges might reasonably be expected when interventions are under consideration for children or adults expected to have difficulties in understanding the relevant information. There is general acceptance that some children and some adults will be unable to understand the potential risks and benefits of some health interventions and hence that they are unable to provide properly informed consent. However, there are major differences between jurisdictions in how these issues are approached. The age at which children are generally regarded as being able to give informed consent, for example, varies substantially between countries (Hein et al., 2015), as do the approaches taken to situations involving adults with neurodegenerative conditions with the potential to affect their capacity to give informed consent (Guzik-Makaruk, Pływaczewski, Mroczko, Olesiuk-Okomska, & Kulczyńska-Przybik, 2018).

The diversity of approaches across jurisdictions, together with the fact that changes in the legal frameworks concerning informed consent frequently arise from changes in the common law (i.e., arise from decisions reached by the courts on individual cases), rather than from changes in statutory law, mean that any attempt to outline an overall framework would have limited generalizability and probably soon be outdated. It is essential that professionals remain up-to-date regarding the law on consent within the jurisdiction in which they are practicing. We outline here the current situation in England and Wales (Scotland and Northern Ireland each having its own, distinct but similar, legislation), simply in order to provide context for the case studies presented in this and later chapters.

4.3 Capacity and Competence to Give Informed Consent

In the USA, competence or competency is the legally defined right to act in a certain matter or to undertake a specific action, e.g., to make a will or to accept or refuse a specific medical intervention. Capacity by contrast refers to the determination, usually by a doctor or other health professional, of whether a person has the cognitive abilities to understand, process, and weigh relevant information in order to arrive at a rational decision (Leo, 1999). In English law the terms capacity and competence have historically been used in almost exactly converse fashion. Thus, in English law, the term capacity was until recently used to refer to the power of an individual to legally undertake a specific action, whereas competence referred to possession of the skills and abilities required to do so (Bielby, 2005). In some cases, the demonstration of competence is not sufficient to confer capacity; a person in England under the age of 18, for example, does not have the capacity to vote in parliamentary elections irrespective of their competence to do so. In recent years however, and particularly since the passing of the Mental Capacity Act (MCA) 2005, "capacity" has been widely used with regard to adults in the English context to denote both capacity and competence, presumably because for adults lack of competence is almost the only legal ground to deny capacity with regard to a particular action. In discussions regarding children however, competence continues to be used specifically to refer to the ability, rather than to the legal right, to undertake specific activities (Wellesley & Jenkins, 2015).

Using the terms in this sense, the law of England and Wales now mandates a presumption of capacity to give or withhold informed consent in medical interventions (and other matters) in anyone aged 16 or over. Professionals are required to assume that their patients/clients have capacity to give or withhold informed consent unless they have specific reason to believe that this may not be the case. Capacity must be considered with regard to the specific decision to be made. Thus, a person may have capacity to give informed consent to one proposed assessment or intervention but not for another. If the professional considers that the person may lack capacity to make the decision, they must offer to assess the person's capacity to do so and should record the process and outcomes of the capacity assessment (UK Department for Constitutional Affairs, 2007). The required assessment of capacity has two stages. The first involves determining whether the person is experiencing a temporary or permanent impairment of, or disturbance in the functioning of, their mind or brain. The second step is to determine whether the person has the capacity to make the specific decision involved. This firstly involves finding out whether the person is able to understand the decision they need to take, why they need to take it, the alternatives available to them, and the likely consequences of each available course of action (including taking no action). Capacity to make an informed decision then requires the person to be able to understand relevant information presented to her/him, retain that information for a sufficient period to make and express a decision, consider and weigh that information in order to come to a reasoned decision, and express that decision to someone else. The MCA requires the professional to assess the person's ability to undertake each of these steps in coming to an informed decision. Should they be unable to successfully complete any of the stages in the decision process, the professional should first make every attempt to provide supports which will enable them to do so. Good practice in undertaking such a capacity assessment requires a collaborative process including the person concerned, significant other people in their lives, and other professionals such as speech and language therapists (US: speech pathologists or speech-language pathologists) who may be able to support the person in the decision-making process. In English law (as is also the case in Scotland and Northern Ireland), if it is decided that the person lacks capacity to give or withhold informed consent, in most cases no other person is able to provide consent on their behalf. The only exceptions to this are if the person, prior to losing capacity, has appointed an "attorney" under a Lasting Power of Attorney which specifically empowers the attorney to take decisions regarding their health and welfare in the event of their losing capacity or if the relevant court has appointed a deputy with similar powers. In all other cases, the professional proposing to undertake the procedure concerned must decide whether to do so would be in the best interests of the person concerned. The MCA "Code of Practice" (UK Department for Constitutional Affairs, 2007) makes it clear that although where a person lacks capacity the decision concerning choice of treatment is wholly the responsibility of the professional concerned, that professional should consult with others involved in coming to their decision. It also requires that "best interests" should not be defined solely in terms of likely medical or behavioral outcome, but in terms of the whole range of factors which are important to the person concerned and would probably influence their decision if they had capacity to make it. Further, the Code of Practice requires professionals making a "best interests" decision concerning treatment of a person lacking capacity to always seek intervention options which involve minimal infringement of the person's rights.

With regard to children under 16, there is no automatic presumption of competence to consent to treatment in any of the British jurisdictions. However, a person under 16 may be competent to give consent provided that they can demonstrate that they possess the maturity and intelligence to fully understand the proposed procedure and its potential risks and benefits (Griffith, 2016). Competence to give consent therefore depends on both the maturity and intelligence of the child and the complexity and seriousness of the specific decision to be made. As is the case for adults, a child with an ID may be able to show such demonstrable task-specific competence to consent to some procedures (Wellesley & Jenkins, 2015). However, even if a professional considers that a child has demonstrated such competence, parents (or, more precisely, adults with "parental responsibility" for the child) should be involved in the decision-making process in all but very exceptional circumstances (Wellesley & Jenkins, 2015). Conversely, if a child is not competent to give consent, they should still be involved in the decision-making process so far as possible. In situations where children are not competent to give consent, it can be given by any one person who has "parental responsibility" for the child as defined by the UK Children Act (1989), provided that they themselves have capacity to consent. The law requires however that this power to give consent should be exercised in the best interests of the child.

Although professionals working in different jurisdictions will be working within different statutory frameworks with regard to capacity and consent, each of these will offer valuable perspectives on how best to approach these issues. Central principles underpinning most of these frameworks include presumption of capacity/competence unless there are specific reasons to doubt this, the importance of providing information in ways accessible to the client, and the need to work cooperatively with clients and other persons significant to them. Even where it is concluded that the client lacks capacity/competence to provide or withhold informed consent, she/he will have views on the procedures being proposed, should be supported and encouraged to express these, and has a right to have these considered in any decision regarding her/his best interests. It should be remembered that not only intervention but also assessment and diagnostic procedures will require informed consent or capacity assessment and "best interests" considerations. Some behavioral assessment procedures such as direct observation and experimental functional analyses, as well as some medical diagnostic procedures, may involve substantial intrusion on privacy and/or discomfort or inconvenience to the client. Above all, the professional must recognize that the goals and values of the client and people important to them may differ from those of the professional. Maintaining this awareness is particularly important in dealing with clients engaging in SIB, where the goal of reducing the behavior may assume such importance that it can obscure the fact that other goals may be of equal or greater importance from the client's perspective.

4.4 Assessing and Managing Short-Term Effects of Self-Injurious Behavior

The professional asked to provide support for a person engaging in SIB, and possibly other people who provide day-to-day support for the person, will naturally want to ensure that any proposed intervention is based on a careful diagnosis and/or assessment of relevant factors. Such diagnostic and/or assessment procedures may take substantial periods of time to complete. Meanwhile, however, the person engaging in SIB and/or the people supporting them will be obliged to cope with the SIB and its consequences as best they can. The background circumstances will differ according to the individual case. The client may be a young child who has only recently started to engage in SIB or whose SIB has recently increased in frequency and/or severity. On the other hand, the referral may concern a person who has been engaging in SIB for a lengthy period of time. In the latter case, the referral may have been prompted by an increase in the frequency and/or severity of the SIB (including possibly a relapse from a period in which it has been rare), or it may have resulted from a routine review identifying that no concerted efforts have been made for some time to help the person with their behavior. In each of these cases, the professional involved, while working through the diagnostic/assessment procedure, should also as a matter of priority identify the immediate consequences of the SIB for the client and find out how the client and those supporting them are dealing with the behavior in the short term.

Depending on the results of these investigations, the professional may need to provide immediate short-term support to the client and/or those who support her/him in how to manage the behavior. If the physical consequences of the behavior in terms of harm to the client are relatively minor, and/or if there is a well-organized and implemented plan already in place to manage the SIB, such interim support may not be necessary. If however the behavior is already causing serious harm and/or if it appears that it is being managed inconsistently, then such interim support may be necessary in order to prevent serious escalation in the frequency and/or severity of the behavior while more thorough diagnosis and assessment is undertaken. It should be remembered that particular sequences of patterns of social interaction can very rapidly increase the strength (including resistance to extinction) of responses such as SIB. Most notable among these are situations in which a behavior initially results in continuous reinforcement which then evolves to a variable ratio schedule. This sequence of events will be rather likely in cases where a person has just started to engage in SIB and/or where there has been a rapid change in its frequency and/or severity.

Pending the completion of initial diagnostic and assessment procedures, such interim support cannot of course be based on an individualized formulation of the factors contributing to SIB in the particular case. It can and should however be based on the current research base concerning correlates of SIB, probable causal factors in specific syndromes (Oliver et al., 2013), and effective interventions for SIB, together with an initial assessment of specific situations in which SIB is more and less likely to occur. For example, if SIB occurs at a particular point in the daily schedule of a school student with an autism spectrum condition (ASC), although the activity concerned is one which she/he seems to enjoy, the fact that insistence on sameness is a correlate of SIB among people with ASCs should prompt examination of possible inconsistencies between different members of school staff in how the activity is organized and managed, where relevant followed by planning to increase consistency.

Such interim measures, even if they prove to be helpful, are of course no substitute for a comprehensive multielement intervention based on a full assessment. They can however prevent unnecessary exacerbation of the person's SIB while diagnosis/assessment is ongoing and can help to persuade people providing direct support to the client not to attempt to improvise interventions unrelated to any evidence base while they are waiting for professional diagnosis/assessment to be completed.

4.5 Supporting Caregivers

As was noted in Chap. 2, a substantial body of research suggests that the family environment impacts significantly on the development of emotional and behavioral difficulties, at least in young people with ASCs and NDCs in which features of ASC are salient. A parallel stream of research has considered factors which may support or impair the abilities of family members and support staff to successfully implement professionally recommended interventions for SIB and other behavioral difficulties (Allen, 1999). This research has delineated two processes which may impede carers in attempts to implement psychosocial interventions. The first involves carers attributing the causes of behaviors such as SIB to factors internal to, or within the control of, the person engaging in the behavior. Such attributions are hypothesized to result in reduced motivation from carers to help the person engaging in the behavior (Weiner, 1980). The second process involves the direct consequences for carers of witnessing people they care for engaging in SIB. The distress of witnessing such behavior is hypothesized in the short term to motivate carers to respond to individual episodes of SIB in ways which bring the episode to an end as soon as possible (Oliver & Head, 1990) and in the long term to cause stress which limits the ability of carers to cooperate with professionals in developing and implementing psychosocial interventions (Allen, 1999). With regard to attributions regarding the causation of behavior such as SIB, there is convincing evidence that these can change as a result of various types of training (Rose, Gallivan, Wright, & Blake, 2014; Williams, Dagnan, Rodgers, & McDowell, 2012) and that carers' behavior can also change as a result of training. There is however only limited evidence that such training results in changes in the behaviors of the people whom carers are supporting (Knotter et al., 2018). Training directly targeting psychological distress and stress in people supporting people with IDs, for example, by encouraging mindfulness-based practice, has shown promise in reducing levels of this distress and stress (Ó Donnchadha, 2018). There is also some evidence of concomitant reduction in aggressive behavior in the people receiving support when such training is combined with training in positive behavior support (Singh, Lancioni, Karazsia, Chan, & Winton, 2016). In one study involving three mothers of children with ASCs, mindfulness-based parent training was also followed by reductions in numbers of events of aggressive behavior in all three children and SIB for the one child who engaged in SIB. The reduction in SIB was however more modest than the reductions in aggression (Singh et al., 2006).

Although such interventions show promise of potential benefit in enabling both family and professional carers to provide more effective support to people who engage in SIB, more research is needed, and the practical difficulties of providing such interventions on a widespread basis should not be underestimated. The training provided by Singh et al. (2016), for example, required seven full days of training and was led by a highly experienced behavior analyst who also was a long-standing practitioner of meditation. Accessing training of this length may be difficult for parents and other relatives of persons with NDCs owing to other family and work commitments, while maintenance of training for professional workforces may be difficult because of staff turnover. Ensuring ongoing fidelity in implementing and maintaining interventions for SIB is clearly a critical issue and one to which we return in Chaps. 6 and 9.

4.6 Monitoring Severity of Tissue Damage and Wound Management

In some individuals who engage in milder forms of SIB, the behavior may result in only transient marking or reddening of the body surface. In other cases, however, the SIB may result in abrasions, contusions, or lacerations. Repeated targeting of the same body site (Symons & Thompson, 1997) may impair wound healing and/or lead to development of scar tissue. In all cases of SIB which result in abrasions or lacerations, there is an obvious possibility of wound infection, which increases in probability if the wound is repeatedly opened or exposed to contamination.

Monitoring of the severity of tissue damage resulting from SIB is an issue which has been relatively little researched in treatment studies. Studies of pharmacological interventions have typically relied on standardized behavior rating scales, while research into behavioral interventions has generally used direct observational measurement of the rate or duration of SIB, or the percentage of time during which SIB occurs, as the preferred outcome measure (Iwata, Pace, Kissel, Nau, & Farber, 1990). The primary argument adduced in favor of using such measures rather than observation of tissue damage is that the latter may be relatively insensitive to changes in responding over time and that it is impossible to determine whether changes in wounds reflect changes in the frequency or in the intensity of self-injurious acts (Iwata et al., 1990). Measuring the tissue damage caused by SIB can sometimes however be useful in several ways. Firstly, the damage itself is usually a primary reason for wishing to help a person reduce their SIB, and thus reduction in such damage is a useful measure of the "social validity" of the extent of change produced by an intervention (Iwata et al., 1990; Wolf, 1978). Assessing the extent and severity of tissue damage which is being caused by a person's SIB can be particularly helpful in deciding whether an intervention which brings with it some costs for the person (perhaps, e.g., the use of protective equipment which limits their engagement in certain activities) is actually resulting in worthwhile change in their SIB. Similarly, such assessment can provide an objective basis for deciding whether a person's SIB is causing such damage that some initial interim intervention is necessary even before their SIB has been fully assessed or whether the damage is sufficiently minor that it can safely be allowed to continue while assessment is being completed and a minimally intrusive intervention developed.

Although a variety of trauma scales have been developed for use in medical settings such as accident and emergency departments, these are usually designed to assess a very broad range of injuries, both in terms of the nature of the injury and its severity, rendering the scales relatively insensitive in discriminating within the (comparatively) limited variety and severity of injuries typical of most cases of SIB (Iwata et al., 1990). Although little research effort has been devoted to the development and validation of measures which are suitable for use in assessment of SIB, Iwata et al. (1990) developed the Self-Injury Trauma (SIT) scale for this purpose. Part One of the SIT scale records current topographies of SIB in which the person concerned engages, together with evidence of past injuries (e.g., scars) which may be indicative of past SIB which may currently be controlled by use of restraints or protective equipment or by avoidance of situations which exacerbate SIB. In addition to topographies of SIB which can produce marked external trauma, Part One also notes whether the person concerned engages in pica, vomiting or rumination, air-swallowing, or hair-pulling. Part Two comprises an assessment of current (unhealed) wounds at each of 21 body locations. A count of the number of wounds at each location where there are injuries is used to generate a score on a three-point scale (1 one wound, 2 two to four wounds, 3 five or more wounds). Then, at each location where there are injuries, the type (contusion or abrasion/laceration) and severity of the most severe wound present are noted, with severity again being rated on a three-point scale. Part Three of the SIT scale then uses the sums of these number and severity ratings to generate two overall indices of the number and severity of wounds which have been observed. Finally, the person completing the SIT scale can complete an estimate of the overall risk to the person resulting from their SIB, which is based on both severity and location of wounds observed, with more severe contusions of the head and lacerations close to the eyes being identified as injuries of particular concern.

Iwata et al. (1990) demonstrated acceptable levels of interrater agreement for the SIT scale, both for judgments of the number, type, and severity of wounds at each body location and for the number and severity index scores and overall risk ratings. They noted however that the scale does not assess internal injuries and that the observed number and severity of injuries do not necessarily correlate highly with the extent and severity of self-injurious behavior. They further stressed that the overall risk ratings which can be derived using the SIT are simply a categorization of the physical damage currently being produced by SIB rather than a prediction of future risk. It should be noted also that full completion of the SIT scale is itself a highly intrusive procedure involving a whole body examination, requiring completion by a suitably qualified professional such as a nurse or physician and the consent of the person concerned or an individual with parental responsibility for that person, or an appropriate "best interests" consideration in the case of an adult lacking capacity to consent. Iwata et al. (1990) propose however that if initial assessment suggests that particular body areas are free from injury, further assessment may sensibly be limited to those areas where injury has been observed. Such a procedure still requires appropriate consent or "best interests" processes, and the involvement of professionals appropriately qualified to perform physical examinations, but reduces the overall intrusiveness of the procedure. In general, if the aim is to monitor whether SIB is increasing or reducing, the use of other methods, discussed in Chap. 6, will be more sensitive to change and hence will be preferred to use of the SIT scale. However, there will be situations where monitoring the extent and severity of wounds resulting from SIB is critical. One example would be where there is concern that use of a relatively non-intrusive intervention, even though it may be gradually reducing the frequency of SIB, is doing so only at the cost of increased tissue damage in the short term. In such a situation, use of the SIT scale may enable objective monitoring of the extent and severity of wounds being experienced by the person concerned.

It may be thought that methods of assessing and recording wound severity have been rendered redundant by digital photography. In situations where it is critical to monitor wound severity, photographs can be useful (Hampton & Kilroy-Findley, 2016). The taking of photographs can itself however be intrusive, and photographs almost always record information concerning the client beyond that which is strictly required for clinical purposes. Consideration of relevant regulations regarding capture and storage of personal data, and local policies on how digital images are stored within clinical notes, will be necessary (Hampton & Kilroy-Findley, 2016). In addition, the gradual changes in wound severity which occur in some cases of SIB are difficult to monitor using photographs taken in normal clinical conditions. For these reasons, if photography is used, it is helpful to have a standardized method of measuring the severity of the wound, to enable comparisons to be made, and to enable the measure to be recorded in clinical notes without the need to store the image itself. Wilson, Iwata, and Bloom (2012) describe a method for computing wound surface area (WSA), a commonly used measure of wound severity, using freely available computer software. The method does require the person engaging in SIB to cooperate in having a photograph of her/his wound taken with a metric ruler also in the shot, but does not require any direct contact with the wound. Measurement of WSA does not take into account the depth of wounds, and the method may be more difficult to apply where SIB results in contusion rather than laceration. In situations where it is important to monitor change in tissue damage however, measuring WSA, for example, at appointments where dressings are being changed, may be a helpful method.

In many situations where a person is engaging in repetitive self-injury which results in actual tissue damage, there will be a significant risk of wounds being repeatedly re-opened together with a significant risk of infection (Kilroy-Findley, 2015). Wound healing may be impaired for a number of reasons, and in such cases, it is important that wound care is overseen by a nurse or medical professional who can monitor changes in wounds and provide advice to the person engaging in SIB and people supporting her/him on managing the wound and minimizing risk of infection.

4.7 Risk Assessment and Management

People without NDCs who engage in NSSI may only infrequently make contact with services, and predicting the risk of recurrence and/or escalation of NSSI is often a major concern for professionals working with them (Quinlivan et al., 2017). This may also be the case for more able people with NDCs. Many people with NDCs will however have been in contact with services from early childhood and will be receiving support from parents, other family members, or professional carers. For these people, the situations which are likely to lead to their engaging in self-injury will probably be reasonably well-known. Although they may unexpectedly engage in SIB in a novel context, in most cases people will be aware of the contexts associated with greater or lesser risk of SIB even if the specific characteristics of the environment which elicit SIB remain unclear. A person, for example, may be more likely to engage in SIB when they are obliged to wait, or when they are unoccupied, or at specific points in personal care routines. In these situations the primary goal of risk assessment and management is to ensure that the person and those supporting them are aware of situations or activities which are likely to lead to SIB, have made a conscious decision as to whether the benefits of participation outweigh the risks associated with the possibility of SIB, and have clear plans as to how to minimize the risk of SIB and how to proceed if the person does begin to self-injure. In all settings, but particularly where many different people are likely to be supporting the person engaging in SIB, it is important that the situations likely to lead to SIB, the associated balance of benefits and risks, and the actions to be taken if the person does engage in SIB have all been clearly documented and explained to those persons providing the support.

Some elements of risk management plans will be straightforward. If having to wait is likely to lead to a person engaging in SIB, for example, the plan may suggest that they do their shopping in small local stores where they are unlikely to have to queue in order to pay for their purchases and/or shop in supermarkets at times which are not normally busy. Sometimes however the risk management plan will specify actions different from those which may be recommended in therapeutic interventions. A person may, for example, be participating in a therapeutic program intended to increase their ability to cope with queueing in which they are encouraged to use various coping strategies to avoid engaging in SIB while being obliged to wait. The risk management plan however may suggest that if the person's SIB reaches a certain level of intensity, they should be encouraged to leave the shop at once. In such situations, particularly those in which many different people are supporting the person with an NDC, it is important that those people are well briefed and trained regarding both the therapeutic program and the risk management plan and understand the contexts in which each should be followed. In some cases, the challenges involved in managing risk may require difficult decisions as to whether the extent of unavoidable "residual risk" is acceptable, either by the person concerned if they have capacity to make an informed decision or by those providing support if the person does not have such capacity. In the latter case, the decision must be made on the basis of a judgment regarding the best interests of the person concerned.

4.8 Use of Protective Equipment and Restraints

Although little systematic information is available regarding their use, there is no doubt that both interpersonal direct restraint and various types of protective equipment and physical/mechanical restraints continue to be used with some people who engage in SIB (Jones et al., 2007). Information is particularly sparse regarding the use of interpersonal direct restraint with people who engage in SIB. Most relevant research has focused on the use of direct and mechanical restraint with children and adults with IDs who engage in "challenging behaviors" without specification of the topography of these behaviors. In a large-scale study of a variety of residential services for adults with IDs in the UK, Emerson et al. (2000) reported that 53% of the people surveyed were reported to have engaged in "moderately serious" or "severe" forms of challenging behavior within the month prior to the survey. Interpersonal physical restraint was reported to have been used with 44% of these people, while mechanical restraint was reported to have been used with 3%. Allen, Hawkins, and Cooper (2006) surveyed parents who were members of a UK charitable organization dedicated to dissemination of knowledge regarding the causes and management of challenging behavior. Over 85% of parents who responded reported having used interpersonal physical restraint with their child with an ID, and 26% reported using mechanical restraints of various kinds. An analysis of administrative records from one organization's community-based habilitation and residential services for adults with IDs in the USA however reported much lower rates of interpersonal physical intervention, with physical restraint used with less than 8% of service users over a 6-month period (Luiselli, Sperry, & Magee, 2011). Lundström, Antonsson, Karlsson, and Graneheim (2011) found a relatively high rate of use of mechanical restraints with adults with IDs living in community group homes, with over 17% having experienced such restraint within a single week. The relatively high rate of mechanical restraint reported by this study appears to be due to the fact that Lundström et al. did not enquire solely about restraint used in response to challenging behavior but also about restraint used to limit people's mobility, including chair belts and chairs with fixed tray tables. There appears to be substantial variability between services in the proportions of service users who experience interpersonal physical or mechanical restraint, with Sturmey (2009) reporting these to vary from 0 to 45% and 0 to 30%, respectively, in English services provided by the UK National Health Service and independent healthcare providers.

Several studies have investigated possible associations between SIB and the use of specific types of restrictive interventions. McGill, Murphy, and Kelly-Pike (2009) asked 100 staff working in services for adults and children with IDs in the UK to provide information on up to 3 service users from their organization with whom restrictive interventions were used, and over 50% of the people reported on were described as engaging in SIB. For over 40% of those people, interpersonal direct restraint was sometimes used in response to SIB, while items of protective equipment (including mechanical restraints) were used with 10%. Using data from a statewide reporting system for services for adults, and some children, with IDs in the Australian state of Victoria, Webber, McVilly, and Chan (2011) showed that mechanical restraints and protective equipment were more frequently used in response to SIB rather than aggression to others or destruction of property. Splints and braces, restrictive clothing such as one-piece suits, protective helmets, socks and gloves, belts and straps, and other methods were all reported to be used, although it appeared that reported use of belts also included use of vehicle seat belts in some cases. Webber et al. (2019) showed that people with a hearing, physical, neurological, communication, or visual impairment, and those with ASCs, were at heightened risk for use of mechanical rather than other forms of restraint, a finding possibly related to these individual factors also being risk factors for SIB.

The use of protective equipment and mechanical restraints with people who engage in SIB may have reduced over recent decades. Taylor, Oliver, and Murphy (2011), following up a group of people with IDs who had been identified as engaging in SIB 20 years earlier, found that despite there having been little change in their SIB, only one of the nine people who had originally used protective equipment or mechanical restraints was still using any form of protection. This man had originally used multiple types of protection/restraint, but at follow-up was being supported by staff who only used cushions to minimize damage resulting from his SIB. There have been frequent calls for reduction in the use of both physical interventions and mechanical restraints in the support of people engaging in SIB (and other behaviors), and a number of individual- and organizational-level interventions have been shown to have some effectiveness in this regard (Deveau & Leitch, 2015; Matson & Boisjoli, 2009; Sturmey, 2009; Williams, 2010; Williams & Grossett, 2011).

It appears however that both interpersonal physical restraint and the use of protective equipment and mechanical restraints continue to be used with some people with NDCs who engage in SIB. While the use of interpersonal direct restraint has increasingly become governed by formal policy guidance, little such guidance exists with regard to the use of protective equipment and mechanical restraints (Jones et al., 2007). This is despite the fact that such methods may be regarded as relatively highly intrusive (Fig. 4.1).

Jones et al. (2007) propose in fact that guidance originally suggested by Spain, Hart, and Corbett (1984) remains relevant. Spain et al. (1984) propose that where reactive management is necessary to reduce harm when people are engaging in SIB, it may sometimes be preferable to use material or mechanical restraints rather than direct interpersonal restraints in order to avoid the possibility of social reinforcement of the SIB. Spain et al. (1984) further suggest that any mechanical restraints should be easily applied and removed. They caution that people should not be left unattended while wearing any form of protective equipment and that the equipment itself should only be provided and maintained by suitably qualified therapists who can adapt it as necessary for the individual. Spain et al. (1984) also suggest that equipment which closely resembles normal attire, and which interferes minimally with the person's ability to engage in activities other than SIB, is always to be preferred and recommend that a plan to reduce the use of such equipment in the long term should be in place from the inception of its use.

Spain et al. (1984) also suggested that in some cases, having protective equipment or mechanical restraints available in case of emergency might increase the confidence of family members or staff supporting people engaging in SIB in using less intrusive interventions, by assuring them that a method of preventing severe harm was available if necessary. One potential difficulty with such equipment is however that its use may become routine. In service settings, psychoactive medication is usually stored in secure locations and accessible only to members of staff who are trained and designated as competent to administer it correctly. Protective equipment and mechanical restraints by contrast are often kept together with the

LEAST RESTRICTIVE

- Distraction (Hastings, 1996)
- Diversion to a reinforcing/compelling event, strategic capitulation (LaVigna and Willis, 2002)
- Verbal commands to stop or other forms of communication such as attempts to reassure and calm the person, touching the person (e.g. Hastings, 1996a,b)
- Adaptations to physical environment – padding furniture and fixtures, using a cushion to prevent injury, e.g. when hitting head against hard surfaces (e.g. Hastings, 1996a,b; Spain et al., 1984)
- Physical or personal restraint, i.e. holding the person in some way (e.g. Harris, 1996; Hastings, 1996a,b)
- Protective devices designed to prevent or reduce injury but not restrain individuals such as helmets (e.g. Dorsey, Iwata, Reid, & Davis, 1982; Duker and Seys, 1997; Murphy et al., 1993; Spain et al., 1984)
- Various types of appliances designed to mechanically restrain individuals to prevent the occurrence of SIB such as arm splints, bed or chair ties (e.g. Dorsey, Iwata, Reid, & Davis, 1982; Duker and Seys, 1997; Murphy et al., 1993; Spain et al., 1984)

MOST RESTRICTIVE

Fig. 4.1 A continuum of management strategies for self-injurious behavior. Reproduced with permission of Sage Publications from Jones, E., Allen, D., Moore, K., Phillips, B., & Lowe, K. (2007). Restraint and self-injury in people with intellectual disabilities: A review. *Journal of Intellectual Disabilities, 11*(1), 105–118. ©2007 Sage Publications

other possessions of the service user, and it is frequently possible that a staff member unaware of the specific circumstances under which their use is recommended may wrongly assume that they should be used as a matter of course.

All of these issues suggest that the use of protective equipment or mechanical restraint should be employed, if at all, only as one component of a structured and closely monitored multielement intervention. Such considerations apply even to apparently less intrusive environmental modifications such as placing padding on hard surfaces against which a person bangs their head. Just as use of arm splints to prevent hand-to-head hitting may result in the person developing an alternative form of SIB, padding hard surfaces may result in head-to-surface banging being redirected to new points, possibly resulting in more severe injury (Harris, 1996). Careful planning and ongoing monitoring for possible untoward consequences are therefore essential in any use of such measures.

4.9 Clinical and Organizational Supports for Good Practice

At least in adults with IDs, probably in adults with ASCs, and possibly in older children with ASCs, SIB appears to be relatively persistent (see Chap. 2). For the person concerned, their families, and support staff and professionals working with them, SIB may appear to be an intractable problem which can only be managed rather than meaningfully ameliorated. Researchers have pointed out that even in adults a substantial minority of people who engage in SIB cease doing so (at least for substantial periods of time) and have urged the need for professionals to avoid slipping into "therapeutic nihilism" (Cooper et al., 2009). Maintaining a focus on long-term change may however be difficult for all concerned when faced either with chronic SIB which shows little sensitivity to environmental changes or with repeated crises in which SIB escalates dramatically for limited periods of time. In everyday practice these difficulties are often compounded by the fact that the person engaging in SIB may also engage in aggression toward other people and experience other emotional and behavioral difficulties which at times may distract all concerned from a primary focus on the SIB.

As noted earlier, episodes of SIB are often distressing not only for the person concerned but also for their families, support staff, and professionals working with them. These feelings are likely to be compounded by anxiety and doubts regarding how best to support the person engaging in SIB. Reflecting on the experiences of healthcare staff working with people without NDCs who engage in SIB, Smith et al. (2015) argued that similar processes could result in a state of dysregulation involving the person engaging in SIB, their families and friends, and healthcare staff working with them. Smith et al. (2015) suggested such a state of dysregulation could lead to an inappropriately narrow focus on risk assessment and short-term management and create a pressure for ad hoc (and therefore often inconsistent) decision-making at the expense of therapeutic engagement and collaborative working.

Awareness of such processes and a willingness to address them in clinical supervision are essential first steps in avoiding or limiting such dysregulation. Even this basic level of support will however often be unavailable to families of people engaging in SIB and may be difficult to access for support staff working directly with them, even though some research suggests that a substantial proportion of staff working with people with ASCs who engage in "challenging behaviors" such as SIB experience potentially clinically significant levels of anxiety (Merrick, Grieve, & Cogan, 2017). As noted earlier, interventions directly targeting emotional responses to behaviors such as SIB (Ó Donnchadha, 2018) may be helpful but can also require significant time investment. Recent research into the effectiveness of positive behavior support suggests that "setting wide" intervention targeting a range of factors including staffing issues can have positive impacts on "challenging behaviors" (McGill et al., 2018). Despite the time demands involved, incorporating training in mindfulness-based practice into such interventions may prove to be a relatively time-efficient approach to maintaining the effectiveness of such interventions in the long term (Singh et al., 2016).

4.10 Case Studies

Rose A

Rose A is 3.5 years old and lives at home with her parents. Her parents were in their mid-30s when she was born, having had a son over 10 years earlier. At antenatal appointments the possibility of screening for Down syndrome had been discussed with them, but they declined this as they were delighted to be having a second child and decided that they would not consider a termination of pregnancy, irrespective of the test results. When Rose was born, she was very floppy, and cytogenetic testing rapidly confirmed a diagnosis of Down syndrome. Rose has substantial general developmental delay, with particular difficulties with expressive language. She has however recently started to use a few words. She is a generally happy and sociable child. Other than periodic concerns about her health, which have included constipation and middle ear infection, her parents' main concern is that she has started to engage in various stereotyped behaviors, including body rocking, which can become more vigorous if she is distressed.

Ayanna B

Ayanna B is 14 years old and lives at home with her parents. She attends a special school, having been diagnosed with an autism spectrum condition and a severe intellectual disability. Ayanna is a lively teenager who enjoys being outside, ball-games, and swimming. She is well liked by the staff supporting her because of the enthusiasm and enjoyment with which she joins in nearly all activities at school. She dislikes however any activity which requires her to sit still for lengthy periods of time, and in such situations she sometimes starts to cry and slap her own face. Ayanna's behavior can upset other students in the class, so if she starts to cry and self-injure, the teaching assistant normally takes her out of the room and takes Ayanna for a short walk around the school grounds to help her calm. Ayanna is quite independent in most self-help skills and participates in basic food preparation. She understands multi-step requests, but has never developed speech. She has however for many years used symbols in order to communicate, although she uses these only to make requests, never to comment on persons or events.

Darren C

Darren C is 8 years old and has a diagnosis of Cornelia de Lange syndrome (CdLS), with a severe intellectual disability. He understands simple requests, although he has no functional vocal expressive language. He communicates by using gestures together with a few formal signs which he has learned since moving to a specialist school for children with intellectual disabilities 2 years ago, having previously spent 2 years in a specialist classroom within a regular first school. Darren sometimes engages in SIB, including biting his hands and hitting his face with his hands, most often when he is asked to transition between activities. This behavior has however improved since the school carefully arranged his activity schedule so that within each third of the school day, his sequence of activities always involved moving through increasingly preferred activities culminating in a snack or meal break. As

Darren would happily transition to a new, less preferred, activity from a break once he had finished his meal or snack, this approach appeared to have helped to substantially reduce his SIB.

Arshad D

Arshad D is 19 years old, lives with his family, and is in his final year at a special school. Arshad has a severe intellectual disability, and when he leaves school, it is planned that he will continue to live with his family while receiving support from a community-based provider of day services and activities for people with intellectual disabilities. He will however be spending much more time in his family home than currently. Arshad's father works long hours in his family's business based in a city approximately 40 miles away from the family home, and in addition to supporting Arshad, his mother also looks after her own mother, who lives with the family, and Arshad's two younger sisters.

Arshad engages in SIB in which he scratches himself, occasionally with such severity that he draws blood, mainly on his forearms and lower legs. For many years, his SIB has been managed by attempting to distract him from the behavior by offering him activities and if necessary putting gloves on him to minimize the injury he can cause. His social worker is concerned that his SIB may escalate when he leaves school because he will probably be less stimulated and engaged at home that he is at school. In a report prepared for a review meeting at Arshad's school, the social worker therefore proposed that implementing a program to reduce Arshad's SIB should be a high priority for his remaining time at school.

At the review meeting, at which the social worker, school staff, and Arshad's mother were present, his mother however expressed the view that helping Arshad to learn to use the toilet independently was a much higher priority than trying to reduce his SIB. From her point of view, the SIB was being successfully managed by the current measures, and since Arshad had engaged in the behavior from a very young age, she thought it unlikely that anything could be done about it. Arshad's independence skills, on the other hand, had improved during his time at school, and Arshad regularly used the toilet appropriately provided that he was reminded to do so. His mother thought however that it would be very helpful if Arshad could learn to go to the toilet completely independently. The meeting came to no conclusion regarding priorities for Arshad, but his teacher agreed to consult with a clinical psychologist who provided support to the school on the feasibility of helping Arshad with his SIB during his remaining time at the school.

Sarah E

Sarah E is 23 years old and has diagnoses of severe intellectual disability and autism. She lives in a community residential service to which she moved soon after she left school, partly because of the difficulties her parents encountered in managing her SIB, which comprises striking her face and head with her hands or knees and also banging her head on hard surfaces. Sarah has very limited independence skills and engages in very little constructive activity, spending much time walking around with no obvious specific purpose. She understands basic requests but has no effective form of conventional expressive communication, although she will indicate things she wants to other people. If, for example, she would like a drink, she will get hold of another person and take them to the kitchen sink or hand them an empty cup. At various times, Sarah has been prescribed antipsychotic medication, an anticonvulsant (prescribed as a mood stabilizer), and naltrexone, but none of these have had any discernible effect on her SIB. She has also been provided with a protective helmet which staff encourage her to wear during periods when she is engaging in head-to-surface SIB.

Nathan F

Nathan F is 21 years old and lives with his mother, who is approaching 60. Nathan's father sadly died following a heart attack years ago. Nathan is small in stature and has a very severe intellectual disability. Although he is independent in basic self-care skills, he has very limited understanding of language and no expressive communication. He participates in activities with a community-based day service three half-days each week, but otherwise stays at home with his mother. With the community group, he enjoys walking and swimming and joins in activities at a local community garden. He has a long history of engaging in self-injury which primarily involves delivering blows to his ears and cheeks with his hands. Most of these blows appear to be relatively low in intensity, but Nathan has been provided with a protective helmet and gloves which his mother encourages him to wear on the rare occasions that his self-injury is more severe.

References

Allen, D. (1999). Mediator analysis: An overview of recent research on carers supporting people with intellectual disability and challenging behaviour. *Journal of Intellectual Disability Research, 43*(4), 325–339. https://doi.org/10.1046/j.1365-2788.1999.00209.x

Allen, D., Hawkins, S., & Cooper, V. (2006). Parents' use of physical interventions in the management of their children's severe challenging behaviour. *Journal of Applied Research in Intellectual Disabilities, 19*(4), 356–363. https://doi.org/10.1111/j.1468-3148.2006.00292.x

Bielby, P. (2005). The conflation of competence and capacity in English medical law: A philosophical critique. *Medicine, Health Care and Philosophy, 8*(3), 357–369. https://doi.org/10.1007/s11019-005-0537-z

Cooper, S.-A., Smiley, E., Allan, L. M., Jackson, A., Finlayson, J., Mantry, D., & Morrison, J. (2009). Adults with intellectual disabilities: Prevalence, incidence and remission of self-injurious behaviour, and related factors. *Journal of Intellectual Disability Research, 53*(3), 200–216. https://doi.org/10.1111/j.1365-2788.2008.01060.x

Department for Constitutional Affairs. (2007). *Mental Capacity Act 2005: Code of practice*. Retrieved from https://www.gov.uk/government/publications/mental-capacity-act-code-of-practice.

Deveau, R., & Leitch, S. (2015). The impact of restraint reduction meetings on the use of restrictive physical interventions in English residential services for children and young people. *Child: Care, Health and Development, 41*(4), 587–592. https://doi.org/10.1111/cch.12193

Dorsey, M. F., Iwata, B. A., Reid, D. H., & Davis, P. A. (1982). Protective equipment: Continuous and contingent application in the treatment of self-injurious behavior. *Journal of Applied Behavior Analysis, 15*(2), 217–230. https://doi.org/10.1901/jaba.1982.15-217

Duker, P. C., & Seys, D. M. (1997). An inventory method for assessing the degree of restraint imposed by others. *Journal of Behavior Therapy and Experimental Psychiatry, 28*(2), 113–121. https://doi.org/10.1016/S0005-7916(97)00010-4

Dunn, M., Fulford, K. W. M., Herring, J., & Handa, A. (2018). Between the reasonable and the particular: Deflating autonomy in the legal regulation of informed consent to medical treatment. *Health Care Analysis, 27*(2), 1–18. https://doi.org/10.1007/s10728-018-0358-x

Edwards, S. D., & Hewitt, J. (2011). Can supervising self-harm be part of ethical nursing practice? *Nursing Ethics, 18*(1), 79–87. https://doi.org/10.1177/0969733010386166

Embregts, P. J. C. M., Negenman, A., Habraken, J. M., de Boer, M. E., Frederiks, B. J. M., & Hertogh, C. M. P. M. (2019). Restraint interventions in people with moderate to profound intellectual disabilities: Perspectives of support staff and family members. *Journal of Applied Research in Intellectual Disabilities, 32*(1), 172–183. https://doi.org/10.1111/jar.12519

Emerson, E., Robertson, J., Gregory, N., Hatton, C., Kessissoglou, S., Hallam, A., & Hillery, J. (2000). Treatment and management of challenging behaviours in residential settings. *Journal of Applied Research in Intellectual Disabilities, 13*(4), 197–215. https://doi.org/10.1046/j.1468-3148.2000.00036.x

Griffith, R. (2016). What is Gillick competence? *Human Vaccines & Immunotherapeutics, 12*(1), 244–247. https://doi.org/10.1080/21645515.2015.1091548

Gutridge, K. (2010). Safer self-injury or assisted self-harm? *Theoretical Medicine and Bioethics, 31*(1), 79–92. https://doi.org/10.1007/s11017-010-9135-z

Guzik-Makaruk, E. M., Pływaczewski, E. W., Mroczko, P., Olesiuk-Okomska, M., & Kulczyńska-Przybik, A. (2018). Consent to medical procedures of patients with neurodegenerative diseases: A comparative study of legal regulations in selected European countries and in the United States. *Journal of Alzheimer's Disease, 63*(1), 53–67. https://doi.org/10.3233/JAD-171176

Hampton, S., & Kilroy-Findley, A. (2016). Taking photographs of wounds and data protection. *Wounds UK, 12*(1), 40–44. Retrieved from https://www.wounds-uk.com/journal.shtml

Harris, J. (1996). Physical restraint procedures for managing challenging behaviours presented by mentally retarded adults and children. *Research in Developmental Disabilities, 17*(2), 99–134. https://doi.org/10.1016/0891-4222(95)00036-4

Hastings, R. P. (1996a). Staff strategies and explanations for intervening with challenging behaviours. *Journal of Intellectual Disability Research, 40*(2), 166–175. https://doi.org/10.1111/j.1365-2788.1996.tb00618.x

Hastings, R. P. (1996b). Erratum: Staff strategies and explanations for intervening with challenging behaviours (Journal of Intellectual Disability Research (40) 166-175). *Journal of Intellectual Disability Research, 40*(4), 384.

Hastings, R. P., & Noone, S. J. (2005). Self-injurious behavior and functional analysis: Ethics and evidence. *Education and Training in Developmental Disabilities, 40*(4), 335–342. Retrieved from http://www.daddcec.org/Publications/ETADDJournal/ETADDArchives/tabid/81/IssueID/25/Default.aspx

Hein, I. M., Troost, P. W., Lindeboom, R., Christiaans, I., Grisso, T., van Goudoever, J. B., & Lindauer, R. J. L. (2015). Feasibility of an assessment tool for children's competence to consent to predictive genetic testing: A pilot study. *Journal of Genetic Counseling, 24*(6), 971–977. https://doi.org/10.1007/s10897-015-9835-7

Heyvaert, M., Saenen, L., Maes, B., & Onghena, P. (2014). Systematic review of restraint interventions for challenging behaviour among persons with intellectual disabilities: Focus on effectiveness in single-case experiments. *Journal of Applied Research in Intellectual Disabilities, 27*(6), 493–510. https://doi.org/10.1111/jar.12094

Heyvaert, M., Saenen, L., Maes, B., & Onghena, P. (2015). Systematic review of restraint interventions for challenging behaviour among persons with intellectual disabilities: Focus on experiences. *Journal of Applied Research in Intellectual Disabilities, 28*(2), 61–80. https://doi.org/10.1111/jar.12095

Iwata, B. A., Pace, G. M., Kissel, R. C., Nau, P. A., & Farber, J. M. (1990). The Self-injury Trauma (SIT) scale: a method for quantifying surface tissue damage caused by self-injurious behavior. *Journal of Applied Behavior Analysis, 23*(1), 99–110. https://doi.org/10.1901/jaba.1990.23-99

Jones, E., Allen, D., Moore, K., Phillips, B., & Lowe, K. (2007). Restraint and self-injury in people with intellectual disabilities: A review. *Journal of Intellectual Disabilities, 11*(1), 105–118. https://doi.org/10.1177/1744629507074006

Kilroy-Findley, A. (2015). The psychology of self-harm and self-injury: Does the wound management differ? *Wounds UK, 11*(1), 16–26. Retrieved from https://www.wounds-uk.com/journal.shtml

Knotter, M. H., Spruit, A., De Swart, J. J. W., Wissink, I. B., Moonen, X. M. H., & Stams, G. J. M. (2018). Training direct care staff working with persons with intellectual disabilities and challenging behaviour: A meta-analytic review study. *Aggression and Violent Behavior, 40*, 60–72. https://doi.org/10.1016/j.avb.2018.03.005

LaVigna, G. W., & Willis, T. (2002). Counter-intuitive strategies for crisis management within a non-aversive framework. In D. Allen (Ed.), *Ethical approaches to physical interventions. Responding to challenging behaviour in people with intellectual disabilities*. Kidderminster: British Institute of Learning Disabilities.

Lefèvre-Utile, J., Guinchat, V., Wachtel, L. E., Cohen, D., Perron, A., Montreuil, M., … Reyre, A. (2018). Personal protective equipment and restraints alternatives in the management of challenging behaviors in inpatients with autism and intellectual disability (part 1: Patients' perspectives). [Équipements de protection individuelle et outils de sécurisation alternatifs à la contention dans la prise en charge des troubles graves du comportement des personnes avec autisme et déficience intellectuelle (partie 1: perspective des patients)]. *Neuropsychiatrie de l'Enfance et de l'Adolescence, 66*(7-8), 443–459. https://doi.org/10.1016/j.neurenf.2018.08.001

Leo, R. J. (1999). Competency and the capacity to make treatment decisions: A primer for primary care physicians. *Primary Care Companion to the Journal of Clinical Psychiatry, 1*(5), 131–141. Retrieved from https://www.psychiatrist.com/PCC/article/Pages/1999/v01n05/v01n0501.aspx

Luiselli, J. K., Sperry, J. M., & Magee, C. (2011). Descriptive analysis of physical restraint (protective holding) among community living adults with intellectual disability. *Journal of Intellectual Disabilities, 15*(2), 93–99. https://doi.org/10.1177/1744629511410831

Lundström, M. O., Antonsson, H., Karlsson, S., & Graneheim, U. H. (2011). Use of physical restraints with people with intellectual disabilities living in Sweden's group homes. *Journal of Policy and Practice in Intellectual Disabilities, 8*(1), 36–41. https://doi.org/10.1111/j.1741-1130.2011.00285.x

Matson, J. L., & Boisjoli, J. A. (2009). Restraint procedures and challenging behaviours in intellectual disability: An analysis of causative factors. *Journal of Applied Research in Intellectual Disabilities, 22*(2), 111–117. https://doi.org/10.1111/j.1468-3148.2008.00477.x

McGill, P., Murphy, G., & Kelly-Pike, A. (2009). Frequency of use and characteristics of people with intellectual disabilities subject to physical interventions. *Journal of Applied Research in Intellectual Disabilities, 22*(2), 152–158. https://doi.org/10.1111/j.1468-3148.2008.00483.x

McGill, P., Vanono, L., Clover, W., Smyth, E., Cooper, V., Hopkins, L., … Deveau, R. (2018). Reducing challenging behaviour of adults with intellectual disabilities in supported accommodation: A cluster randomized controlled trial of setting-wide positive behaviour support. *Research in Developmental Disabilities, 81*, 143–154. https://doi.org/10.1016/j.ridd.2018.04.020

Merrick, A. D., Grieve, A., & Cogan, N. (2017). Psychological impacts of challenging behaviour and motivational orientation in staff supporting individuals with autistic spectrum conditions. *Autism, 21*(7), 872–880. https://doi.org/10.1177/1362361316654857

Morse, R. J., & Wilson, R. F. (2016). Realizing informed consent in times of controversy: Lessons from the SUPPORT study. *The Journal of Law, Medicine & Ethics, 44*(3), 402–418. https://doi.org/10.1177/1073110516667938

Murphy, G., Oliver, C., Corbett, J., Crayton, L., Hales, J., Head, D., & Hall, S. (1993). Epidemiology of self injury, characteristics of people with severe self injury and initial treatment outcome. In C. Kiernan (Ed.), *Research into Practice? Implications of Research on the Challenging Behaviour of People with Learning Disability* (pp. 1–35). Kidderminster: Kidderminster: British Institute of Learning Disabilities.

Newell, K. M., Challis, J. H., Boros, R. L., & Bodfish, J. W. (2002). Further evidence on the dynamics of self-injurious behaviors: Impact forces and limb motions. *American Journal on Mental Retardation, 107*(1), 60–68+74. https://doi.org/10.1352/0895-8017(2002)107<0060:FEOTDO>2.0.CO;2

Newell, K. M., Sprague, R. L., Pain, M. T., Deutsch, K. M., & Meinhold, P. (1999). Dynamics of self-injurious behaviors. *American Journal on Mental Retardation, 104*(1), 11–21. https://doi.org/10.1352/0895-8017(1999)104<0011:DOSB>2.0.CO;2

Ó Donnchadha, S. (2018). Stress in caregivers of individuals with intellectual or developmental disabilities: A systematic review of mindfulness-based interventions. *Journal of Applied Research in Intellectual Disabilities, 31*(2), 181–192. https://doi.org/10.1111/jar.12398

Oliver, C., Adams, D., Allen, D., Bull, L., Heald, M., Moss, J., … Woodcock, K. (2013). Causal models of clinically significant behaviors in Angelman, Cornelia de Lange, Prader-Willi and Smith-Magenis syndromes. *International Review of Research in Developmental Disabilities, 44*, 167–211. https://doi.org/10.1016/B978-0-12-401662-0.00006-3

Oliver, C., & Head, D. (1990). Self-injurious behaviour in people with learning disabilities: Determinants and interventions. *International Review of Psychiatry, 2*(1), 101–116. https://doi.org/10.3109/09540269009028276

Oliver, C., Licence, L., & Richards, C. (2017). Self-injurious behaviour in people with intellectual disability and autism spectrum disorder. *Current Opinion in Psychiatry, 30*, 97–101. https://doi.org/10.1097/YCO.0000000000000313

Pickard, H., & Pearce, S. (2017). Balancing costs and benefits: A clinical perspective does not support a harm minimisation approach for self-injury outside of community settings. *Journal of Medical Ethics, 43*(5), 324–326. https://doi.org/10.1136/medethics-2017-104152

Quinlivan, L., Cooper, J., Meehan, D., Longson, D., Potokar, J., Hulme, T., … Kapur, N. (2017). Predictive accuracy of risk scales following self-harm: Multicentre, prospective cohort study. *British Journal of Psychiatry, 210*(6), 429–436. https://doi.org/10.1192/bjp.bp.116.189993

Rose, J., Gallivan, A., Wright, D., & Blake, J. (2014). Staff training using positive behavioural support: The effects of a one-day training on the attributions and attitudes of care staff who work with people with an intellectual disability and challenging behaviour. *International Journal of Developmental Disabilities, 60*(1), 35–42. https://doi.org/10.1179/2047387713Y.0000000020

Singh, N. N., Lancioni, G. E., Karazsia, B. T., Chan, J., & Winton, A. S. W. (2016). Effectiveness of caregiver training in mindfulness-based positive behavior support (MBPBS) vs. training-as-usual (TAU): A randomized controlled trial. *Frontiers in Psychology, 7*, 1549. https://doi.org/10.3389/fpsyg.2016.01549

Singh, N. N., Lancioni, G. E., Winton, A. S. W., Fisher, B. C., Wahler, R. G., McAleavey, K., … Sabaawi, M. (2006). Mindful parenting decreases aggression, noncompliance, and self-injury in children with autism. *Journal of Emotional and Behavioral Disorders, 14*(3), 169–177. https://doi.org/10.1177/10634266060140030401

Smith, M. J., Bouch, J., Bradstreet, S., Lakey, T., Nightingale, A., & O'Connor, R. C. (2015). Health services, suicide, and self-harm: Patient distress and system anxiety. *The Lancet Psychiatry, 2*(3), 275–280. https://doi.org/10.1016/S2215-0366(15)00051-6

Spain, B., Hart, S. A., & Corbett, J. (1984). The use of appliances in the treatment of severe self-injurious behaviour. In G. Murphy & B. Wilson (Eds.), *Self-injurious behaviour: a collection of published papers on prevalence, causes, and treatment in people who are mentally handicapped or autistic* (pp. 262–271). Kidderminster: British Institute of Mental Handicap.

Sturmey, P. (2009). Restraint, seclusion and PRN medication in English services for people with learning disabilities administered by the National Health Service: An analysis of the 2007 national audit survey. *Journal of Applied Research in Intellectual Disabilities, 22*(2), 140–144. https://doi.org/10.1111/j.1468-3148.2008.00481.x

Sullivan, P. J. (2017). Should healthcare professionals sometimes allow harm? The case of self-injury. *Journal of Medical Ethics, 43*(5), 319–323. https://doi.org/10.1136/medethics-2015-103146

Symons, F. J., & Thompson, T. (1997). Self-injurious behaviour and body site preference. *Journal of Intellectual Disability Research, 41*(6), 456–468. https://doi.org/10.1111/j.1365-2788.1997.tb00737.x

Taylor, L., Oliver, C., & Murphy, G. (2011). The chronicity of self-injurious behaviour: A long-term follow-up of a total population study. *Journal of Applied Research in Intellectual Disabilities, 24*(2), 105–117. https://doi.org/10.1111/j.1468-3148.2010.00579.x

Webber, L. S., McVilly, K. R., & Chan, J. (2011). Restrictive interventions for people with a disability exhibiting challenging behaviours: Analysis of a population database. *Journal of Applied Research in Intellectual Disabilities, 24*(6), 495–507. https://doi.org/10.1111/j.1468-3148.2011.00635.x

Webber, L. S., Richardson, B., White, K. L., Fitzpatrick, P., McVilly, K., & Forster, S. (2019). Factors associated with the use of mechanical restraint in disability services. *Journal of Intellectual and Developmental Disability, 44*(1), 116–120. https://doi.org/10.3109/13668250.2017.1310814

Weiner, B. (1980). A cognitive (attribution)-emotion-action model of motivated behavior: An analysis of judgments of help-giving. *Journal of Personality and Social Psychology, 39*(2), 186–200. https://doi.org/10.1037/0022-3514.39.2.186

Wellesley, H., & Jenkins, I. (2015). Consent in children. *Anaesthesia and Intensive Care Medicine, 16*(12), 632–634. https://doi.org/10.1016/j.mpaic.2015.09.007

Wilkins, D. (2012). Ethical dilemmas in social work practice with disabled people: The use of physical restraint. *Journal of Intellectual Disabilities, 16*(2), 127–133. https://doi.org/10.1177/1744629512444986

Williams, D. E. (2010). Reducing and eliminating restraint of people with developmental disabilities and severe behavior disorders: An overview of recent research. *Research in Developmental Disabilities, 31*(6), 1142–1148. https://doi.org/10.1016/j.ridd.2010.07.014

Williams, D. E., & Grossett, D. L. (2011). Reduction of restraint of people with intellectual disabilities: An organizational behavior management (OBM) approach. *Research in Developmental Disabilities, 32(6)*, 2336–2339. https://doi.org/10.1016/j.ridd.2011.07.032

Williams, S., Dagnan, D., Rodgers, J., & McDowell, K. (2012). Changes in attributions as a consequence of training for challenging and complex behaviour for carers of people with learning disabilities: A systematic review. *Journal of Applied Research in Intellectual Disabilities, 25*(3), 203–216. https://doi.org/10.1111/j.1468-3148.2011.00654.x

Wilson, D. M., Iwata, B. A., & Bloom, S. E. (2012). Computer-assisted measurement of wound size associated with self-injurious behavior. *Journal of Applied Behavior Analysis, 45*(4), 797–808. https://doi.org/10.1901/jaba.2012.45-797

Wolf, M. M. (1978). Social validity: the case for subjective measurement or how applied behavior analysis is finding its heart. *Journal of Applied Behavior Analysis, 11*(2), 203–214. https://doi.org/10.1901/jaba.1978.11-203

Chapter 5
Assessment of Self-Injurious Behavior

5.1 Overview of the Assessment Process

Figure 5.1 provides an overview of the assessment process which we will outline in this chapter. The goals of assessment are twofold: first, to define the characteristics of the self-injurious behavior (SIB) engaged in by the individual client and to identify which of the stages (or "subtypes") of SIB outlined in Chap. 3 the client's SIB most closely resembles in terms of its patterning and dynamics and second, to undertake specific further assessment relevant to each stage/subtype of SIB. Before describing this process in detail, we must enter several caveats. Firstly, the "subtypes" of SIB which we described in Chap. 3 are of course the various possible stages in, or endpoints of, the evolutionary process described in that chapter, which is itself, at the moment, hypothetical. We believe however that the evidence reviewed in Chap. 3 provides reasonable grounds to believe that the processes described there provide at least a partial description of the processes involved in the development of SIB. Secondly, the model presented in Chap. 3 posits that these "subtypes" are not distinct categories nor even distinct branches from a common stem, but rather different stages in one continuous process. As such, it will be expected that each person with a history of SIB will be at some stage in this process, including the possibility of being in transition with regard to the predominant causal process. Further, we assume that the evolutionary process is one in which differing causal factors become more or less predominant, but with all prior factors remaining involved to some degree at later stages. Thus, we assume that Pavlovian conditioning of new conditional stimuli which may then elicit SIB continues to occur even after SIB acquires goal-directed (operant) functions, and we assume that operant processes continue to have some influence on SIB even after S-R processes have become predominant in its control.

We also stress that Fig. 5.1 is not proposed as a "pathway" for the assessment process, but rather is intended to outline a series of issues to be addressed and

F. Furniss, A. B. Biswas, *Self-Injurious Behavior in Individuals with Neurodevelopmental Conditions*, Autism and Child Psychopathology Series,
https://doi.org/10.1007/978-3-030-36016-0_5

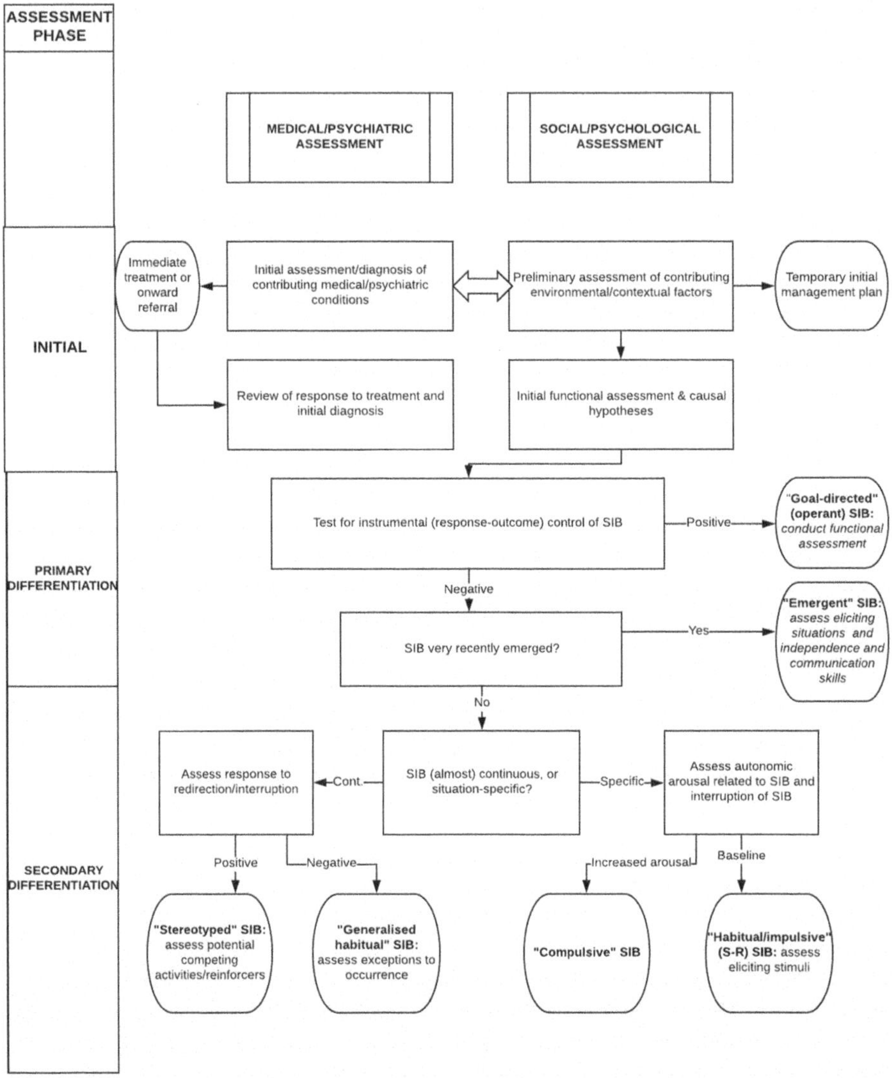

Fig. 5.1 Assessment process for self-injurious behavior

questions to be asked which may prove to be of heuristic value in interpreting the information gathered in the course of assessment. The remainder of this chapter will however be structured around the three main phases which we propose for the assessment process, namely, an initial phase followed by phases of primary and secondary differentiation. Following pre-assessment preparation (see Sect. 5.2 below), the initial phase of assessment will require both medical/psychiatric and social/psychological input and is focused on defining the behaviors of concern and assessing physical and social/environmental factors which may be contributing to the causation of SIB. The aim is to provide a foundation not only for further assessment but also for relevant medical treatment and (if relevant) development of an initial, temporary, behavior management plan to stabilize the situation and prevent or limit serious harm. The second phase of assessment (primary differentiation) is focused on detailed functional assessment of the antecedents and possible maintaining factors influencing the person's SIB, followed by a test of whether the behavior is primarily controlled by instrumental/operant (response-reinforcer) processes or is impulsive/habitual in nature (controlled primarily by S-R processes). If the behavior appears to be under operant control, additional functional assessment/analysis may then be undertaken. The third phase of assessment (secondary differentiation) is applicable only if the SIB appears to be primarily under S-R control and involves further assessment aimed at differentiating habitual/impulsive, stereotyped, and compulsive forms of SIB.

5.2 Pre-assessment

Whether the client is an infant who has only recently started to engage in SIB, a child whose SIB has recently increased in frequency and/or severity, or an adult who has engaged in SIB for many years, several issues must be addressed even before assessment commences. Firstly, either informed consent to the assessment process or an appropriate decision that assessment is in the person's best interests must be in place. As noted in Chap. 4, the clinician must therefore have shared information regarding the purposes, methods, and possible risks of the assessment process (and, in broad terms, the range of interventions which might be identified as relevant) with the client and/or the people with legal authority to give consent for the process. In doing so, she/he must have taken into account the values and interests of the persons concerned as well as the general body of professional and scientific knowledge regarding the methods to be used. Although it might seem premature to be raising these issues at the very beginning of the assessment process, the client and her/his significant others will very probably and very reasonably wish to know what benefit is likely to arise from the assessment process and whether it will be of significant value in identifying opportunities for effective intervention. It will also be useful for the clinician to have some understanding of the values and priorities of the person concerned from the outset of the process. If, for example, the client and/or people able to give consent to treatment on her/his behalf are in principle opposed to the use of pharmacological treatments, it will be of use to the clinician to be aware of this from the outset of the process. Ball, Bush, and Emerson (2004), Cooper, Heron, and Heward (2007), and Goldiamond (1974) suggest a number of issues which may usefully be raised during discussions on this and similar issues. Firstly, what benefits (other than the immediate reduction in physical harm) do the client and her/his significant others expect would result from a reduction in the client's SIB? Do they anticipate that this behavior change will increase the client's access to environments and social opportunities which will enhance her/his quality of life and support her/his development? What degree of risk do they consider the behavior poses? On the assumption that the SIB has some function for the person, what alternative behavior do she/he and significant others think could achieve the same outcomes for the person? Are necessary resources in place to complete the assessment and to sustain likely possible interventions? Finally, what is the history of previous change attempts? Although the clinician will probably wish to return to this issue later in the process of assessment and intervention, some level of awareness of previous assessments and interventions which have been undertaken, and the client's perspective on their outcomes, is extremely helpful in considering the plan for the assessment process. If it is proposed to repeat assessments which have previously been undertaken, careful discussion with the client and those who support her/him of the purpose and anticipated value of such repetition is both fundamental to gaining informed consent and vital to supporting the client's commitment to the assessment process. Thorough initial discussion on these issues, together with an open invitation to the client and relevant others to return to these throughout the course of assessment and intervention, will both provide valuable information and establish a context of collaborative working and respect for the views of the client and her/his significant others from the outset of the process.

5.3 Initial Assessment

5.3.1 Defining the Behavior(s) of Concern

A critical first step in assessment is to reach a common understanding, together with everyone involved in the assessment process, as to what behavior or behaviors are to be assessed. Although this may seem to be a straightforward problem, in practice defining what is meant by SIB for an individual person can be as difficult as defining the term in general (Rojahn, Schroeder, & Hoch, 2008). Definitions of a behavior may be based on function or topography (Cooper, Heron, & Heward, 2007). Function-based definitions identify the target behavior as any behavior which produces a specific effect on the environment (including the person's own body). Taylor, Oliver, and Murphy (2011), for example, defined SIB as "repeated, self-inflicted, nonaccidental injury producing bruising, bleeding, or other temporary or permanent tissue damage, and repetitive behaviours that had the potential to do so if preventative measures (e.g. protective devices, restraints) were not taken" (Taylor et al., 2011, pp. 106–107). Topographically based definitions identify the target behavior by describing its form or (often) by providing a general description of a class of behaviors (e.g., "hand-to-head hitting") together with specific descriptions of behaviors which are to be recorded as members of the class. It may be useful or necessary to define SIB in terms of both topography and function, e.g., it may be necessary to define self-injury as any contact between the person's hand and face which results in reddening of the skin. However the SIB is defined, if it is to be accurately recorded, its definition must be phrased in terms of observable aspects of the behavior and its consequences, so that different observers can agree as to whether a particular behavioral episode does or does not constitute an example of the SIB.

From the behavior analytic perspective, an operant is a class of responses which have a common relationship with a reinforcing consequence, and meaningful relationships between a person's behavior and environmental events will become clear only if the behavior is defined in terms of operant classes. A person's hand-to-head hitting may be one member of an operant class which also includes hitting others; on the other hand, different self-injurious behaviors may be members of different operant classes. In principle, assessment (and especially functional assessment) of individual topographically defined behaviors prior to deriving hypotheses about operant class membership from the results of these assessments is to be preferred (Rojahn et al., 2008). This process can however be laborious, both for the clinician and for the client and people supporting the client, who may be asked the same questions repeatedly for each topographically defined behavior. Alternatively, a hypothesis may be formed early in assessment as to which topographically dissimilar behaviors may be members of a single operant class, with investigation of factors influencing SIB undertaken for the hypothesized operant class rather than for each individual topographically defined behavior. Frequent co-occurrence of target behaviors and consistent occurrence in a particular sequence are indicators of possible common functional class membership. Such co-occurrence is however only a limited indicator of functional identity, and the clinician taking this path needs to remain alert to the possibility that relationships between SIB and environmental events and other influencing factors may be obscured by the fact that specific topographies have different relationships with the factors being considered.

5.3.2 Clinical History

Assessment of SIB should begin with the clinician obtaining a full clinical history, by reference to previous clinical notes and discussion with the client and/or the people supporting her/him. In many cases it will be difficult to obtain a clear account of the development of SIB. The behavior concerned will often have emerged at a relatively young age and may not have been regarded as particularly problematic until it started to result in tissue damage. Particularly if the client has limited language skills, it will often be the case that family members, for example, will only have limited information regarding relevant events which may have occurred during school years, since much of their knowledge of such events will have been gained from discussions with educational staff some time after the relevant events occurred. The client may have interacted throughout her/his life with multiple health and social care agencies and sometimes with separate divisions within such agencies, and some relevant information may be difficult or impossible to obtain.

In addition to developmental and medical history, the clinician should enquire regarding possibly relevant life events, including those with traumatic potential. Although research is limited, traumas such as abuse and bereavement, and overall extent of potentially stressful life experiences, are known to be associated with increased levels of a range of behavioral and affective difficulties in people with intellectual disabilities (IDs) (Bond et al., 2019; Byrne, 2018; Hulbert-Williams et al., 2014; Hulbert-Williams & Hastings, 2008; O'Dwyer et al., 2018; Vervoort-Schel et al., 2018). Studies of groups of adults with IDs who have experienced sexual abuse or bereavement have shown that by comparison with control groups matched for gender, age, and ability, those with histories of sexual abuse experience elevated levels of behavioral disturbance, sexualized behavior, mental health problems, and symptoms of post-traumatic stress disorder (PTSD), while those who have been parent-bereaved experience increased levels of behavioral disturbance, "caseness" for depression and anxiety, and higher rates of additional life events such as moves of home (Hollins & Esterhuyzen, 1997; Sequeira, Howlin, & Hollins, 2003).

With regard to a broader range of life events, Hatton and Emerson (2004) reported that children with IDs who had experienced two or more potentially stressful life events were more likely to experience emotional and conduct disorders and also that children with IDs were more likely than those without IDs to experience a range of adverse life events. In a series of population-based studies of adults with IDs, Cooper, Smiley, and their colleagues have demonstrated that the number of life experiences during the previous 12 months is associated with mental ill-health (including behavior problems). They also found that experience of abuse, neglect, or exploitation during adult life predicted incidence of mental ill-health (excluding challenging behaviors and dementia and delirium) at 2-year follow-up and that parental divorce in childhood and a higher number of life events in the preceding 12 months predicted incident episodes of challenging behavior at 2-year follow-up. Finally, for participants with profound intellectual disabilities, the number of life events also predicted the incidence of mental health problems (including behavior problems) over a 2-year period (Cooper et al., 2007; Cooper, Smiley, Morrison, Williamson, & Allan, 2007; Smiley et al., 2007).

It should not be assumed that engaging in SIB (or experiencing any other kind of emotional or behavioral disturbance) is necessarily an indicator that a person has experienced abuse or other trauma (Rojahn et al., 2008). Owen et al. (2004) found that the number of life events experienced in the previous 12 months by people living in institutional settings (as reported by carers) correlated significantly with frequency of aggressive/destructive behaviors, but not stereotyped behavior or SIB. Nevertheless, consideration of the possibility of a history of serious trauma, or of a series of lesser traumas, will alert the clinician to the possibility of other emotional and behavioral difficulties possibly relevant to the person's SIB and also may assist with understanding of unexpectedly severe reactions to apparently innocuous stimuli or settings.

5.3.3 *Assessment of Current Physical Health and Psychiatric Status*

A wide variety of physical health problems may contribute to SIB (Petty, Bacarese-Hamilton, Davies, & Oliver, 2014), and initial assessment should include enquiries about pain in any part of the body, headache, migraine, and menstrual pain and about other sources of discomfort such as hay fever, coughs and colds, and constipation and other gastrointestinal problems. Medical and dental examination needs to include the ear, nose, throat, and eye, together with consideration of any dental issues which need to be appropriately treated. History taking for gluten sensitivity, lactose intolerance, or other allergic conditions is important, as symptoms and discomfort arising from these may also contribute to SIB. The possibility of iatrogenic factors including side effects from existing medications should be explored, including those arising from excipients in addition to those arising from active ingredients. Tablets may, for example, contain lactose as an excipient, which may cause problems for people with lactose intolerance.

Psychiatric examination will obviously include assessment of ID and ASC and consideration of the possibility of genetic syndromes associated with SIB including Cornelia de Lange syndrome, fragile X syndrome, Lesch-Nyhan syndrome, Prader-Willi syndrome, Rett syndrome, Smith-Magenis syndrome, and tuberous sclerosis. Assessment should also consider the possible presence of other potentially treatable psychiatric disorders which may contribute to causation and/or persistence of SIB, including anxiety disorders, mood disorders, post-traumatic stress disorder, and psychotic disorders.

Allowing sufficient time to take a detailed history and awareness of probable difficulties in obtaining a complete and accurate history are crucial, as is consideration of the person's developmental level and how this may affect their presentation; for adults with IDs, use of adapted criteria for diagnosis of psychiatric disorders which take account of these issues may be helpful (Cooper & Simpson, 2006; Simpson, Mizen, & Cooper, 2016).

5.3.4 *Assessment of Relevant Comorbid Conditions*

5.3.4.1 Sleep Difficulties

As noted in Chap. 2, several studies have found associations between SIB and disturbed or variable (nighttime) sleep in children and adults with IDs and/or autism spectrum conditions (ASCs). Sleep difficulties are common in children and adults with ASCs and/or IDs, and a variety of behavioral and other interventions have been reported to be helpful in improving the extent and/or quality of sleep (Cuomo et al., 2017; Delemere & Dounavi, 2018; Kirkpatrick, Louw, & Leader, 2019; Sanberg, Kuhn, & Kennedy, 2018; Shanahan, Palod, Smith, Fife-Schaw, & Mirza, 2019; Van de Wouw, Evenhuis, & Echteld, 2012). Although improvement in sleep duration or quality will not necessarily reduce SIB, pharmacological interventions to improve sleep have been reported to be associated with reductions in SIB in several studies (Rojahn et al., 2008), and case studies of behavioral interventions to improve sleep (or to address consequent fatigue) have been reported to improve behavioral difficulties including SIB in several cases (DeLeon, Fisher, & Marhefka, 2004; Horner, Day, & Day, 1997; O'Reilly, 1995; Smith, Carr, & Moskowitz, 2016). Initial assessment of SIB should therefore include enquiries regarding sleep difficulties, which if treated might result in a reduction in the extent and/or severity of SIB.

5.3.4.2 Pain

Although findings regarding the association between chronic pain and SIB at a group level have been variable (see Chap. 2), there is little doubt that pain or significant discomfort may contribute to SIB in individual cases. Otitis media (Luiselli, Cochran, & Huber, 2005; O'Reilly, 1997), constipation (Christensen et al., 2009), and elevated intracranial pressure (Hartman, Gilles, McComas, Danov, & Symons, 2008) have all been demonstrated to exacerbate SIB in individual cases, and Pary and Khan (2002) suggested that migraines or cluster headaches might be another factor to do so.

Identification of possibly relevant medical conditions will most often best be achieved by taking a careful history, sometimes including a family history, by careful attention to signs and symptoms observed by the clinician or reported by the client or people close to them, and by referral to appropriate specialists as necessary. Many children and adults with neurodevelopmental conditions (NDCs) will be able to accurately self-report pain they are experiencing. Others may be able to use some of the methods which have been developed to assist typically developing children to report pain (Manworren & Stinson, 2016).

For people with some NDCs, such as Rett syndrome, pain appears to be a common experience (Barney, Feyma, Beisang, & Symons, 2015; Symons, Byiers, Tervo, & Beisang, 2013), and there may be suspicion that a person with limited communication skills is experiencing pain from an unknown cause. In such cases the use of pain rating scales may be helpful. Four examples are briefly described in Box 5.1. Others are described in reviews by Cascella, Bimonte, Saettini, and Muzio (2019) and Doody and Bailey (2017), while De Knegt et al. (2013) review broader research into behavioral indicators of pain in people with IDs. Although the developers of some assessment tools report suggested "cutoff" scores for identification of pain, it should be remembered that ratings of behavioral indicators of pain are not equivalents of subjective self-report of pain experienced and use of these scales should form only one part of a comprehensive clinical assessment (Herr, Coyne, McCaffery, Manworren, & Merkel, 2011).

Box 5.1 Assessment Toolkit: Assessment of Pain in People with Limited Communication

The **Paediatric Pain Profile** (PPP) (Hunt et al., 2004, 2007) is a 20-item behavior rating scale designed to assess pain in children with severe neurological disability. The rater, after observing the child for a defined period of time, rates each item on a four-point scale (observed "not at all," "a little," "quite a lot," or "a great deal"). The internal consistency of the scales is good (Cronbach's $\alpha = 0.75$ for the child "at her/his best" and 0.82 when she/he is experiencing the most significant pain), interrater reliability is acceptable, and the PPP total score correlates significantly with other ratings of pain and is sensitive to the effects of analgesia. Engaging in SIB is one of the items rated.

The **Revised Face Legs Activity Cry and Consolability** (r-FLACC) pain assessment tool (Malviya, Voepel-Lewis, Burke, Merkel, & Tait, 2006) was developed for use with children with cognitive impairments (CI) and assesses pain by observational ratings of facial expression, leg position and activity, overall activity, crying, and response to caregiver attempts to comfort the young person. Each is rated on a 3-point scale, with 0 indicating no signs of pain and 2 maximum distress. The scale can be partly individualized by adding behaviors reported by caregivers to be indicators of pain to the standard indicators used on the r-FLACC. Malviya et al. reported that the r-FLACC showed high interrater reliability (intraclass correlation coefficient = 0.9 for total score), that r-FLACC scores showed moderate to high correlations with parental ratings of children's pain (and ratings by the children themselves where they could give them), and that r-FLACC scores reduced significantly following administration of analgesia. Kochman et al. (2017) have replicated findings of high interrater reliability and sensitivity for the tool.

The **Non-communicating Children's Pain Checklist-Revised (NCCPC-R)** (Breau, McGrath, Camfield, & Finley, 2002) was also developed for use with children with CI and has seven subscales (vocal, eating/sleeping, social, facial, activity, body/limb, physiological signs) each comprised of two to six items. The facial subscale, for example, includes the items "A furrowed brow" and "Turning down of mouth, not smiling," while the physiological signs subscale includes the items "Shivering" and "Tears." In the initial evaluation of the NCCPC-R, caregivers were asked for each item to rate how often it was observed during a 2-h period (24-h period for eating/sleeping items). The ratings for each item ("not at all," "just a little," "fairly often," or "very often") are converted to scores from 0 to 3, giving a maximum possible score of 90 for the 30-item scale. The NCCPC-R shows high internal consistency (Cronbach's $\alpha = 0.93$). Total scores correlate significantly (Pearson's $r = 0.46$) with caregiver overall ratings of severity of pain, do not differ significantly for children across episodes of pain, but are significantly higher during episodes of pain than during periods believed by caregivers to be pain-free (Breau et al., 2002).

The **Non-communicating Adults Pain Checklist-Revised (NCAPC)** (Lotan et al., 2009) was developed from the NCCPC-R for use with adults with intellectual and developmental disabilities. It comprises 18 items assessing 6 "sub-dimensions" of pain behaviour: vocal reaction, emotional reaction, facial expression, body language, protective reaction, and physiological reaction. Cronbach's α for the NCAPC is 0.773 (Lotan et al., 2009), and scale scores have been shown to be stable within and across non-pain situations, but are significantly higher during healthcare procedures involving some degree of pain or discomfort (influenza vaccinations and dental hygiene treatment) than during non-pain situations (Lotan et al., 2009; Lotan, Moe-Nilssen, Ljunggren, & Strand, 2010).

5.3.4.3 Overactivity and Impulsivity

Overactivity/impulsivity is an important correlate of SIB, and the model we proposed in Chap. 3 suggests that relative discounting of delayed reinforcement, leading to a general aversion to delay of reinforcement, is likely to contribute to the development of SIB. Since behavioral interventions can increase tolerance of delayed reinforcement (Vessells, Sy, Wilson, & Green, 2018), it may be possible to reduce SIB by such interventions. Although a plethora of assessment instruments are available for the assessment of symptoms of attention deficit hyperactivity disorder (ADHD) (Collett, Ohan, & Myers, 2003), few have been developed to assess such symptoms in people with IDs. The Scale of Attention in Intellectual Disability (Teacher version) (T-SAID; Freeman, Gray, Taffe, & Cornish, 2015) is a 44-item scale intended for use by teachers of children with IDs. It has four subscales: hyperactivity/impulsivity, inattention, verbal communication, and following instructions. Each item is rated as being observed "never/rarely," "sometimes," or "often." The subscales of the T-SAID show high internal consistency and correlate positively with corresponding subscales from other scales for assessing ADHD symptoms. The scale also has good test-retest reliability (Freeman et al., 2015). The Activity Questionnaire (AQ; Burbidge et al., 2010) is a rating scale comprising 18 items, each scored on a 5-point scale ranging from 0 (never/almost never) to 5 (always/almost all of the time). The AQ has three subscales, overactivity, impulsivity, and impulsive speech. The subscales show high internal consistency and strong interrater and test-retest reliability, with interrater reliability coefficients of 0.70 or greater and test-retest reliability coefficients of 0.87 or greater. Although neither of these scales as yet has representative normative data, the T-SAID and AQ may usefully supplement clinical judgment regarding the severity of an individual's difficulties with impulsivity.

Current developments including computerized tests and diagnostic interviews such as the Diagnostic Interview for ADHD in Adults with Intellectual Disability

(DIVA-5-ID) resulting from burgeoning interest in diagnosis of ADHD in adults (Kooij et al., 2019) may also prove helpful in individual cases.

5.3.5 *Preliminary Assessment of Contributing Environmental/Contextual Factors*

The final element in initial assessment is assessment of environmental and contextual factors influencing SIB. This assessment will naturally continue into the initial functional assessment, and the two will normally be undertaken as one process. The natural starting point will be to interview either the client or someone who knows her/him well, regarding the contexts in which SIB is more or less likely to occur, and the effects of the behavior on the client's social environment. A number of semi-structured interview formats, such as the Functional Assessment Interview (FAI; O'Neill, Albin, Storey, Horner, & Sprague, 2015), are available to guide this process. Semi-structured interview schedules provide a format for the clinician to gather a wide range of descriptions of the form, interrelationships, context, consequences, and history relating to a challenging behavior, together with information on the client's communicative abilities and possible socially appropriate behaviors which might be reinforced as functional alternatives to challenging behavior. The FAI includes questions on the topography, frequency, duration, and intensity of the behaviors to be assessed, their co-occurrence (as an indicator of potential operant class co-membership), motivating operations, antecedents, and possible maintaining consequences. The relative efficiency of the challenging behavior (in terms of the effort it involves, the rate at which it results in hypothesized reinforcement, and the immediacy of that reinforcement) is also considered. Although the FAI process commences with a series of questions regarding the characteristics of topographically described behaviors, completion of the rest of the process requires the clinician to decide whether to pursue the interview with reference to a single topography of SIB or with reference to a hypothetical functional class. If the former option is chosen, the interview should focus on the most serious and frequent topography of SIB. The FAI also includes questions on prosocial behaviors hypothesized to be functionally equivalent to the challenging behavior, the client's usual methods of communicating various needs and desires, possible general reinforcers, and the history of attempts to reduce the frequency and/or severity of SIB. The FAI does not provide decision rules for developing hypotheses regarding the functions of target behaviors, leaving the user to interpret the informant's answers and to develop "summary statements" outlining hypotheses regarding functional relationships. Presumably for this reason, there has been little research on the psychometric properties of the FAI. Reese, Richman, Belmont, and Morse (2005) however, using the FAI in a comparison of functions of challenging behavior in children with and without autism, conducted the FAI with the parents of 46 children presenting challenging behaviors. The interviewer then reviewed the parents' recorded answers and categorized the functions of the challenging behaviors into six categories, three "standard" functions (gain attention, escape demand, or gain tangible item) and three hypothesized "autism-specific" functions (e.g., escape sensory stimulation). For 27 cases, a second trained rater independently repeated the categorization on the basis of the recorded interviews. Occurrence reliability was 81% for the "gain attention" function, 84% for "escape demand," and 93% for "gain item." Although these figures are not directly comparable to measures of interrater reliability where two different informants are used, these data do suggest that experienced personnel (raters were psychologists or psychology postdoctoral fellows with experience/training in functional assessment) achieve conventionally acceptable levels of agreement on hypotheses regarding behavioral function given responses from an FAI interview.

5.3.6 Development of a Temporary Management Plan

At the completion of this initial phase of assessment, the medical/psychiatric assessment will have evaluated medical or psychiatric conditions which may be contributing to the client's SIB, and there may be initial evidence from response to medical treatment to suggest the relevance or otherwise of the conditions identified. The social/psychological assessment may have led to the development of hypotheses regarding the function or functions of the client's SIB, but will certainly at least have identified contexts in which the behavior is more or less likely to occur. Depending on the severity of the client's SIB and the risk of harm, it may be appropriate to put in place a temporary management plan based on the results of these assessments. In many cases the most robust approach will be to avoid, so far as is possible, situations which evoke SIB. In some cases this can be done with little or no impact on the client's quality of life. In other cases however (e.g., where SIB is highly likely to occur during transitions from one place or activity to another), such an avoidance strategy may be highly disruptive to the person's education or work and social and recreational activities. In these situations strategies such as providing the person with additional information regarding transitions, or modifying the density of reinforcement provided in situations to which they are moving, may be helpful (Castillo et al., 2018). However successful or otherwise such a temporary management plan may be in terms of reducing the occurrence of SIB, it should not substitute for a comprehensive assessment-based intervention. The same caveat applies in cases where treatment of medical conditions reduces SIB. Although successful medical treatment of painful conditions will significantly reduce SIB in some cases, a person not provided with other supports will be at risk of relapse into SIB if faced with comparable stressors in the future.

5.4 Primary Differentiation: Distinguishing Between Goal-Directed (Operant) and Stimulus-Response Control by Testing for Operant Control of Self-Injurious Behavior

5.4.1 Initial Functional Assessment and Development of Causal Hypotheses

5.4.1.1 Experimental Functional Analysis (EFA)

Completion of the FAI will have provided information needed to formulate hypotheses regarding the function or functions of the client's SIB. Completion of the "summary statements" regarding behavioral function is a helpful exercise in thinking through the range of possible intervention options. These hypotheses however will generally be based on information from one informant, may be based on a hypothesis regarding operant class membership, and at best will be based on careful observation by the informant which necessarily cannot provide information regarding functional causality. It is, for example, almost certain that SIB will evoke a reaction from other people which may appear to be a plausible reinforcer for the behavior, but the mere fact that this reaction consistently follows SIB does not demonstrate that it causes the behavior. For almost the last 40 years, the solutions proposed by applied behavior analysts to address this problem have been developed from the experimental functional analysis (EFA) methodology initially described by Iwata, Dorsey, Slifer, Bauman, and Richman (1982). An EFA briefly exposes the person engaging in SIB to a systematically arranged (analogue) social environment in which certain antecedent conditions are reliably present, and the specified behavior (or class of behaviors) comprising the client's SIB is reliably followed by a specified consequence. The approach assumes that that observation of high levels of SIB in response to a particular contingency during the EFA indicates that similar contingencies maintain SIB in the person's everyday environment. Table 5.1 outlines the four conditions developed by Iwata et al. (1982) to assess the processes maintaining SIB in children with developmental disabilities, with one ("unstructured play") being a control condition and the others ("social disapproval," i.e., contingent attention; "task demand," i.e., contingent escape from task demands; and "alone") being designed to evaluate which of three possible reinforcement processes described by Carr (1977) is primarily responsible for maintaining the person's SIB. In EFAs modelled directly on the example of Iwata et al. (1982), each condition is typically presented for 15 min. The possibility of "carryover" effects (as might arise if a condition in which SIB was reinforced was always immediately followed by one in which SIB was not reinforced, resulting in "extinction bursts" of SIB in the second condition) may be minimized by presenting conditions in varying orders, or by presenting conditions in a fixed specific order designed to minimize such effects, and by including breaks between conditions. Levels of SIB are recorded (as frequency or duration as most appropriate) in each session. In Iwata et al.'s (1982)

Table 5.1 Outline of functional analysis conditions used by Iwata et al. (1982)

Condition label	Hypothesis regarding the function of SIB to be tested	Antecedent condition (motivating operation)	Consequences delivered contingent on SIB
"Social disapproval"	SIB maintained by contingent carer attention	Toys available to the child. Carer present but does not interact with the child, busies him/herself with an activity	Adult verbally expresses concern and/or disapproval of the SIB paired with brief, nonpunitive physical contact (e.g., puts hand on the child's shoulder)
"Academic demand"	SIB maintained by contingent escape from task demands	Adult uses three-step (verbal, modelling, physical guidance) least-to-most prompting to engage the child in challenging educational activities	Adult terminates the current task demand and turns away from the child for 30 s, with additional 30 s suspension of demands for repeated SIB
"Alone"	SIB maintained by automatic reinforcement (e.g., sensory stimulation)	Child is left alone in room with no toys/activities available and observed from outside room	None
"Unstructured play"	Control condition	Variety of toys are available. The adult remains close to the child, does not block/restrict any child behavior, periodically offers toys to child while making no demands, gives social praise and brief physical contact at least once in every 30 s provided the child is not engaged in SIB	None

original paper, sessions were repeated until higher levels of the target behavior were consistently observed in one condition than in the others.

The results of experimental analyses by convention are typically plotted as illustrated, using hypothetical data, in Fig. 5.2. A consistently higher level of SIB in the "social disapproval" (contingent attention) condition is interpreted as supporting a hypothesis that the target behavior is maintained by positive social reinforcement in the person's everyday environment. A consistently higher level of the behavior in the "task demand" (contingent escape from task demand) condition is taken to indicate a corresponding function for the behavior in the natural environment, while a higher level of the behavior in the "alone" condition is generally interpreted as suggesting that the behavior is maintained by automatic reinforcement. An undifferentiated pattern of responding (similar levels of the target behavior in all conditions)

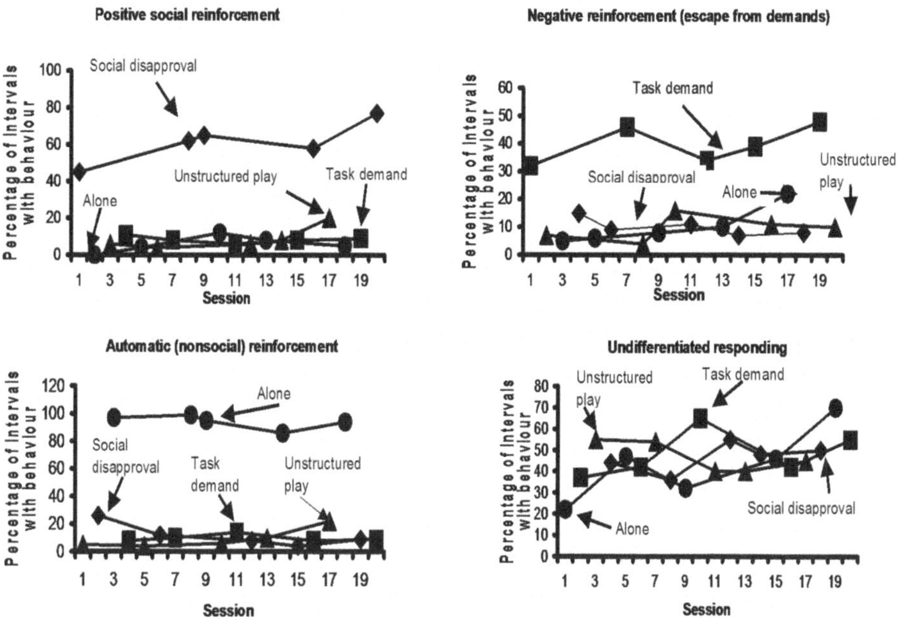

Fig. 5.2 Patterns of responding consistent with alternative functional hypotheses in experimental functional analyses. (Reprinted/adapted by permission from Springer Nature: Springer Science + Business Media LLC, *Applied behavior analysis for children with autism spectrum disorders* by Johnny L. Matson (Editor), © Springer Science + Business Media LLC, 2009)

may indicate that the behavior is genuinely multifunctional, that it is maintained by automatic reinforcement, or that it is maintained by some other process not modelled by the analogue conditions.

In order to specify which conditions should be included in an EFA, the clinician must first of course have developed some hypotheses regarding the function of SIB and may need to design additional conditions to those originally described by Iwata et al. (1982) in order to test those hypotheses. A hypothesis that challenging behavior is reinforced by contingent access to items with which a person engages in repetitive behaviors, for example, may be tested by a condition in which the items are present but the person is given access to them only contingent on occurrence of SIB (Roscoe, Schlichenmeyer, & Dube, 2015). Also, if there is no suggestion from preliminary assessment that the challenging behavior is maintained by a particular reinforcement process (e.g., positive social reinforcement), the corresponding condition ("social disapproval") may be omitted from the experimental analysis. Use of EFAs, particularly for assessment of potentially seriously harmful target behaviors such as SIB, poses a number of technical and ethical challenges. Conducting and interpreting the results of EFAs requires substantial time and skilled and knowledgeable personnel. The assessments must be thoroughly planned, and results subject to careful review, to ensure that artifacts of the assessment process, such as the specific materials used, sequencing of conditions, and variability in motivating operations across sessions, do not confuse the interpretation of data. The most immediate ethical issue is that EFAs intentionally seek to evoke high rates of SIB. In the case of potentially seriously harmful SIB, therefore, either a priori decision rules governing conditions in which a condition will be terminated, or the presence of an independent appropriately qualified judge to call a halt if unacceptable harm is occurring, or both, must be arranged (Iwata et al., 1982). Particularly in the case of extended EFAs, caution must be exercised with regard to the possibility that repeated exposure to systematic reinforcement conditions may further strengthen SIB or even establish a new function for the target behavior not previously learned in the person's natural environment (Neef & Peterson, 2007). In recent years, substantial efforts have been made to revise EFA methodology so as reduce the time required to conduct EFAs (see Box 5.2). Studies have also begun to investigate the degree of risk of negative impact of EFAs on the behaviors under assessment and develop ways to avoid or minimize this risk (see Box 5.3).

Box 5.2 Improving the Efficiency and Validity of EFAs

In recent years applied behavior analysts have devoted substantial attention to adapting EFA methodology to the time and resource constraints typical of clinical settings. The brief EFA method developed by Wacker et al. (1994) typically comprises a single session using methods derived from those of Iwata et al. (1982) followed by a brief evaluation of hypotheses derived from that analysis in a mini-reversal or multielement design. The initial EFA tests individualized hypotheses based partly on rating scales completed by caregivers, i.e., the EFA will generally not include all four of the conditions described by Iwata et al. (1982), and conditions are generally presented for 5–10 min. Derby et al. (1992), reporting a case series of children and adults with IDs assessed using brief EFAs, found that for clients referred for assessment of SIB, the behavior was observed in 70%, and a distinct maintaining condition identified in the initial brief EFA for only 54%, of the people assessed. Muething et al. (2017) asked expert panels to make consensus judgements on the functions of challenging behaviors of 19 children, mostly with ASCs, using data from brief EFAs and data from "standard" EFAs. Agreement on function between the two types of assessment was found for only 26% of cases. Further research is therefore needed to determine whether brief EFAs of this type can be used as an effective substitute for more extended EFAs.

Despite this limitation, methods for conducting brief EFAs continue to be researched. Call, Zangrillo, Delfs, and Findley (2013) compared the functions identified by brief EFAs developed on Derby et al.'s (1992) model with a variation in which only antecedent conditions varied across EFA conditions. No consequences (e.g., attention, brief cessation of task demands) were programmed to follow challenging behavior, although dangerous behavior was prevented with minimal interaction. Functions identified from such A-B brief EFAs generally matched those from A-B-C brief EFAs for five young children.

Badgett and Falcomata (2015) replicated this finding with four children with ASCs, demonstrating also that a further variation of A-B brief EFA methodology, in which latency to the first occurrence of challenging behavior, rather than frequency of the behavior, was measured also generally produced results concordant with those from the other methods. Falcomata, Muething, Roberts, Hamrick, and Shpall (2014) demonstrated that interventions based on functions of challenging behavior identified by such latency-based A-B brief EFAs were effective in reducing these behaviors in young children with ASCs.

Analyses conducted in settings and by people who are not part of the client's normal social environment may fail to identify the function of SIB because specific motivating operations, discriminative stimuli, and reinforcers evoking and maintaining SIB in the natural environment are not replicated in the EFA (see, e.g., Carr, Yarbrough, & Langdon, 1997; Richman & Hagopian, 1999; Ringdahl & Sellers, 2000). Carr et al. (1997) and Vollmer and Smith (1996) suggest using descriptive analyses to identify relevant stimuli for incorporation into experimental analyses.

Hanley, Jin, Vanselow, and Hanratty (2014) used interviews with parents/caregivers to design interview-informed synthesized contingency analyses (IISCAs) in which a single test condition involving evocative contexts, materials, and putative reinforcers individualized for the person concerned is compared with a test condition which is identical except for the reinforcement contingency. Jessel, Ingvarsson, Metras, Kirk, and Whipple (2018) showed that FCT interventions based on IISCAs were highly effective in reducing challenging behaviors (including SIB) in 25 children with ASCs or Tourette syndrome in an extended outpatient service.

Box 5.3 Risks from EFAs and Their Mitigation

Ethical concerns regarding the use of EFAs to assess functions of SIB center on two issues. The first is the possibility of a person causing themselves serious harm during the assessment itself. Iwata (Iwata et al., 1982, 1994) described the use of medical/nursing supervision of assessments, and a priori decision rules governing conditions in which an assessment condition would be terminated, to minimize such risk. With such protections in place, although injuries do occur more frequently (in terms of rate per hour) during EFAs than at other times, the overall rate of injury is low (averaging less than one per 10 h involvement in EFA), and most injuries (over 75%) are minor (Kahng et al., 2015). However, many published reports of EFA use do not mention specific safeguards (although these may have been in place: Weeden, Mahoney, & Poling, 2010).

Brief EFAs, and especially those using latency measures, in which conditions are terminated following the first occurrence of SIB, would obviously be expected to reduce the risk of harm (LaRue et al., 2010). An alternative method of reducing harm is to conduct EFAs with contingencies applied not to SIB, but to behaviors which are reliable precursors of SIB. Fritz, Iwata, Hammond, and Bloom (2013) used observational methods to identify precursors to challenging behavior (including SIB) engaged in by people with IDs. The results of EFAs using precursor behaviors agreed with those using the more serious behaviors of concern in seven out of eight cases, and interventions based on the results of precursor-based EFAs are successful in reducing challenging behaviors (Hoffmann, Sellers, Halversen, & Bloom, 2018).

A second cause for concern when using EFAs is that reinforcing SIB during an EFA may increase SIB in other situations or even (with extended functional analyses) establish a new function for the behavior not previously learned in the person's everyday environment (Neef & Peterson, 2007). It is often argued that there is little risk of such generalization when EFAs are conducted in settings, and by personnel, distinct from those in the person's natural environment. However, the risk would presumably be increased if EFA conditions more closely resemble those the person encounters in everyday life. Empirical evidence on this question is limited, but the few studies which have been conducted suggest that participating in an EFA generally has little or no effect on levels of the behavior assessed subsequently observed in the person's natural environment (Call, Findley, & Reavis, 2012; Davis, Durand, Fuentes, Dacus, & Blenden, 2014; Shabani et al., 2013), but that some individuals do engage in challenging behaviors with increased or decreased frequency after the behavior has been assessed using EFA (Call et al., 2017). The conditions under which such effects are seen, and causal mechanisms, remain unclear.

However, in view of the technical and ethical issues involved in conducting EFAs with individuals engaging in serious SIB, such assessments should only be conducted by the rapidly growing number of clinicians with appropriate professional qualifications in applied behavior analysis (Greer & Kodak, 2018).

5.4.1.2 Indirect and Observational Methods for Functional Assessment

For the clinician who is not a board-certified behavior analyst, other assessment tools are available to progress functional assessment of SIB from the basis provided by the FAI. These include rating scales to be completed by (or using interview information from) the client and/or others who know them well and direct observational methods. For the clinician working in an outpatient clinic, completion of a rating scale is the logical next step to support or disconfirm the hypotheses regarding the function of SIB derived from completion of the FAI.

5.4.1.3 Rating Scales for Functional Assessment

The Motivation Assessment Scale (MAS) developed by Durand and Crimmins (1988) is a 16-item questionnaire with the likelihood of challenging behavior occurring in various situations rated on a 7-point Likert-type scale. Originally designed to assess the influence of social attention, tangible, escape, and sensory consequences on self-injury, the questionnaire has since been used with other topographies of challenging behavior (Duker & Sigafoos, 1998). Early evaluations of the psychometric properties of the scale suggested that the MAS had acceptable internal consistency, construct validity, test-retest and interrater reliability, and predictive validity (Bihm, Kienlen, Ness, & Poindexter, 1991; Durand & Crimmins, 1988). However, subsequent studies on the MAS, with one exception (Koritsas & Iacono, 2013), have found indices of interrater reliability substantially lower than those reported by Durand and Crimmins in 1988 (Duker & Sigafoos, 1998; Newton & Sturmey, 1991; Shogren & Rojahn, 2003; Sigafoos, Kerr, & Roberts, 1994; Spreat & Connelly, 1996; Virues-Ortega, Segui-Duran, Descalzo-Quero, Carnerero, & Martin, 2011; Zarcone, Rodgers, Iwata, Rourke, & Dorsey, 1991). It may be argued that correlations between subscale scores are less important than agreement as to which subscale receives the highest score, suggesting the primary function of the behavior. Here the reported performance of the MAS varies widely between studies, with the percentage of pairs of raters who agree ranging from 29.1% (Zarcone et al., 1991) to 73.9% (Virues-Ortega et al., 2011). Findings on test-retest reliability however suggest that this is acceptable, with Shogren and Rojahn (2003) reporting intraclass correlation coefficients (ICCs) between subscale scores ranging from 0.71 to 0.88 when the MAS was completed on the behavior of 20 adults with IDs by 31 respondents at an interval of 2 weeks, and Barton-Arwood, Wehby, Gunter, and Lane (2003) reporting agreement on primary function in 70% of cases when the MAS was completed with information from teachers of 30 children with emotional or behavioral disorders at an interval of 1 week. With regard to internal consistency, Duker and Sigafoos (1998) reported values of Cronbach's alpha ranging from 0.68 to 0.87; Shogren and Rojahn (2003) values between 0.8 and 0.96; Freeman, Walker, and Kaufman (2007) values between 0.6 and 0.87; Koritsas and Iacono (2013) values from 0.73 to 0.87; and Virues-Ortega et al. (2011) values between 0.65 and 0.82, for the four subscales of the MAS. Newton and Sturmey (1991) and Virues-Ortega et al. (2011) however found levels of internal consistency for the entire MAS comparable to those of the subscales, raising the possibility that the high levels of consistency for the subscales may be an artifact resulting from a factor such as perceived problem severity affecting ratings given for items throughout the scale. With regard to construct validity, findings have been mixed. Duker and Sigafoos (1998) performed principal component analyses separately on maladaptive (e.g., stereotypic and self-injurious), disruptive (e.g., screaming), and destructive (e.g., aggressive) behaviors, finding the greatest correspondence between emergent factors and the subscale structure of the MAS for destructive behaviors, with two factors showing high loadings for items from the escape and tangible subscales, respectively. Kearney, Cook, Chapman, and Bensaheb (2006) performed a confirmatory factor analysis on data from 335 completions of the MAS. Acceptable fit with the a priori subscale structure was achieved only in a second analysis excluding all items from the sensory subscale together with three items from other subscales, suggesting particular difficulties with the items intended to evaluate potential automatic reinforcement. Virues-Ortega et al. (2011) identified three factors corresponding to the attention, tangible, and sensory subscales of the MAS but found that items from the escape subscale tended to load on to the factor identified with the tangible subscale. Koritsas and Iacono (2013) identified four factors, but of these only one (corresponding to the attention subscale) was well-determined. Overall therefore no consistent factor structure has emerged from these studies.

The Questions About Behavioral Function (QABF) scale (Vollmer & Matson, 1995) is a 25-item questionnaire designed to identify the function of any challenging behavior in people with IDs. The five subscales of the assessment relate to five possible functions: reinforcement by attention, reinforcement by escape from situations or task demands, non-social reinforcement, tangible reinforcement, and physical (i.e., behavior associated with pain or physical discomfort). Each function has five corresponding items on the scale, which informants rate on a Likert-type scale from 0 (never) to 3 (often), with respect to how often the behavior occurs in particular contexts. Two summary scores are obtained for each subscale. The item endorsement score is the number of items in that subscale endorsed (i.e., with a score greater than 0). The severity score is obtained by summing the ratings given for the five items for the subscale (maximum score 15).

Paclawskyj, Matson, Rush, Smalls, and Vollmer (2000) examined the test-retest reliability of the QABF in a sample of 34 people with profound or severe intellectual disabilities presenting a variety of challenging behaviors. Pearson correlation coefficients for the five QABF subscales with assessments repeated with the same informant over intervals from 1 to 3 weeks ranged from 0.795 upward, and conventionally acceptable levels of reliability using a number of indices (Spearman correlations, percent agreement, and kappa) were also found for individual scale items. The interrater reliability of the QABF was examined for a total sample of 57 participants, again with diverse challenging behaviors. Pearson correlation coefficients for subscale scores were from 0.79 upward, with measures of individual item interrater reliability lower than for test-retest reliability, but still generally adequate. To assess the internal reliability and construct validity of the scale, Paclawskyj et al. (2000) collected QABF data on challenging behaviors of 243 residents of a state institution with predominantly profound IDs and behaviors including SIB, aggression, and property destruction. Cronbach's alpha for the subscales ranged from 0.9 to 0.928, and an exploratory factor analysis produced a solution with five factors corresponding to the five QABF subscales and accounting for over 76% of the variance shared by test items. Furthermore, alpha for the total QABF scale (0.6) was substantially lower than for the subscales, suggesting that the internal reliabilities of the subscales were not simply an artifact of generalized response tendencies affecting the whole scale. Shogren and Rojahn (2003) however examined the psychometric properties of the QABF in assessing functions of challenging behaviors of 20 individuals with IDs and found that while Pearson correlations for subscale score test-retest reliability for the QABF ranged from 0.62 to 0.93, and subscale Cronbach's alpha values for the attention, escape, non-social, and tangible subscales all exceeded 0.8, alpha for the physical subscale was only 0.24 and Pearson correlations for subscale interrater reliability ranged from 0.46 to 0.60. Thus, not only did Shogren and Rojahn (2003) find lower levels of test-retest and interrater reliability and internal consistency for the QABF than those reported by the scale's developers, but the levels of interrater reliability in particular were only modest. Nicholson, Konstantinidi, and Furniss (2006) examined QABFs completed by pairs of raters evaluating 118 challenging behaviors presented by 40 children and young adults with severe IDs. Pearson correlations assessing interrater reliability for subscale severity scores were 0.54 for attention, 0.57 for escape, 0.62 for non-social, 0.52 for physical, and 0.42 for tangible. The values of Cronbach's alpha were 0.85 for the attention subscale, 0.88 for the escape subscale, 0.79 for the non-social subscale, 0.92 for the physical subscale, 0.88 for the tangible subscale, and 0.83 for the total QABF. Principal axis factoring with varimax rotation suggested a 6-factor solution accounting for 73% of the variance in item scores, with 4 factors showing high loadings from items from the QABF subscales physical, attention, tangible, and escape, respectively, a fifth factor showing high loadings from 4 of the 5 items in the QABF non-social subscale, and item 18 from the non-social subscale ("engages in the behavior in a highly repetitive manner, ignoring his/her surroundings") being the single item loading highly on the sixth factor. This study therefore supported earlier research suggesting good construct validity of the QABF, but found lower levels of (particularly) interrater reliability than those reported by the scale's developers, and high levels of internal consistency for the whole scale as well as subscales. Further studies, including some of German and Spanish translations of the QABF, have confirmed that the scale demonstrates a five-factor structure corresponding well with its subscale structure and that the internal consistencies of the subscales are fair to good (Bienstein & Nussbeck, 2009; Freeman et al., 2007; Koritsas & Iacono, 2013; Simó-Pinatella et al., 2013; Zaja, Moore, Van Ingen, & Rojahn, 2011). Wallace, Vega, and Hernandez (2015) however found poor internal consistency for the non-social subscale, for which unsatisfactory internal consistency was also found in the German version. Simó-Pinatella et al. (2013) also found, consistent with the findings of Paclawskyj et al. (2000), that Cronbach's alpha was higher for the subscales than for the scale as a whole. With regard to interrater reliability of the QABF, further studies have found interrater ICCs from 0.56 to 0.95 for subscales of the QABF, with 14 of 20 ICCs reported exceeding 0.75 (Bienstein & Nussbeck, 2009; Koritsas & Iacono, 2013; Simó-Pinatella et al., 2013; Zaja et al., 2011). The high test-retest reliability of the QABF has also been confirmed, with Spearman correlation coefficients for subscale scores reported to range from 0.649 to 1.0 for assessments conducted at an interval of 7–20 days (Simó-Pinatella et al., 2013) and ICCs to range from 0.76 to 0.87 over a mean interval of 7.8 weeks (Zaja et al., 2011). With regard to the MAS and the QABF, therefore, the research reviewed above strongly suggests that the QABF is substantially the more psychometrically robust of the two options.

As with semi-structured interviews, a number of other functional analysis checklists are available, e.g., the Problem Behavior Questionnaire (Lewis, Scott, & Sugai, 1994) and the Functional Analysis Screening Tool (Iwata, Deleon, & Roscoe, 2013). None to date have demonstrated advantages in terms of reliability or validity by comparison with the MAS and QABF with the possible exception of the Functional Assessment for Multiple Causality (FACT: Matson et al., 2003). This assessment was developed to evaluate the relative importance of different sources of reinforcement when SIB (or other challenging behaviors) have more than one function. Its subscale structure corresponds to that of the QABF, but it has 35 forced-choice items asking respondents which (if either) of two situations is more associated with the behavior being assessed. The limited research to date shows the FACT to have a factor structure corresponding to its subscale structure, high internal consistency for its subscales, and measures of test-retest and interrater reliability generally higher than those for the QABF (Matson et al., 2003; Zaja et al., 2011). A shorter form of the QABF has also been developed (Singh et al., 2009). The Contextual Assessment Inventory (CAI: McAtee, Carr, & Schulte, 2004) takes a broader approach to assessing the extent to which a range of contextual variables may be functionally related to challenging behavior. Initial data presented by the scale's developers suggest however that item-by-item "test-retest" reliability is satisfactory but that interrater reliability is modest. Carr, Ladd, and Schulte (2008) found however that contexts identified by the CAI as being associated with challenging behaviors for 17 people with developmental disabilities were also recorded as such in service records and confirmed as such by direct observation for five of those people. The CAI may therefore be useful in providing a wide-range overview of contexts associated with SIB.

5.4.1.4 Convergent Validity of Rating Scales for Functional Assessment with EFA Outcomes

Since EFA has become regarded as the "gold standard" for identifying the function of operant SIB, it is important to know the proportion of cases in which the function identified by an interview such as the FAI, or by a rating scale such as the QABF, is also that identified by an EFA. Toogood and Timlin (1996) conducted functional assessments/analyses on 121 challenging behaviors presented by 20 adults with severe IDs. For each participant, they completed an informant-based interview and the MAS and carried out four EFA sessions. Structured decision criteria were used in ascribing functions based on interpretation of results from the experimental analyses. The percentage of behaviors for which functional hypotheses could be developed was 74 using interview data, 70 using the MAS, and 41 using EFA data. Considering only those behaviors where both methods in a pair identified a function, the greatest probability of agreement on the primary function of behaviors between methods was 0.55 (MAS with interview). The probability of both indirect methods agreeing with the hypothesis developed from the experimental analysis was 0.41. The proportion of agreements on function irrespective of whether that was the primary function identified was also highest for the MAS with the interview (0.88), while the probability of the indirect methods identifying any function also identified by experimental analysis was 0.76 (interview) and 0.63 (MAS). Cunningham and O'Neill (2000) compared conclusions reached on the basis of administration of the FAI and MAS, and EFAs, regarding functions of challenging behaviors in three young children with autism. For two of the children, all three methods agreed on the primary function of the behavior; for the third, the FAI and experimental analysis identified the same function. Girolami and Scotti (2001) used the same assessment approaches to identify possible functions of mealtime problem behaviors in three children with developmental disabilities. All three methods agreed on primary function for two children, and the MAS agreed with the EFA on primary function for the third child. Alter, Conroy, Mancil, and Haydon (2008) again used the FAI, MAS, and EFAs to assess the functions of challenging behaviors presented by four young boys who were not diagnosed with any NDC. The MAS and EFA agreed on the function of the behavior for two of the boys, whereas functions identified by the FAI and MAS were identical for one boy only, as was also the case for functions identified by the FAI and EFA.

Research has also been conducted on the concurrent validity of the QABF. Paclawskyj, Matson, Rush, Smalls, and Vollmer (2001) evaluated the convergent validity of QABF assessments by comparison with EFAs and the MAS with 13 participants with primarily profound IDs and target behaviors including SIB, aggression, and stereotypy. The QABF identified a total of 16 functions for the challenging behaviors assessed, with the challenging behavior of 3 participants assessed as having 2 major functions. The EFAs identified a total of 13 functions for the behaviors assessed, failing to suggest a function in 3 cases owing to low frequencies of observed behavior and suggesting 2 functions in 3 of the remaining 10 cases. Of the 16 functions identified by the QABF, 9 (56%) were also identified by the experimental analyses (which for one case also identified a second function not identified by the QABF). If the 3 cases for which the experimental analysis failed to identify a function were excluded, the QABF identified 12 functions in the remaining 10 cases, with 9 (75%) of these confirmed by the experimental analyses, which also identified 1 additional function in the case already mentioned. The MAS identified a single function for 12 participants and 2 functions for the remaining participant. Of the 14 functions identified by the MAS, 7 were also identified by the EFAs, which in 2 cases also identified an additional function not indicated by the MAS. Excluding the 3 undifferentiated experimental analyses, in the remaining 10 cases, the MAS identified 11 functions, 7 of which were also identified by the experimental analyses. Spearman rank-order correlations between QABF and MAS subscale scores did not indicate unique relationships between subscales from the two instruments purportedly examining the same function. Scores on the MAS sensory subscale correlated significantly with scores on the QABF non-social and tangible subscales, and scores on the MAS tangible subscale correlated significantly with scores on the QABF non-social, physical, and tangible subscales. Freeman et al. (2007) however found Pearson correlations ranging from 0.66 upward between total scores on corresponding MAS and QABF subscales (attention, escape, MAS sensory/QABF non-social, and tangible). The highest correlations between non-corresponding subscales were 0.58 (MAS escape with QABF tangible) and 0.55 (MAS tangible with QABF escape); however, high correlations had also been found for these subscales within the two rating scales. Hall (2005) used the QABF and experimental analyses to assess functions of challenging behaviors of four adults with severe IDs. The experimental analyses identified one case each in which non-social reinforcement, escape from demands, attention, and access to tangibles maintained challenging behavior. The QABF results concurred with those of the EFA in three cases and identified an escape function in the case where the experimental analysis had suggested attention as the reinforcer. Working with seven children with diagnoses of autism, Tarbox et al. (2009) found that the QABF (completed by interview of caregivers) identified exactly the same function or functions as EFAs for the target behaviors of three of the children. For three of the other four children, the QABF and EFA both identified at least one function in common. Healy, Brett, and Leader (2013) assessed the functions of SIBs, stereotyped behaviors, and aggressive/destructive behaviors engaged in by 32 children and adolescents diagnosed with ASCs, some of whom were also diagnosed with ID, using the QABF and extended or brief EFAs. The QABF and EFA identified exactly the same function or functions for 24 participants, identified at least 1 function in common for 6 others, and failed to agree for 1 (for the remaining participant, the QABF did not identify a function). Wallace et al. (2015) adopted a different approach to assessing the validity of the QABF by creating videos in which pairs of actors role-played interactions in which one engaged in challenging behavior and the second responded in ways which would be expected if the behavior were maintained by positive social reinforcement, tangible reinforcement, escape from task demands, or non-social reinforcement (e.g., in the video depicting positive social reinforcement, the second actor interacted with the first contingent on the first actor engaging in challenging behavior). Wallace et al. (2015) then asked 80 students enrolled in introductory psychology or counselling courses to complete the QABF having the viewed one of the videos. Of the 80 QABFs completed, 66 identified the behavioral function which the video was designed to illustrate.

Smith, Smith, Dracobly, and Pace (2012) used both the MAS and the QABF to assess the functions of 42 challenging behaviors engaged in by 27 adults with (mainly very severe) IDs. The MAS and QABF were completed by graduate and undergraduate students interviewing staff of the residential service in which participants lived. Five (or, in one case, four) different staff members were interviewed regarding each behavior. If the sensory subscale was the highest scoring MAS subscale, and on the QABF either the nonsocial or physical subscale was the highest scoring, this was taken to be an agreement. Considering all the subscales (social attention, tangible, escape, and sensory for the MAS and attention, tangible, escape, non-social, and physical for the QABF), the proportion of behaviors for which assessments completed with at least four of the five respondents were in agreement with respect to the function of the behavior was 57% for the QABF and 52% for the MAS. For seven of the participants for whom there was agreement from least four QABF completions regarding behavioral function (for six of whom there was similar agreement within the MAS results), an EFA was then completed to identify the function of the behavior concerned. The function identified by the QABF was also identified as the maintaining function by the EFA for six of these seven people. In the seventh case, the participant's behavior in different EFA conditions was not sufficiently differentiated to allow a function to be identified. The functions identified by the MAS corresponded with those from the EFA in four cases.

Overall, then, the substantial studies of Smith et al. (2012) and Healy et al. (2013) suggest that the results of a functional assessment using the QABF can be expected to concur with those from an EFA in somewhere between 75% and 86% of cases. The level of agreement between results from the MAS and EFAs appears to be somewhat lower, and this, together with the data on the interrater reliability and internal consistency of the two instruments, reviewed in Sect. 5.4.1.3 above, strongly suggests that the QABF is to be preferred in assessing the functions of challenging behaviors in people with NDCs. Several cautions should however be borne in mind when using the QABF in assessing the functions of SIB. Research into the psychometric properties of the QABF, and into its convergent validity with outcomes from EFAs, has been conducted with groups of participants engaging in challenging behaviors varying widely in both form and severity, and the interrater reliability of the QABF may vary both with type of behavior being assessed and with the frequency with which that behavior occurs (Nicholson et al., 2006). From a clinical perspective, it should also be remembered that the reliability and validity of the scale will probably also depend on the way it is administered. The studies which have reported higher levels of reliability and concurrent validity for the QABF (e.g., Healy et al., 2013; Paclawskyj et al., 2000, 2001; Smith et al., 2012) all used a procedure in which experienced psychologists or behavior analysts (or students working under their supervision) completed the scales by interviewing informants who were familiar with the clients concerned. A study in which school personnel were asked to complete QABFs with minimal supervision (May, Sheng, Chitiyo, Brandt, & Howe, 2014) found low levels of interrater reliability and internal consistency for the scale. It is therefore recommended that the QABF should be completed by the clinician interviewing informants who know the client well rather than by asking the informants to complete the scale independently. Clinical experience is also required in the interpretation of QABF results, since there are no definitive decision rules. Matson, Bamburg, Cherry, and Paclawskyj (1999) identified a function if one subscale had an endorsement score of 4 or greater and no other subscale had an endorsement score of more than 2. Vollmer and Matson (1995) also suggested an endorsement score of 4 or 5 as indicating a clear function, but noted that scores for other subscales should be interpreted in the light of the possibility that the behavior assessed may have several functions. Other researchers (e.g., Smith et al., 2012) have taken the QABF subscale with the highest severity score to indicate primary function. Finally, although Smith et al. (2012) note that there was no specific rationale for choosing five respondents to interview, it will probably be helpful to interview a minimum of two informants independently when using the QABF, selecting informants other than the person interviewed in completing the FAI. Such a procedure gives the clinician information on potential function of the SIB from three informants (e.g., a parent, teacher, and involved therapist), enabling provisional conclusions to be drawn regarding the consistency with which functions are identified using information from different sources.

5.4.1.5 Observational Methods for Functional Assessment

Even in situations where there appears to be a high level of agreement between different sources of indirect assessment regarding the function of SIB, collecting some data by direct observation will often be valuable. The direct observation may be carried out by the clinician, the client, or people who work with or support the client. Although the clinician will already have obtained consent (or come to a "best interests" decision) for the indirect procedures described above, appropriate consent or "best interests" processes need to be considered separately where use of observational methods is being considered. Direct observation is intrusive, and the principles of using the least intrusive method feasible, and carefully balancing the likely value of the information to be gained against the degree of intrusion involved, should be applied. In the context of functional behavioral assessment, it should be remembered that analyses conducted on the basis of observational assessments show relatively low levels of agreement with those using EFAs (Thompson & Iwata, 2007). In fact, levels of agreement on function between methods using direct observation and EFAs have often been found to be substantially lower than those between rating scales and EFAs (e.g., Toogood & Timlin, 1996), even when sophisticated analytic methods have been used in interpreting the observational data (Hall, 2005). A challenging problem for observational methods is that a person engaging in SIB, especially if the SIB is severe, will almost always draw some kind of response from other people present, which may or may not function as a reinforcer for the SIB. The clinician should therefore be conservative in estimating the likely contribution of information to be gained from direct observation to the functional assessment process. There will however be situations where observational methods will be helpful, for example, situations in which the client and/or other people familiar with them find themselves unable to answer assessment questions because they perceive the SIB as occurring continuously or as being apparently unrelated to any environmental events. In such cases the clinician will need to consider whether useful information can be obtained by asking the client or persons supporting them to observe and record their behavior or whether it is necessary for the clinician to observe directly. In the latter case, observation should wherever possible be carried out in situations where it can be done unobtrusively and without unnecessarily drawing the attention of others to the fact that the client is being observed. It will be necessary to plan in advance what limits to the observation will be put in place, for example, the areas into which the observer will not follow the client or circumstances in which the observer will cease observation.

Prior to undertaking direct observation, useful information may be obtained by asking the client or people supporting him/her to complete a scatterplot record (Touchette, MacDonald, & Langer, 1985) for several days. The scatterplot (see

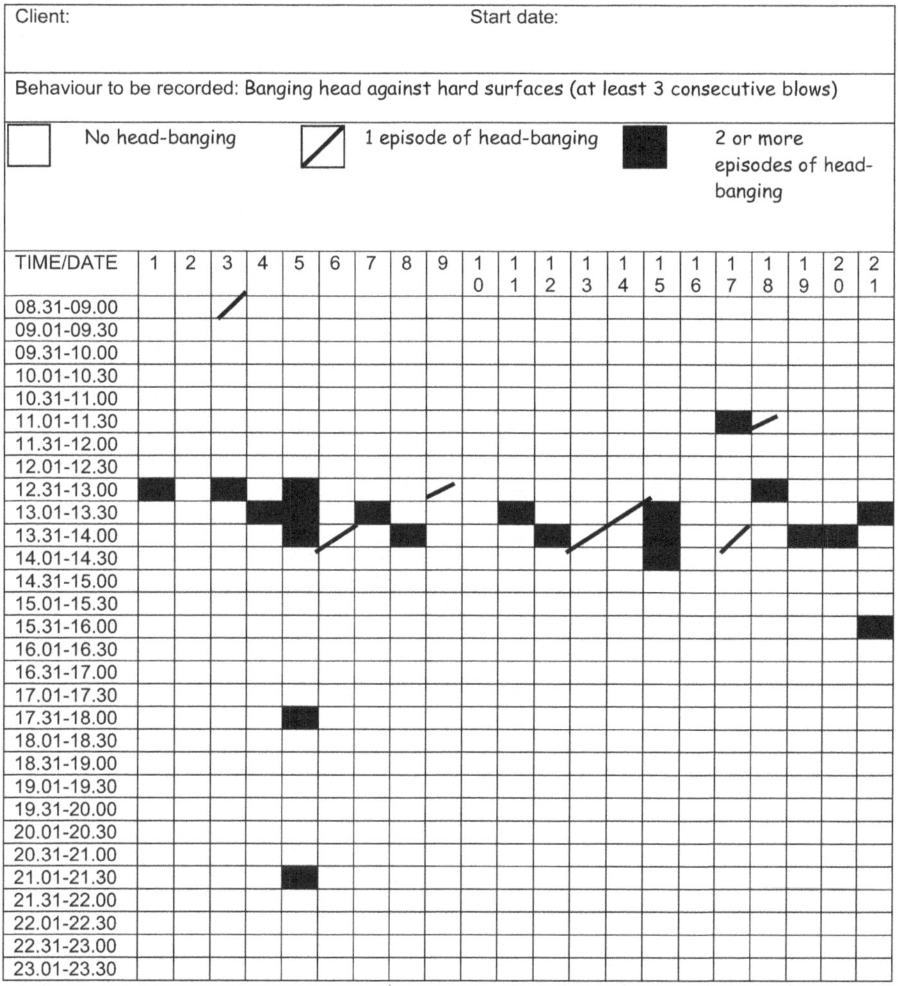

Fig. 5.3 Example of scatter plot record (Touchette et al., 1985). (Reprinted/adapted by permission from Springer Nature: Springer Science + Business Media LLC, *Applied behavior analysis for children with autism spectrum disorders* by Johnny L. Matson (Editor), © Springer Science + Business Media LLC, 2009)

example at Fig. 5.3) is a recording form which divides the person's waking day into a series of intervals, usually of 30 to 60 min, on which the person keeping the record notes either whether or not the SIB occurred during that period or alternatively records whether the SIB occurred extensively, to a limited extent, or not at all. The results of scatterplots may themselves suggest hypotheses regarding functions of SIB. If SIB occurs most frequently during periods when household chores are typically performed, for example, a hypothesis of reinforcement by escape from such chores may be suggested for further evaluation. Where people responding to interviews describe SIB as happening "all the time," scatterplots may identify regular periods in which the person briefly stops self-injuring, possibly suggesting that relevant establishing operations or discriminative stimuli controlling the behavior are absent at these times. Scatterplots can also be practically useful in planning direct observations by indicating times of day at which such observation is most likely to effectively capture occurrences of the target behavior. There is however little evidence regarding the reliability, validity, and utility of scatterplot records. Kahng et al. (1998), collecting scatterplot data on challenging behaviors of 20 children and adults with developmental disabilities living in residential facilities, found poor interobserver reliability in 5 cases and were unable (without statistical analysis) to discern reliable temporal patterns of responding in all the other cases. It might be expected that scatterplot analysis would be most useful where clients participate in tightly timetabled schedules such as may be found in schools, but factors influencing the utility of scatterplots remain to be investigated.

Another alternative to the clinician directly observing the client's behavior is to request the client, or people supporting her/him, to complete antecedent-behavior-consequence (ABC) records of her/his SIB (and possibly other behaviors believed to be possible members of the same operant class). Such records, variously called descriptive (Miltenberger 2001) or narrative (Cooper, Heron, & Heward, 2007) ABC records, involve the observer recording a description (including time of occurrence) of each occurrence of SIB together with events occurring immediately before and after the behavior. A four-column recording sheet such as that shown in Fig. 5.4 is often used. Unless the clinician is in a position to train and support people in

ABC recording sheet Client's name:			
Date and time	**Antecedents.** Describe what happened just *before* the behaviour. What was X doing? Who else was present? What were they doing? What else was happening, etc.?	**Behaviour.** What exactly did X do? Be as specific as possible.	**Consequences.** What happened immediately *following* the behaviour. What did you do? What did X do? What did other people do? What else happened?
01/09/18, 5.34 p.m.	X was sitting at the kitchen table playing a game on his tablet computer. For some reason the game "froze"	X looked at me and then put the tablet down and started to bang his head hard against the table	I told X several times to stop banging his head and I would re-start the game programme. Eventually he stopped and I got the game going again.

Fig. 5.4 Example of a completed narrative ABC recording sheet. (Reprinted/adapted by permission from Springer Nature: Springer Science + Business Media LLC, *Applied behavior analysis for children with autism spectrum disorders* by Johnny L. Matson (Editor), © Springer Science + Business Media LLC, 2009)

completing such records however, observers with limited training in behavioral observation and recording may well record rather vague descriptions of the person's emotional or behavioral state (e.g., "became anxious" or "became upset"), rather than environmental events, as antecedents to the target behavior.

One approach to this problem is to use checklist ABC records (Miltenberger, 2001) in which antecedents, behaviors, and consequences of interest are pre-specified. In such checklist records, each column of the ABC recording sheet has a list of events of possible interest, and the observer marks the columns to specify which behaviors, antecedents, and consequences were observed at each occurrence of the target behavior. Such charts may include a wide range of antecedents, behaviors, and consequences and be used for exploratory data collection and analysis if there is as yet no hypothesis regarding the function of the SIB (see Fig. 5.5 for an example).

Exploratory ABC Chart					
Client's name: X		**Staff initials:**		**Date:**	**Time:**
✓	**What happened just before the behaviour?**	✓	**Behaviour**	✓	**What happened immediately after?**
	X appeared to be in physical discomfort/pain		Hit own head or face with closed fist		Received more social contact/attention
	Environment was noisy		Slapped own head or face with open hand		Received less social contact/attention
	X had no social interaction for over 5 minutes		Banged elbow hard on furniture		Went to quieter and/or less crowded area
	X had nothing to do for over 5 minutes		Banged head against hard surface		Was given something to eat or drink
	X was having to wait to do something		Pushed or hit another person		Was given an activity to do
	A particular individual entered the room		Called/asked for help from staff		Demands or requests were withdrawn/reduced
	X was changing activity or location				Was given more help to complete task/activity
	X had been asked to do something				Was taken out for walk
	X had just begun a task or activity				Was spoken to about behaviour
	X had just finished a task or activity				Sensory input was reduced
	X was asked to stop doing something				Other people were asked to leave the area
	X was unable to obtain a desired item				Was asked to move away from other people within area
	Other (specify):		Other (specify):		Other (specify):

Fig. 5.5 Exploratory checklist ABC recording sheet. (Reprinted/adapted by permission from Springer Nature: Springer Science+Business Media LLC, *Applied behavior analysis for children with autism spectrum disorders* by Johnny L. Matson (Editor), © Springer Science + Business Media LLC, 2009)

Hypothesis-testing ABC chart											
Client's name:											
Please record date, time, your initials, and tick all boxes which apply each time you observe SIB or when X asks for help from support workers											
Date	Time	Initials	ANTECEDENTS			BEHAVIOUR			CONSEQUENCES		
			Transition	Noisy env.	Task demand	Hit head	Slap face	Ask for help	Go for walk	Task ended	Given help

Fig. 5.6 Hypothesis-testing checklist ABC recording sheet. (Reprinted/adapted by permission from Springer Nature: Springer Science+Business Media LLC, *Applied behavior analysis for children with autism spectrum disorders* by Johnny L. Matson (Editor), © Springer Science + Business Media LLC, 2009)

Alternatively, the recording sheet may list only specific antecedents, behaviors, and consequences hypothesized to be of interest as a result of a prior indirect assessment (O'Neill et al., 2015; see Fig. 5.6 for an example).

Use of ABC records can enable the clinician to estimate how frequently topographically distinct target behaviors co-occur, facilitating identification of possible operant classes. The ABC record can also be used to tally the frequency with which particular antecedents and consequences precede and follow SIB. However, the relative frequencies with which individual antecedents and consequences are observed do not necessarily indicate their functional relevance to the person's SIB.

In developing hypotheses regarding behavioral function from ABC records, consideration should be given to the internal coherence of such hypotheses. That is, even if social interaction initiated by other people is a frequent consequence when a person engages in SIB, caution should be exercised in hypothesizing that social reinforcement is maintaining the SIB unless experiencing reduced levels of social interaction, or the cessation of such interaction, is also a common antecedent for SIB. Sometimes however a particular consequence (e.g., termination of requests by other people to participate in self-care routines) necessarily implies the antecedent presence of such requests, and so ABC records may therefore give an impression of a coherent antecedent-SIB-reinforcement sequence in situations where there is no functional relationship between the SIB and the environmental events surrounding it. When ABC records are completed only when SIB has occurred, a further difficulty is that no account is taken of the overall level of occurrence of the relevant antecedents and consequences (Lerman & Iwata, 1993). With this type of recording, task demands are likely, for example, to be recorded as a frequent antecedent to SIB for a child with an ASC participating in an intensive educational program simply because such demands are frequently being placed on the child.

This problem can only be overcome by observing the person's SIB continuously for a period of time. Such observation raises several ethical and practical issues. It is unlikely that the person engaging in SIB, or persons supporting them such as parents, teachers, or support staff, will be able to undertake such observations in the course of their daily activities, and so the clinician is likely to have to undertake the observation personally. As noted earlier, such observation will to a lesser or greater extent be intrusive and possibly disruptive to the person's normal routines. Given that conclusions based on descriptive assessments usually show lower agreement with those from EFAs than those drawn from the QABF, consideration should be given to the likelihood that useful information will be obtained sufficient to warrant the degree of intrusion which will be involved. There will however be situations where continuous direct observation can be helpful, especially where SIB is evoked by establishing operations acting over extended periods of time. Where a person, for example, starts to engage in SIB in response to the absence of social interaction from other people, this relationship may not be apparent to a person who is keeping an ABC record while also busy with other activities.

Direct observation is likely to be time-consuming (Lerman & Iwata, 1993), and prior review of information from previous assessments such as FAIs and scatterplots can help in scheduling observation during situations and times of day in which SIB is likely to be observed. Observations can be recorded using standard four-column ABC charts, or by using a checklist-style recording form, and recording all occurrences of antecedents and consequences of interest irrespective of whether the target behavior has occurred. Such ABC continuous recording (Cooper, Heron, & Heward, 2007) can however be laborious, and if the clinician is interested in specific antecedents and consequences, partial-interval recording may be preferred. In this method the observation period is divided into a series of brief time intervals (typically 5–20s in duration). For each interval, the observer records at the end of the interval whether or not SIB and any environmental events of interest (whether as possible antecedents or consequences) were observed at any time during the interval, i.e., the person is recorded as engaged in SIB during a 10-s interval even if SIB occurred for only 1 s during the interval.

Given such data, the conditional probability of a behavior given the occurrence of an antecedent can be compared with the unconditional (overall) probability of the behavior (see Fig. 5.7 for an example). Similarly, the conditional probability of a consequence following a behavior can be compared with the unconditional probability of the consequence. In the example given, the conditional probability of the person being observed head-hitting increases (over the unconditional probability for the whole period of observation) when she/he is unoccupied and conversely reduces when she/he is occupied. The probability of carer-initiated social interaction however remains the same whether or not the person being observed is head-hitting. Conditional probabilities of one event occurring together with another do not indicate the direction of causality (if any) between the two; their calculation can however suggest specific relationships for further investigation.

Partial-interval behaviour recording sheet					
Interval duration: 10s					
Client's name: X			**Date/time of observation**:		
Behaviours/Events to be Recorded: Behaviour/event A: Hitting head with closed fist Behaviour/event B: Occupied with game or other activity Behaviour/event C: Unoccupied Behaviour/event D: Parent or carer initiated interaction					
Interval Number	**Time Period**	**Behaviour A**	**Behaviour B**	**Behaviour C**	**Behaviour D**
1	0-10s	√	0	√	0
2	11-20s	0	√	0	0
3	21-30s	0	√	0	0
4	31-40s	√	0	√	0
5	41-50s	√	0	√	0
6	51-60s	√	0	√	√
7	61-70s	0	√	0	0
8	71-80s	0	0	√	0
9	81-90s	√	0	√	0
10	91-100s	√	√	0	√
11	101-110s	0	0	√	√
12	111-120s	0	0	√	√
INTERVALS WITH BEHAVIOUR/EVENT RECORDED		6	4	8	4
PERCENTAGE INTERVALS WITH BEHAVIOUR/EVENT RECORDED		6/12x100%= 50%	4/12x100%= 33%	8/12x100%= 67%	4/12x100%= 33%

UP (head-hitting) (6/12 intervals) = 0.5

CP (head-hitting when occupied) (1/4 intervals) = 0.25

CP (head-hitting when unoccupied) (5/8 intervals) = 0.625

UP (parent-initiated interaction) (4/12 intervals) = 0.33

CP (parent-initiated interaction while head-hitting) (2/6 intervals) = 0.33

UP: unconditional probability

CP: conditional probability of behaviour/event X given behaviour/event Y

Fig. 5.7 Partial-interval recording behavior observation sheet with conditional probability calculations. (Reprinted/adapted by permission from Springer Nature: Springer Science + Business Media LLC, *Applied behavior analysis for children with autism spectrum disorders* by Johnny L. Matson (Editor), © Springer Science + Business Media LLC, 2009)

5.4.1.6 Functional Assessment: From Causal Hypotheses to Possible Interventions

Having completed an FAI with a primary informant, completed QABFs by interviewing other people who know the client well, possibly asked the client or other people to complete scatterplot or ABC records, and if necessary completed direct observations, the final step in an initial functional assessment of SIB is to review the information gathered and develop a hypothesis of the processes involved in maintaining the client's SIB. Throughout the process it should be borne in mind that the quality and utility of the functional assessment process will depend not only on the assessment instruments chosen but also on the expertise and experience of the clinician in undertaking functional assessments and interpreting results within a behavioral conceptual framework (Dracobly, Dozier, Briggs, & Juanico, 2018; Lanovaz, Argumedes, Roy, Duquette, & Watkins, 2013). The analysis should identify relevant establishing operations, discriminative stimuli, and reinforcement processes, together with alternative behaviors, currently in the client's behavioral repertoire or which the client could learn, which would result in the same consequences as the SIB. Phrasing the summary of the analysis in plain language (Kern, Sokol, & Dunlap, 2006) can assist in discussing the hypothesis with the client and/or caregivers. Theoretical clarity regarding the processes involved is however also valuable. It is particularly important in considering antecedent events to distinguish between motivating operations and discriminative stimuli, since options for intervention differ between motivational and stimulus control processes. Two examples of completed summary analyses are given in Table 5.2.

This analysis of the processes currently maintaining the target behavior should then be used to develop a range of options for intervention which should preferably both reduce SIB and strengthen (or first teach and then strengthen) positive functionally equivalent behaviors. Such interventions may include interventions targeting each stage of the hypothesized causal process (motivating operation, discriminative stimuli, functional alternatives to SIB, and reinforcement contingencies). The process of defining and selecting intervention options is discussed further at the end of this chapter.

Table 5.2 Examples of statements of hypothetical behavioral functions of SIB

Motivating operation	Discriminative stimulus	Behavior	Reinforcement
When nobody talks to Lauren D for more than 5 min	And other people are visibly present	She slaps her face repeatedly	And people then ask her what is wrong
		[a]She could call out [b]She could learn to raise her hand	
When Dean M is dealing with a telephone call from a customer who becomes confrontational	And his supervisor is present but talking with another worker	He scratches his face	And his supervisor then picks up the call from Dean, ending the confrontation
		[a]He could tell the customer that someone will call them back and then terminate the call [b]He could learn how to put the customer on hold and gesture to his supervisor to come over to take the call	

[a]Possible functionally equivalent behavior already in the person's repertoire
[b]Possible functionally equivalent behavior which the person could learn

5.4.2 Testing for Operant Control of Self-Injurious Behavior

At this stage in the assessment process, the clinician will have a preliminary hypothesis (or hypotheses) regarding the function of the client's SIB. This hypothesis will be based on available information regarding the antecedents and consequences of the behavior. At this stage however, the relative importance of behavior-consequence and antecedent stimulus-behavior relationships in the causation of the SIB will be unclear, and the next stage in assessment is to evaluate the relative dominance of the goal-directed (action-outcome learning) and habit (stimulus-response learning) systems described in Chap. 3 in the maintenance of the client's SIB.

If the clinician holds a BCBA qualification (or is able to refer on to a person thus qualified), one possible way of determining whether the behavior is primarily goal-directed in nature (i.e., under operant control) is to undertake an EFA. If the standard conditions developed by Iwata et al. (1982) are employed, an EFA will conclude that the SIB is maintained by positive social reinforcement, negative social reinforcement, or "automatic" reinforcement or may conclude that the source of reinforcement cannot be identified. In situations where an EFA identifies "automatic" reinforcement as maintaining SIB, our model would suggest that various non-operant processes may also be involved, and we return to this point in our discussion of "secondary differentiation" later in this chapter. If social or other external sources of reinforcement are identified by an EFA as maintaining SIB, this should be taken as a strong indication that the behavior is under operant control. It should however be considered that standard EFA conditions involve manipulation of antecedents to, as well as consequences of, behavior and may make "false positive" identifications of operant control. The standard "task demand" condition, for example, involves a high rate of requests to the person to undertake challenging tasks. If such requests elicit habitual/impulsive SIB, the "task demand" condition will thus result in a high level of SIB even though the behavior is not primarily under operant control. Such false positive results from EFA may account for the proportion of cases, which appears to be approximately 6–11%, where function-based treatments do not effectively reduce SIB even where external (non-automatic) consequences have been identified as maintaining SIB (Iwata et al. 1994).

If however the clinician is not in a position to undertake an EFA, or wishes to further evaluate whether SIB is being maintained by external reinforcement identified by an EFA, an alternative method of testing whether the SIB is under operant control is available. The methodology for undertaking this evaluation is in principle straightforward and involves processes and procedures identical to those originally used by Dickinson (1985; see Chap. 3) in differentiating goal directed from habitual behavior. The processes available to differentiate these two sources of control are devaluation of the reinforcer and disruption of the response-reinforcer contingency. The most reliable procedure available to implement these processes is to initiate a time-limited trial of the behavioral intervention, usually described as "noncontingent reinforcement" (NCR), in which a reinforcer is delivered on a schedule independent of the behavior presumed to be maintained by that reinforcer. Such interventions will be described further in the next chapter, but typically involve the putative reinforcing event being provided on a fixed-time or variable-time schedule, usually with the proviso that the reinforcer is not provided immediately following occurrence of the SIB or other challenging behavior involved. Provided that the reinforcer is delivered in sufficient quantity and with sufficient frequency, such interventions should both devalue its power to reinforce SIB (through satiation) and disrupt the SIB-reinforcer contingency (by frequently making the reinforcer available when no SIB has occurred). Kahng, Iwata, Thompson, and Hanley (2000), investigating the use of NCR with three adults with severe IDs who engaged in SIB and aggression, found that use of NCR with a reinforcer which had been identified through an EFA produced rapid reductions in the SIB and aggression of the people concerned. Kahng et al. (2000) showed that both devaluation of the reinforcer and disruption of the behavior-reinforcer contingency contributed to the effects of NCR. Interventions using NCR typically begin by delivering the reinforcer on a fixed-time (FT) schedule with the interval between reinforcers equal to the mean baseline interval between instances or episodes of SIB and then progressively thin the schedule so that the reinforcer is delivered at longer intervals (see Chap. 6 for further details). Where SIB is believed to be maintained by positive reinforcement (e.g., by contingent social interaction or provision of tangibles), implementing NCR is normally straightforward. Where SIB is believed to be maintained by negative reinforcement (e.g., by escape from aversive situations), NCR can also be delivered by providing breaks from the aversive situation on a fixed-time schedule (Vollmer, Marcus, & Ringdahl, 1995). In this case however, the intervention may need to begin from a starting point of continuous escape from the situation, a procedure which would be expected to reduce SIB irrespective of its predominant source of control (S-R or response-reinforcer). It is only when the schedule has then been modified to the point where the person is again experiencing the aversive situation that it will be possible to assess whether the provision of noncontingent breaks is substantially reducing SIB. Interventions which work by reducing the aversiveness of the situation, e.g., by reducing the aversiveness of a noisy situation through the use of sound-attenuating headphones (Kettering, Fisher, Kelley, & LaRue, 2018), although they may be helpful to the person concerned, likewise will not provide an adequate test of whether the SIB is predominantly controlled by S-R or by operant processes. Where the SIB is hypothesized to be maintained by "automatic reinforcement," the assessment process will be further complicated by the fact that the precise nature of such reinforcement can rarely be specified and NCR interventions at best use forms of stimulation hypothesized to resemble the effective reinforcer (Richman, Barnard-Brak, Grubb, Bosch, & Abby, 2015).

NCR typically produces substantial reductions in levels of challenging behaviors (Richman et al., 2015), and an evaluation of its effectiveness in reducing SIB may be carried out either by implementing an intervention during discrete test periods (e.g., Kahng et al., 2000) or by more extended intervention in the person's everyday environment (e.g., Tomlin & Reed, 2012). To use the impact of NCR intervention as an indicator of whether SIB is predominantly under S-R or operant control, however, two conditions must be met. The first, obviously, is that the reinforcer used in the NCR intervention must be the reinforcer maintaining the SIB. The objection may be raised that whether this is the case or not can only be determined by carrying out an EFA. Doing so would undoubtedly strengthen confidence in any conclusion which may be drawn from the trial of NCR. However, NCR interventions using hypothesized reinforcers identified on the basis of descriptive assessments alone can be effective (e.g., Tomlin & Reed, 2012). Equally important however is the fact that NCR interventions, at least in their initial stages, typically completely abolish the motivating operation establishing reinforcer effectiveness, i.e., positive reinforcers are provided almost continuously or escape from aversive situations is continuously permitted. During this phase of the intervention, an NCR intervention is likely to reduce levels of SIB whatever the predominant controlling influences. It is only when the NCR schedule has been sufficiently thinned that the person is being substantially exposed to conditions which previously evoked SIB that it will be possible to see whether devaluing the reinforcer and disrupting the SIB-reinforcer contingency is effectively reducing levels of SIB. Even then, care must be taken in evaluating the effectiveness of the intervention. Even after schedule thinning, the percentage of time in which the person is faced with the conditions which previously elicited SIB may be lower than was the case prior to intervention. In such situations, pre-intervention and during-intervention rates of SIB must be compared only for periods of time in which the person is actually coping with conditions which previously led to SIB (Roscoe, Iwata, & Rand, 2003).

With these caveats in mind, a relatively brief trial of NCR using the best available evidence regarding the reinforcer responsible for maintaining the SIB will often provide a good indication as to the relative importance of S-R and operant processes in maintaining the behavior. If a well-planned and well-implemented NCR program substantially reduces SIB, this is a strong indicator that the behavior is largely under operant control and suggests that operant interventions such as NCR and functional communication training should be effective in reducing the behavior. In this case, such interventions should be considered, possibly following further functional assessment or EFA in order to confirm the effective reinforcer. If NCR does not have an impact on levels of SIB (after correcting for proportion of time spent in the evoking conditions), this is an indicator that the behavior may predominantly be controlled by S-R and other processes. This does not mean that operant processes are not influencing the behavior or that operant interventions may not contribute to its reduction. It does suggest however that other, non-operant, behavioral interventions such as systematic desensitization to SIB evoking conditions may additionally be necessary to substantially reduce the behavior. Such interventions are discussed in the next chapter.

5.5 Secondary Differentiation (Distinguishing Between Non-operant Subtypes of Self-Injurious Behavior)

If the previous stage of assessment has led to the conclusion that SIB is not predominantly controlled by operant processes, further assessment may be necessary in order to identify controlling processes. Our model assumes that the changes in the relative importance of different sources of control for SIB occur in an evolutionary manner, i.e., some sources of control become less important, and others more important, over time. This does not however imply that that factors which become less important in influencing SIB become irrelevant nor that SIB can usefully be divided into operant and "biological" subtypes. Further assessment should be used as a means to identify additional interventions which may increase the overall positive impact of operant interventions, not as a substitute for them. A series of questions may usefully be addressed however to find indicators of which processes may be predominant in each individual case.

5.5.1 Emergent Self-Injurious Behavior

Occasionally, particularly if the clinician is working with young children, SIB which does not respond to the test of operant control provided by NCR may represent "emergent" SIB which has yet to come under operant control (Kurtz et al., 2003). In this situation, further assessment should be directed to identifying precisely the situations or other factors which are eliciting SIB. Our model assumes that these will predominantly be aversive situations involving either pain or frustration or rapid situational transitions (Berkson, 2002). Further assessment should be focused therefore on re-consideration of the possibility of any painful medical conditions, delineation of the transitions or frustrating situations which elicit SIB, and assessment of the child's communication, self-help, and coping skills relevant to overcoming these frustrations. Once these are defined, appropriate intervention may comprise any necessary medical treatment, providing the child with additional information regarding transitions, or modifying the density of reinforcement provided in situations to which they are moving (Castillo et al., 2018), and teaching the child self-help and/or communication skills (or providing her/him with resources such as augmentative communication to compensate for difficulties in these areas) necessary to cope with situational challenges. It may also be appropriate to provide parents or other caregivers with support on behavior management to minimize the likelihood of the SIB developing operant functions.

5.5.2 "Habitual/Impulsive" Self-Injurious Behavior

With an older child or adult who has a long history of engaging in SIB, failure of the SIB to respond to the test of operant control provided by NCR suggests that operant processes may have become less important in the maintenance of the SIB, which may predominantly be controlled by S-R or other processes. One important question is whether the SIB is episodic, occurring in discrete bursts, or whether it occurs continuously or almost continuously. If the SIB is episodic, the next focal point for assessment should be the antecedent conditions under which it occurs. Much of this assessment may already have been undertaken during the preliminary functional assessment. Further assessment, including direct observation, may however be necessary if either no antecedents have been identified or if antecedents have been identified only in general terms (e.g., mealtimes, change points in routines, particular social situations, and so on). If no antecedents have been identified, further consideration should firstly be given to the possibility that the SIB is evoked at some point by an ongoing process (e.g., extended exposure to challenging academic work, busy social situations, noise, etc.) so that there appears to be no immediate change in antecedent conditions just prior to the person beginning to engage in SIB. If antecedents to SIB have been identified only in general terms, assessment should focus on defining which aspects or elements of the situations evoke SIB. This may be done by discussion with the person engaging in SIB and/or supporting others or by direct observation. The assessment can usefully follow the model of assessment of specific fears and phobias in persons with NDCs (e.g., Koegel, Openden, & Koegel, 2004) in identifying the earliest point in a routine at which SIB is seen, what parameters of the situation affect the probability or severity of SIB, what situations most reliably evoke SIB, and whether there are apparently related situations which do not evoke SIB. For example, for a person who engages in SIB at mealtimes, it will be useful to know at exactly what point in the sequence of events leading up to mealtimes SIB usually commences, whether variability in the situation (e.g., location, people present, time of day, etc.) affects the probability or severity of SIB, and whether there are any mealtime or related situations (e.g., picnics) which do not usually evoke SIB. It should be remembered that Pavlovian conditioning processes may have led to SIB being evoked by antecedents which have been associated with the original eliciting stimulus by temporal contiguity only, so that SIB may, for example, be evoked by the theme music to a television program which happened to have been playing when a person experienced choking during a mealtime. In people with substantial language skills, such networks of association may be further extended by semantic processes so that stimuli which have never been physically associated with an evoking stimulus may nevertheless gain the ability to evoke SIB (Dymond, Dunsmoor, Vervliet, Roche, & Hermans, 2015). If situations or specific stimuli are identified which reliably evoke SIB which is however not responsive to NCR, it is probable that the behavior is primarily controlled by the habit (S-R) system. Potentially useful behavioral interventions will include progressive exposure/systematic desensitization, and further assessment should focus on developing a "hierarchy" of situations ranging from those minimally likely to evoke SIB to those extremely likely to evoke severe SIB, as is used in intervention with phobias (Koegel et al., 2004).

5.5.3 "Compulsive" Self-Injurious Behavior

Within the model we propose for the development of SIB, the progression from habitual/impulsive to compulsive SIB represents one of the final possible stages in the development of SIB, and making the distinction between habitual/impulsive and compulsive forms of SIB for the individual person may be challenging. There are however two clinical signs which may be indicative of compulsivity in SIB. Elevated levels of anxiety are believed to constitute one factor contributing to the development of compulsivity (see Chap. 3), and one potential indicator is a person's level of autonomic arousal, anxiety, and agitation when engaging in SIB and when attempts are made to persuade them to stop doing so. A high level of autonomic arousal when engaging in SIB, which may escalate further in response to attempts to persuade the person to stop, may suggest a compulsive aspect to the SIB. Despite recent developments in the assessment of anxiety in people with NDCs, particularly adults with IDs and children with ASCs (Bearss et al., 2016; Hallett et al., 2013; Hermans, van der Pas, & Evenhuis, 2011; Hermans, Wieland, Jelluma, Van der Pas, & Evenhuis, 2013; Lecavalier et al., 2014), most available methods assess long-term anxiety rather than dynamic "state" anxiety (Vigneau & Cormier, 2008). Moskowitz et al. (2013) however have described a multimethod approach to assessing anxiety in children with ASCs and IDs using observation of individually defined "anxious behaviors," an overall anxiety rating, heart rate measures, and observation of challenging behaviors associated with anxiety. Most studies to date of the dynamic relationships between autonomic arousal and SIB have used heart rate (HR), or heart rate variability (HRV), to measure arousal (Cohen, Yoo, Goodwin, & Moskowitz, 2011; Hall, Hammond, & Hustyi, 2013; Hoch, Symons, & Sng, 2013; Jennett, Hagopian, & Beaulieu, 2011; Lydon, Healy, & Dwyer, 2013). Although the ongoing development of relatively noninvasive methods for heart-rate monitoring may make it possible to monitor HR and HRV clinically for some individuals (Nuske et al., 2019), in many cases arousal associated with SIB can currently only be assessed by clinical observation. The second clinical sign which may be indicative of compulsivity in SIB is the presence of self-restraint (SR). If the person engages in SR (see Chap. 7), and especially if they become highly aroused, anxious, or agitated when SR is interrupted (or if externally applied restraints are removed), this also may be indicative of compulsivity in their SIB (Hyman, Oliver, & Hall, 2002).

5.5.4 "Stereotyped" and "Generalized Habitual" Self-Injurious Behavior

If initial assessment suggests that a person engages in SIB continuously or almost continuously throughout their waking day, it is useful first of all to verify (or otherwise) these reports by discussion with additional informants and/or direct observation. Reports that a person engages in SIB "all the time" may actually indicate that she/he engages in SIB in many different situations, but she/he may also refrain from doing so for extended periods. Some people do however engage in SIB for very high proportions of their waking day. In such situations a useful next step in assessment is to find out how the person responds when another person attempts to engage them in another activity. A person's response will obviously often depend on the alternative activity suggested, and it may be necessary to try a wide variety of alternatives. For some people it may be necessary to carry out a systematic stimulus preference assessment (see Box 5.4) in order to identify a suitably interesting activity or item. For some people it will however be found that although they may normally engage in SIB for very extended periods of time, offering a suitably stimulating alternative activity will reliably gain their interest and interrupt SIB. For people who experience such stereotyped SIB, further assessment should focus on systematic assessment of activities and reinforcers with which they will prefer to engage rather than engaging in SIB.

Box 5.4 Assessing Stimulus Preferences and Likely Effectiveness of Potential Reinforcers

When trying to interest people who engage in stereotyped SIB in other activities, a systematic assessment may be necessary to identify activities and stimuli which are sufficiently reinforcing to compete with the SIB. This assessment is typically undertaken in two stages. In the first stage, a pool of relatively preferred activities and stimuli are identified and, where possible, ranked in order of preference. One approach to such preference assessment is to ask the person her-/himself, or other people who know them well, to identify preferred stimuli using open-ended questions or survey schedules (e.g., Fisher, Piazza, Bowman, & Amari, 1996). Such reported preferences may however show limited correspondence with those suggested by direct observation of the person's behavior toward such stimuli. The second stage in assessment is therefore to directly assess which of the activities and stimuli identified in the first stage are more highly preferred by the individual.

There are two broad approaches to such direct assessment of stimulus/activity preferences. In "free-operant" assessment, the person can freely access all the items and activities to be assessed, if necessary having previously been encouraged to "sample" each item/activity. During the assessment, the amount of time which she/he spends engaging with each activity/stimulus is recorded (Roane, Vollmer, Ringdahl, & Marcus, 1998). In "trial-based" preference assessments, the person's preferences for items/activities from the pool of items are assessed by systematically observing either choices when items are presented simultaneously, in pairs (Fisher et al., 1992) or larger groupings (Deleon & Iwata, 1996), or alternatively by observing the person's behavior toward items when they are presented individually (DeLeon, Iwata, Conners, & Wallace, 1999). Relative preference for each item can be assessed by measuring levels of "approach" responses (e.g., looking toward the item), physical contact with the item, or active engagement with/use of the item.

Stimulus preferences change over time and are dependent on contextual factors, and it will often be necessary to frequently re-assess preferences. Choices between sources of stimulation also do not depend solely on the characteristics of the stimulation, but also on factors such as the level of effort required to access the stimulation (Shore, Iwata, DeLeon, Kahng, & Smith, 1997). Items and activities identified as highly preferred in choice-based assessments may therefore not reduce stereotyped SIB in the person's everyday environment unless they can be readily accessed with low effort.

Where necessary, activities and items being considered as potential reinforcers can be directly assessed for their effectiveness in reducing SIB in a "competing items assessment" (Groskreutz, Groskreutz, & Higbee, 2011; Ringdahl, Vollmer, Marcus, & Roane, 1997) in order to identify the most effective items/activities to be used in an intervention program.

Other people who engage in extended SIB will however be disinterested in all attempts to engage them in competing activities and will immediately recommence SIB if they are briefly interrupted (e.g., by someone asking the person to stop hitting themselves and momentarily holding their hands). Such a pattern of responding may be indicative of a process which might be called "generalized habitual" SIB. For some people, this pattern of SIB may have developed from habitual/impulsive (S-R) SIB through a process in which Pavlovian conditioning has led to a wide range of stimuli acquiring the power to elicit SIB. The SIB of a school student may, for example, have initially been evoked by presentation of demanding academic tasks in the classroom, and then through an extended process of Pavlovian conditioning come to be evoked by the classroom environment, then by the whole school environment, then by the appearance of the school bus, and so on until the person starts to engage in SIB as soon as they are asked to come out of their bedroom in the morning. Such situations represent a particularly difficult therapeutic challenge. Further assessment should focus on identifying the possibly very limited range of situations in which the person does not engage in SIB, which may provide a basis for behavioral intervention, based on models provided by behavioral treatment of generalized avoidance behaviors (Dymond, 2019). As is the case with habitual/impulsive SIB which is elicited by specific antecedents, generalized habitual SIB may show a greater or lesser degree of compulsivity. Again, compulsivity may be indicated by the person's level of arousal and anxiety when engaging in SIB or by their engaging in self-restraint. Particular attention should be given to the possibility that in situations where the person does not engage in SIB, they are in fact engaging in very specific forms of self-restraint. Where a person, for example, refrains from self injury only in their own bedroom, this may be because the room is the only situation which has not become associated with aversive events, or it may be that the person makes specific use of bedclothes to engage in self-restraint.

5.5.5 *Secondary Differentiation of Self-Injurious Behavior: Correspondence with Current Operant Perspectives*

Although we doubt the utility of insisting that all forms of SIB are maintained entirely by reinforcement processes, or of attempting to differentiate "operant" and "biologic" types of SIB, the subtypes of SIB which we have labelled "stereotyped," "generalized habitual," and "compulsive" may well correspond to three subtypes of "automatically reinforced" SIB described by Hagopian (Hagopian, Rooker, & Yenokyan, 2018; Hagopian, Rooker, & Zarcone, 2015; Hagopian, Rooker, Zarcone, Bonner, & Arevalo, 2017). If so, where a person has been engaged in a comprehensive EFA including at least an "alone" and "play" (control) conditions, it may also be possible to differentiate between these subtypes of SIB on the basis of the criteria proposed by Hagopian and his colleagues. These are described in detail by Hagopian et al. (2015) and (2017). Briefly, however, Hagopian's "automatically reinforced SIB Subtype 1" is characterized by high levels of SIB in the "alone" condition of an EFA relative to the "play" condition, "automatically reinforced SIB Subtype 2" is characterized by high and variable levels of SIB across all EFA conditions, and "automatically reinforced SIB Subtype 3" is also characterized by high and variable levels of SIB across all EFA conditions, but with the presence also of self-restraint (SR). If data from an EFA are available, therefore, high levels of SIB in the "alone" condition of an EFA relative to the "play" condition may be taken as an indicator of "stereotyped" SIB which may well respond to intervention by provision of suitable forms of stimulation. High and variable levels of SIB across all conditions of an EFA may indicate the presence of "generalized habitual" SIB, and the same pattern of responding accompanied by self-restraint may indicate "generalized habitual" SIB with compulsive features.

5.6 From Assessment to Stages (or "Subtypes") of Self-Injurious Behavior to Intervention

Figure 3.4, presented at the end of Chap. 3, summarized the stages through which SIB may progress, some neural and environmental drivers which contribute to this progression, and behavioral interventions which may both impact positively on SIB at each stage and disrupt progression of SIB to a further stage. The assessment process described in this chapter provides a methodology for identifying the predominant causal processes in individual cases of SIB. Table 5.3 summarizes key stages in the evolution of SIB, together with key indicators associated with each stage, and outlines options for behavioral intervention at each stage, behavioral intervention which may inhibit progression of SIB to later stages, and, where relevant, potential medical and pharmacological interventions which may be considered at each stage. It should be emphasized once again that for each individual at a given moment, SIB will be at some point in its development through the stages identified and hence that

Table 5.3 Key indicators of the stage of SIB and potential interventions (under specialist supervision)

Stage of SIB: key indicators	Behavioral intervention	Behavioral intervention to disrupt progression	Potential medical or psychiatric intervention
Emergent Recently developed, does not appear to be under operant control	Functional communication training (FCT) and independence skill training Treatment to increase tolerance of routine changes & delay		Treatment of painful medical conditions
	Ditto		
Goal-directed (operant) Identified as reinforced by external reinforcers by EFA and/or responds positively to "noncontingent reinforcement" (NCR)	Contingency management, FCT, NCR		Treatment of painful medical conditions
		FCT (multiple mands)	
Habitual/impulsive (S-R) Identified as "automatically reinforced" by EFA and/or does not respond to NCR	Differential reinforcement of other/alternative behavior	Systematic desensitization to SIB-evoking stimuli	Low-dose dopamine receptor blockers
Stereotyped Responds to intervention with competing stimuli	NCR with preferred stimulation	N/A	Not indicated
Generalized Habitual No/limited response to competing stimuli	Behavioral intervention for generalized avoidance[a]	N/A	Low-dose dopamine receptor blockers
Compulsive Elevated arousal/anxiety, self-restraint	Behavioral relaxation[a] Systematic desensitization to SIB-evoking stimuli[a]	N/A	Beta blockers[a] Mood stabilizers[a] SSRIs[b]

EFA **experimental functional analysis,** *SSRI* **selective serotonin reuptake inhibitor,** *beta blocker* **beta-adrenergic receptor blocker**

[a]Denotes interventions for which evidence for efficacy is particularly limited and/or of relatively poor quality

[b]Denotes interventions for which efficacy is particularly limited and/or of limited quality AND which are not recommended for use with children with ASCs

interventions targeting more than one stage/"subtype" of SIB might be helpful. Intervention options are discussed further in Chap. 6, but Table 5.3 highlights three issues of immediate relevance when considering options for intervention with SIB. The first is that many potential interventions should be undertaken only by (or under specialist supervision from) appropriately qualified and specialized professionals in medicine, psychiatry, clinical psychology, or applied behavior analysis. The second issue is that for more complex cases involving generalized habitual or compulsive SIB, the evidence for efficacy of both behavioral and pharmacological interventions is very limited in both quantity and quality. The third issue is that indications for treatment may differ between children and adults and between diagnostic groups. The use of selective serotonin reuptake inhibitors to treat SIB, for example, may be considered (with caution) for adults with IDs, but is not recommended for children with ASCs owing to lack of evidence of effectiveness, frequent occurrence of adverse reactions, and uncertainties regarding appropriate dosage (Lamy & Erickson, 2018; Posey, Erickson, Stigler & McDougle, 2006). We discuss these issues further in Chap. 6.

5.7 Case Studies

Rose A

During a recent episode of ear infection, Rose was sitting on the floor in the sitting room of her house playing with one of her favorite toys and gently body-rocking. For no apparent reason however, she then became very distressed, holding her hand to her right ear, and began to rock more vigorously. In the course of doing so, she struck the back of her head against the nearby wall, which distressed her even further. Her mother immediately went to comfort her and, since the ear infection was being treated, thought no more of the matter until the next week, when a curious incident occurred. Rose was again sitting on the floor playing while her mother worked at a table in the same room. At one point her mother was surprised to see that Rose first looked at her and then banged her head against the wall. She showed none of the distress which had accompanied the first incident, and the force of the blow appeared much reduced from that which had occurred on the first occasion. Her mother decided to carry on with her work, but a few minutes later moved Rose away from the wall and interested her in a new activity. When her mother took Rose to see her speech and language therapist shortly afterward, she discussed the incident with the therapist, who encouraged her to deal with any further episodes in the same way. At the next appointment a month later, the therapist enquired as to whether Rose had banged her head again, but no further incidents had occurred.

Ayanna B

Although Ayanna's self-injury is not regarded as a major problem, as she has grown older, the extent of the disruption which it causes has increased. Having attended a 2-day workshop on positive behavior support, Ayanna's teacher used antecedent-behavior-consequence (ABC) charts to record details of her SIB and the circumstances in which it occurred for a period of 2 weeks. The ABC records showed that Ayanna engaged in SIB almost exclusively during specific group activities in which she had to sit and wait for her turn to contribute. Ayanna's teacher hypothesized that Ayanna found the waiting involved in these activities aversive and that her SIB was reinforced by her being taken out of such activities to go for a walk. Following a discussion with the speech and language therapist supporting the school regarding the possibility of a functional communication intervention to help Ayanna to replace her SIB with a communicative alternative, and consultation with her parents, her class teacher decided to introduce a symbol to enable Ayanna to request to leave group activities. Because of her relatively good understanding of language, the teacher thought that Ayanna would be able express her views on the idea of using a symbol to ask to leave activities, and so she also explained the proposed intervention to Ayanna. When asked if she would like to have an "I want to leave" symbol, Ayanna was enthusiastic about the idea. She rapidly learned to use the symbol following a brief explanation and demonstration of its meaning. If Ayanna held up her "I want to leave" symbol, the teaching assistant left the classroom with Ayanna and took her for a short walk. Following the introduction of the symbol at the beginning of the spring school term, Ayanna's episodes of SIB rapidly reduced in frequency.

Darren C

During the last school term, Darren's behavior showed an unexpected change. He started to engage in SIB when asked to go for his dinner. Over a period of weeks, his hand-biting and face-hitting when he was asked to go to dinner both increased in severity and began to occur at an earlier point in the process. Initially, Darren started to self-injure when he was actually eating his meal, then when asked to choose his meal in the school dining room, and then on entering the dining room, until after 6 weeks he was beginning to self-injure in the classroom when told it was dinnertime. Although staff persisted in trying to encourage him to have his dinner, they increasingly found themselves having to let Darren leave, or avoid entering, the dining room because of the severity of his behavior. Knowing that people with Cornelia de Lange syndrome can suffer from gastroesophageal reflux, Darren's teacher wondered if this could be causing him distress and contacted his parents to ask them to take him to see his general practitioner (GP). The GP referred Darren to a dietician for advice and also prescribed omeprazole, a medication which inhibits the secretion of gastric acid. Once Darren had seen the dietician, the school modified his meals in line with the dietician's advice. Unfortunately, these measures had no effect on Darren's SIB. In fact, his SIB continued to worsen, and his accompanying distress became such that even if he could be persuaded to enter the dining room, he ate very little. As he was continuing to happily eat a snack in his classroom in the morning, his teacher wondered if the level of noise in the dining room might be a factor in his behavior and, following consultation with Darren's parents, arranged for him to eat in the classroom, supervised by a teaching assistant. The teacher was surprised to see that Darren ate his meal happily without engaging in SIB.

After some weeks during which Darren had been taking his meal in the classroom without difficulties, his teacher decided that he should once again try asking Darren to go to the dining room to have his dinner. Darren became extremely distressed, crying, biting his hand, and hitting his face. His teacher was perplexed by the intensity of Darren's reaction to the suggestion that he should go to the dining room. He had asked the teaching assistant to have Darren's dinner ready for him, and as soon as he saw that Darren was becoming distressed, the teacher had immediately shown Darren that he could have his meal in the classroom after all. Darren however had continued to self-injure for over 10 min before he finally calmed. Not wanting to repeat this experience, his teacher discussed his situation with an educational psychologist who visited the school periodically to offer an informal advice clinic for teachers. The psychologist, having enquired carefully about the circumstances in which Darren engaged in SIB and the history of his difficulties, suggested that the problem might have originated because Darren had been experiencing reflux, but that this aversive experience might then have become progressively associated with the sequence of steps which lead up to that experience. Further, she surmised, although the behavior might originally have been reinforced by Darren escaping from or avoiding these aversive experiences, his self-injury might have become a habitual response to any suggestion that he should go to the dining room. She suggested that assuming that Darren's discomfort had been successfully treated by the dietary changes and omeprazole, it should be possible to enable him to return to the dining room by using a program of progressive exposure with reinforcement.

Arshad D

Following the review meeting, the teacher explained the discussion which had taken place to the clinical psychologist. Since Arshad was an adult, the psychologist first arranged to meet with him to introduce herself and explain that she had been asked to try to help him with his SIB. Arshad however had very limited language skills, and concluding that he would be unable to give informed consent to her involvement, the clinical psychologist decided that it would be in Arshad's best interests for her to undertake initial assessment on the basis of information from people who knew Arshad well. The clinical psychologist therefore discussed Arshad's SIB with his mother and with school staff, completed a Functional Assessment Interview (FAI) with his teacher, and completed "Questions About Behavioral Function" (QABF) assessments with information from Arshad's mother and from a teaching assistant who frequently worked with Arshad at school. The information gathered from the FAI suggested that Arshad was less likely to engage in SIB when he was actively involved in activities, but otherwise identified no specific antecedents to episodes of SIB. The usual consequence of Arshad engaging in SIB was identified as people attempting to distract him. For both QABF assessments, the non-social subscale received the highest severity score (11 with the teaching assistant and 10 with Arshad's mother, out of a maximum 15). The tangible subscale received a severity score of 9 in the assessment with the teaching assistant and 6 in the assessment with Arshad's mother. No other subscale (attention, escape, or physical) received a severity score over 4 in either assessment. Following further discussion with the teaching assistant, the clinical psychologist hypothesized that the high score on the tangible scale probably reflected the fact that activities, or sometimes edibles, were often used to distract Arshad from his SIB and that the behavior was primarily maintained by automatic reinforcement. However, the specific nature of the reinforcer maintaining the behavior was not clear, and it seemed likely that any noncontingent reinforcement intervention would have to use a reinforcer chosen on the basis of a stimulus preference or competing items assessment. Having concluded that Arshad did not have capacity to give informed consent to being observed, and following consultation with his mother and his teacher, the psychologist concluded that it would be in his best interests for her to directly observe his behavior in class so that she could give specific advice regarding the schedule to be used in any intervention. Observing Arshad's behavior during two 30-min sessions, she recorded that he spent approximately 30% of his time scratching himself in each session. Based on time intervals between episodes in which he was scratching, she concluded that to have a reasonable chance of success, a noncontingent reinforcement program would have to schedule reinforcement at an average interval of 60 s.

Sarah E

The local government's adult social care service in the area where Sarah lives established a positive behavior support (PBS) service 3 years ago, and a newly appointed manager at Sarah's residential service referred her to the PBS service for assessment and possible treatment of her SIB. Having met Sarah and concluded that she would not be able to understand the purpose of, or give informed consent to, the proposed assessment, the board-certified behavior analyst (BCBA) who had been assigned to work with Sarah initially completed assessments, including a Functional Assessment Interview (FAI) and "Questions About Behavioral Function" assessments (QABFs), which could be undertaken by meeting members of staff who supported Sarah without any intrusion into Sarah's normal routines. The BCBA was however unable to come to any clear conclusions regarding the function(s) of her behavior. Some of Sarah's episodes of self-injury appeared to be responses to her being asked to engage in activity and resulted in participation in the activity being avoided or at least postponed. There were however many other occasions on which she started to self-injure in the absence of any obvious antecedents. Following a formal capacity assessment and detailed consultation with Sarah's family, the manager of the residential service, and the consultant psychiatrist who was involved with Sarah, the BCBA decided that it would be in Sarah's best interests for her to be involved in a limited number of sessions of experimental functional analysis (EFA), with the purpose of identifying the function of Sarah's SIB. As completion of the FAI and QABF had yielded no hypotheses regarding the functions of Sarah's behavior, the EFA used the standard conditions described by Iwata et al. (1982), except that it was considered neither possible nor appropriate to leave Sarah alone in a room while still observing her. A modified "alone" condition was therefore used in which the observer was in the room with Sarah, but did not interact with her. The EFA sessions were carried out with Sarah wearing her helmet in order to reduce the risk that she would seriously harm herself during the assessment. After three 20-min sessions of EFA, conducted in the course of a week, a clear, but rather unexpected, pattern of results emerged. In all three sessions, the "task demand" and "unstructured activity" conditions evoked comparable, and moderately high, levels of hand to head-hitting, with lower levels in the "social disapproval" and "alone" conditions. The "unstructured activity" EFA condition, which was conceived as a control condition against which others are compared, nevertheless shares with the "task demand" condition a procedure in which if a person engages in SIB, the person conducting the assessment briefly ceases to interact with them. The BCBA concluded that for Sarah, even the gentle encouragement to engage in activity presented in the "unstructured activity" was functionally identical to task demand, and hence she concluded that Sarah's SIB was probably maintained by escape from, or avoidance of, task demands.

Nathan F

Because Nathan's SIB usually does not result in physical harm beyond temporary reddening of the area he hits, and because he has engaged in the behavior for such a long time, there has been no systematic attempt to intervene with his self-injury since he was at school. He was recently referred however to the local positive behavior support service by a social worker who was reviewing his case. The BCBA assigned to work with Nathan initially met with Nathan, his mother, and staff from the day service. It was immediately apparent that Nathan rarely engaged in SIB when involved in activities with the day service, and the BCBA decided to focus her further work mainly on his situation at home. As she did not consider that Nathan would have capacity to give informed consent to the assessment process, the BCBA decided to begin the assessment with minimally intrusive methods and completed "Questions About Behavioral Function" (QABF) assessments both with Nathan's mother and with day service staff. These revealed a possible difference in the function of his behavior in the two settings. In the QABF assessment completed with Nathan's mother, the non-social subscale clearly received the highest score, with its severity score of six being twice that for any other subscale. The QABF assessment completed with day service staff also revealed a relatively high severity score of 8 on the non-social subscale, but an even higher score of 10 on the "tangible" subscale. Further discussions with the day service staff revealed that they believed that although Nathan's SIB was largely self-stimulatory, they thought that he also engaged in the behavior because when he did so the staff gave him one of several highly preferred items (one being a set of musical bells) with which Nathan would then amuse himself. It thus appeared possible that although Nathan's SIB might initially have been automatically reinforced, it might also at the day service have developed a socially mediated function of obtaining materials with which to engage in self-stimulating activity.

References

Alter, P. J., Conroy, M. A., Mancil, G. R., & Haydon, T. (2008). A comparison of functional behavior assessment methodologies with young children: Descriptive methods and functional analysis. *Journal of Behavioral Education, 17*(2), 200–219. https://doi.org/10.1007/s10864-008-9064-3

Badgett, N., & Falcomata, T. S. (2015). A comparison of methodologies of brief functional analysis. *Developmental Neurorehabilitation, 18*(4), 224–233. https://doi.org/10.3109/17518423.2013.792298

Ball, T., Bush, A., & Emerson, E. (2004). *Psychological interventions for severely challenging behaviours shown by people with learning disabilities: clinical practice guidelines*. Leicester: British Psychological Society. Retrieved from https://www.bps.org.uk/member-microsites/dcp-faculty-people-intellectual-disabilities/resources

Barney, C. C., Feyma, T., Beisang, A., & Symons, F. J. (2015). Pain experience and expression in Rett syndrome: Subjective and objective measurement approaches. *Journal of Developmental and Physical Disabilities, 27*(4), 417–429. https://doi.org/10.1007/s10882-015-9427-3

Barton-Arwood, S. M., Wehby, J. H., Gunter, P. L., & Lane, K. L. (2003). Functional behavior assessment rating scales: Intrarater reliability with students with emotional or behavioral disorders. *Behavioral Disorders, 28*(4), 386–400. https://doi.org/10.1177/019874290302800402

Bearss, K., Taylor, C. A., Aman, M. G., Whittemore, R., Lecavalier, L., Miller, J., … Scahill, L. (2016). Using qualitative methods to guide scale development for anxiety in youth with autism spectrum disorder. *Autism, 20*(6), 663–672. https://doi.org/10.1177/1362361315601012

Berkson, G. (2002). Early development of stereotyped and self-injurious behaviors: II. Age trends. *American Journal on Mental Retardation, 107*(6), 468–477. https://doi.org/10.1352/0895-8017(2002)107<0468:EDOSAS>2.0.CO;2

Bienstein, P., & Nussbeck, S. (2009). Reliability and validity of a German version of the Questions about Behavioral Function (QABF) scale for self-injurious behavior in individuals with intellectual disabilities. *Journal of Mental Health Research in Intellectual Disabilities, 2*(4), 249–260. https://doi.org/10.1080/19315860903061809

Bihm, E. M., Kienlen, T. L., Ness, M. E., & Poindexter, A. R. (1991). Factor structure of the Motivation Assessment Scale for persons with mental retardation. *Psychological Reports, 68*(3-Supplement), 1235–1238. https://doi.org/10.2466/pr0.1991.68.3c.1235

Bond, L., Carroll, R., Mulryan, N., O'Dwyer, M., O'Connell, J., Monaghan, R., … McCarron, M. (2019). The association of life events and mental ill health in older adults with intellectual disability: Results of the wave 3 Intellectual Disability Supplement to the Irish Longitudinal Study on Ageing. *Journal of Intellectual Disability Research, 63*(5), 454–465. https://doi.org/10.1111/jir.12595

Breau, L. M., McGrath, P. J., Camfield, C. S., & Finley, G. A. (2002). Psychometric properties of the Non-Communicating Children's Pain Checklist-revised. *Pain, 99*(1-2), 349–357. https://doi.org/10.1016/S0304-3959(02)00179-3

Burbidge, C., Oliver, C., Moss, J., Arron, K., Berg, K., Furniss, F., … Woodock, K. (2010). The association between repetitive behaviours, impulsivity and hyperactivity in people with intellectual disability. *Journal of Intellectual Disability Research, 54*(12), 1078–1092. https://doi.org/10.1111/j.1365-2788.2010.01338.x

Byrne, G. (2018). Prevalence and psychological sequelae of sexual abuse among individuals with an intellectual disability: A review of the recent literature. *Journal of Intellectual Disabilities, 22*(3), 294–310. https://doi.org/10.1177/1744629517698844

Call, N. A., Findley, A. J., & Reavis, A. R. (2012). The effects of conducting a functional analysis on problem behavior in other settings. *Research in Developmental Disabilities, 33*(6), 1990–1995. https://doi.org/10.1016/j.ridd.2012.06.001

Call, N. A., Reavis, A. R., Clark, S. B., Parks, N. A., Cariveau, T., & Muething, C. S. (2017). The effects of conducting a functional analysis on problem behavior in other settings: A descriptive study on potential interaction effects. *Behavior Modification, 41*(5), 609–625. https://doi.org/10.1177/0145445517696052

Call, N. A., Zangrillo, A. N., Delfs, C. H., & Findley, A. J. (2013). A comparison of brief functional analyses with and without consequences. *Behavioral Interventions, 28*(1), 22–39. https://doi.org/10.1002/bin.1353

Carr, E. G. (1977). The motivation of self-injurious behavior: A review of some hypotheses. *Psychological Bulletin, 84*(4), 800–816. https://doi.org/10.1037/0033-2909.84.4.800

Carr, E. G., Ladd, M. V., & Schulte, C. F. (2008). Validation of the Contextual Assessment Inventory for problem behavior. *Journal of Positive Behavior Interventions, 10*(2), 91–104. https://doi.org/10.1177/1098300707312543

Carr, E. G., Yarbrough, S. C., & Langdon, N. A. (1997). Effects of idiosyncratic stimulus variables on functional analysis outcomes. *Journal of Applied Behavior Analysis, 30*(4), 673–686. https://doi.org/10.1901/jaba.1997.30-673

Cascella, M., Bimonte, S., Saettini, F., & Muzio, M. R. (2019). The challenge of pain assessment in children with cognitive disabilities: Features and clinical applicability of different observational tools. *Journal of Paediatrics and Child Health, 55*(2), 129–135. https://doi.org/10.1111/jpc.14230

Castillo, M. I., Clark, D. R., Schaller, E. A., Donaldson, J. M., DeLeon, I. G., & Kahng, S. (2018). Descriptive assessment of problem behavior during transitions of children with intellectual and developmental disabilities. *Journal of Applied Behavior Analysis, 51*(1), 99–117. https://doi.org/10.1002/jaba.430

Christensen, T. J., Ringdahl, J. E., Bosch, J. J., Falcomata, T. S., Luke, J. R., & Andelman, M. S. (2009). Constipation associated with self-injurious and aggressive behavior exhibited by a child diagnosed with autism. *Education and Treatment of Children, 32*(1), 89–103. https://doi.org/10.1353/etc.0.0041

Cohen, I. L., Yoo, J. H., Goodwin, M. S., & Moskowitz, L. (2011). Assessing challenging behaviors in autism spectrum disorders: Prevalence, rating scales, and autonomic indicators. In J. L. Matson & P. Sturmey (Eds.), *International handbook of autism and pervasive developmental disorders*. New York: Springer Science+Business Media LLC.

Collett, B. R., Ohan, J. L., & Myers, K. M. (2003). Ten-year review of rating scales. V: Scales assessing attention-deficit/hyperactivity disorder. *Journal of the American Academy of Child and Adolescent Psychiatry, 42*(9), 1015–1037. https://doi.org/10.1097/01.CHI.0000070245.24125.B6

Cooper, J. O., Heron, T. E., & Heward, W. L. (2007). *Applied behavior analysis* (2nd ed.). Upper Saddle River, NJ: Pearson.

Cooper, S.-A., & Simpson, N. (2006). Assessment and classification of psychiatric disorders in adults with learning disabilities. *Psychiatry, 5*(9), 306–311. https://doi.org/10.1053/j.mppsy.2006.06.009

Cooper, S.-A., Smiley, E., Finlayson, J., Jackson, A., Allan, L., Williamson, A., … Morrison, J. (2007). The prevalence, incidence, and factors predictive of mental ill-health in adults with profound intellectual disabilities. *Journal of Applied Research in Intellectual Disabilities, 20*(6), 493–501. https://doi.org/10.1111/j.1468-3148.2007.00401.x

Cooper, S.-A., Smiley, E., Morrison, J., Williamson, A., & Allan, L. (2007). Mental ill-health in adults with intellectual disabilities: Prevalence and associated factors. *British Journal of Psychiatry, 190*(1), 27–35. https://doi.org/10.1192/bjp.bp.106.022483

Cunningham, E., & O'Neill, R. E. (2000). Comparison of results of functional assessment and analysis methods with young children with autism. *Education and Training in Mental Retardation and Developmental Disabilities, 35*(4), 406–414. Retrieved from www.jstor.org/stable/23879867

Cuomo, B. M., Vaz, S., Lee, E. A. L., Thompson, C., Rogerson, J. M., & Falkmer, T. (2017). Effectiveness of sleep-based interventions for children with autism spectrum disorder: A meta-synthesis. *Pharmacotherapy, 37*(5), 555–578. https://doi.org/10.1002/phar.1920

Davis, T. N., Durand, S., Fuentes, L., Dacus, S., & Blenden, K. (2014). The effects of a school-based functional analysis on subsequent classroom behavior. *Education and Treatment of Children, 37*(1), 95–110. https://doi.org/10.1353/etc.2014.0009

De Knegt, N. C., Pieper, M. J. C., Lobbezoo, F., Schuengel, C., Evenhuis, H. M., Passchier, J., & Scherder, E. J. A. (2013). Behavioral pain indicators in people with intellectual disabilities: A systematic review. *The Journal of Pain, 14*(9), 885–896. https://doi.org/10.1016/j.jpain.2013.04.016

Delemere, E., & Dounavi, K. (2018). Parent-implemented bedtime fading and positive routines for children with autism spectrum disorders. *Journal of Autism and Developmental Disorders, 48*(4), 1002–1019. https://doi.org/10.1007/s10803-017-3398-4

DeLeon, I. G., Fisher, W. W., & Marhefka, J.-M. (2004). Decreasing self-injurious behavior associated with awakening in a child with autism and developmental delays. *Behavioral Interventions, 19*(2), 111–119. https://doi.org/10.1002/bin.154

Deleon, I. G., & Iwata, B. A. (1996). Evaluation of a multiple-stimulus presentation format for assessing reinforcer preferences. *Journal of Applied Behavior Analysis, 29*(4), 519–533. https://doi.org/10.1901/jaba.1996.29-519

DeLeon, I. G., Iwata, B. A., Conners, J., & Wallace, M. D. (1999). Examination of ambiguous stimulus preferences with duration-based measures. *Journal of Applied Behavior Analysis, 32*(1), 111–114. https://doi.org/10.1901/jaba.1999.32-111

Derby, K. M., Wacker, D. P., Sasso, G., Steege, M., Northup, J., Cigrand, K., & Asmus, J. (1992). Brief functional assessment techniques to evaluate aberrant behavior in an outpatient setting: A summary of 79 cases. *Journal of Applied Behavior Analysis, 25*(3), 713–721. https://doi.org/10.1901/jaba.1992.25-713

Dickinson, A. (1985). Actions and habits: The development of behavioural autonomy. *Philosophical Transactions of the Royal Society of London B, 308*, 67–78.

Doody, O., & Bailey, M. E. (2017). Pain and pain assessment in people with intellectual disability: Issues and challenges in practice. *British Journal of Learning Disabilities, 45*(3), 157–165. https://doi.org/10.1111/bld.12189

Dracobly, J. D., Dozier, C. L., Briggs, A. M., & Juanico, J. F. (2018). Reliability and validity of indirect assessment outcomes: Experts versus caregivers. *Learning and Motivation, 62*, 77–90. https://doi.org/10.1016/j.lmot.2017.02.007

Duker, P. C., & Sigafoos, J. (1998). The Motivation Assessment Scale: Reliability and construct validity across three topographies of behavior. *Research in Developmental Disabilities, 19*(2), 131–141. https://doi.org/10.1016/S0891-4222(97)00047-4

Durand, V. M., & Crimmins, D. B. (1988). Identifying the variables maintaining self-injurious behavior. *Journal of Autism and Developmental Disorders, 18*(1), 99–117. https://doi.org/10.1007/BF02211821

Dymond, S. (2019). Overcoming avoidance in anxiety disorders: The contributions of Pavlovian and operant avoidance extinction methods. *Neuroscience and Biobehavioral Reviews, 98*, 61–70. https://doi.org/10.1016/j.neubiorev.2019.01.007

Dymond, S., Dunsmoor, J. E., Vervliet, B., Roche, B., & Hermans, D. (2015). Fear generalization in humans: Systematic review and implications for anxiety disorder research. *Behavior Therapy, 46*(5), 561–582. https://doi.org/10.1016/j.beth.2014.10.001

Falcomata, T. S., Muething, C. S., Roberts, G. J., Hamrick, J., & Shpall, C. (2014). Further evaluation of latency-based brief functional analysis methods: An evaluation of treatment utility. *Developmental Neurorehabilitation, 19*(2), 88–94. https://doi.org/10.3109/17518423.2014.910281

Fisher, W., Piazza, C. C., Bowman, L. G., Hagopian, L. P., Owens, J. C., & Slevin, I. (1992). A comparison of two approaches for identifying reinforcers for persons with severe and profound disabilities. *Journal of Applied Behavior Analysis, 25*(2), 491–498. https://doi.org/10.1901/jaba.1992.25-491

Fisher, W. W., Piazza, C. C., Bowman, L. G., & Amari, A. (1996). Integrating caregiver report with systematic choice assessment to enhance reinforcer identification. *American Journal of Mental Retardation, 101*(1), 15–25.

Freeman, K. A., Walker, M., & Kaufman, J. (2007). Psychometric properties of the Questions About Behavioral Function scale in a child sample. *American Journal on Mental Retardation, 112*(2), 122–129. https://doi.org/10.1352/0895-8017(2007)112[122:PPOTQA]2.0.CO;2

Freeman, N. C., Gray, K. M., Taffe, J. R., & Cornish, K. M. (2015). Development of a new attention rating scale for children with intellectual disability: The Scale of Attention in Intellectual Disability (SAID). *American Journal on Intellectual and Developmental Disabilities, 120*(2), 91–109. https://doi.org/10.1352/1944-7558-120.2.91

Fritz, J. N., Iwata, B. A., Hammond, J. L., & Bloom, S. E. (2013). Experimental analysis of precursors to severe problem behavior. *Journal of Applied Behavior Analysis, 46*(*1*), 101–129. https://doi.org/10.1002/jaba.27

Girolami, P. A., & Scotti, J. R. (2001). Use of analog functional analysis in assessing the function of mealtime behavior problems. *Education and Training in Mental Retardation and Developmental Disabilities, 36*(2), 207–223. Retrieved from www.jstor.org/stable/23879736

Goldiamond, I. (1974). Toward a constructional approach to social problems: Ethical and constitutional issues raised by applied behavior analysis. *Behaviorism, 2*(1), 1–84. Retrieved from http://www.jstor.org/stable/27758809

Greer, B. D., & Kodak, T. (2018). Introduction to the special issue on applied behavior analysis. *Learning and Motivation, 62*, 1–3. https://doi.org/10.1016/j.lmot.2017.03.005

Groskreutz, M. P., Groskreutz, N. C., & Higbee, T. S. (2011). Response competition and stimulus preference in the treatment of automatically reinforced behavior: A comparison. *Journal of Applied Behavior Analysis, 44*(1), 211–215. https://doi.org/10.1901/jaba.2011.44-211

Hagopian, L. P., Rooker, G. W., & Yenokyan, G. (2018). Identifying predictive behavioral markers: A demonstration using automatically reinforced self-injurious behavior. *Journal of Applied Behavior Analysis, 51*(3), 443–465. https://doi.org/10.1002/jaba.477

Hagopian, L. P., Rooker, G. W., & Zarcone, J. R. (2015). Delineating subtypes of self-injurious behavior maintained by automatic reinforcement. *Journal of Applied Behavior Analysis, 48*(3), 523–543. https://doi.org/10.1002/jaba.236

Hagopian, L. P., Rooker, G. W., Zarcone, J. R., Bonner, A. C., & Arevalo, A. R. (2017). Further analysis of subtypes of automatically reinforced SIB: A replication and quantitative analysis of published datasets. *Journal of Applied Behavior Analysis, 50*(1), 48–66. https://doi.org/10.1002/jaba.368

Hall, S. S. (2005). Comparing descriptive, experimental and informant-based assessments of problem behaviors. *Research in Developmental Disabilities, 26*(6), 514–526. https://doi.org/10.1016/j.ridd.2004.11.004

Hall, S. S., Hammond, J. L., & Hustyi, K. M. (2013). Examining the relationship between heart rate and problem behavior: A case study of severe skin picking in Prader-Willi syndrome. *American Journal on Intellectual and Developmental Disabilities, 118*(6), 460–474. https://doi.org/10.1352/1944.7558-118.6.460

Hallett, V., Lecavalier, L., Sukhodolsky, D. G., Cipriano, N., Aman, M. G., McCracken, J. T., … Scahill, L. (2013). Exploring the manifestations of anxiety in children with autism spectrum disorders. *Journal of Autism and Developmental Disorders, 43*(10), 2341–2352. https://doi.org/10.1007/s10803-013-1775-1

Hanley, G. P., Jin, C. S., Vanselow, N. R., & Hanratty, L. A. (2014). Producing meaningful improvements in problem behavior of children with autism via synthesized analyses and treatments. *Journal of Applied Behavior Analysis, 47*(1), 16–36. https://doi.org/10.1002/jaba.106

Hartman, E. C., Gilles, E., McComas, J. J., Danov, S. E., & Symons, F. J. (2008). Clinical observation of self-injurious behavior correlated with changes in scalp morphology in a child with congenital hydrocephalus. *Journal of Child Neurology, 23*(9), 1062–1065. https://doi.org/10.1177/0883073808314155

Hatton, C., & Emerson, E. (2004). The relationship between life events and psychopathology amongst children with intellectual disabilities. *Journal of Applied Research in Intellectual Disabilities, 17*(2), 109–117. https://doi.org/10.1111/j.1360-2322.2004.00188.x

Healy, O., Brett, D., & Leader, G. (2013). A comparison of experimental functional analysis and the Questions About Behavioral Function (QABF) in the assessment of challenging behavior of individuals with autism. *Research in Autism Spectrum Disorders, 7*(1), 66–81. https://doi.org/10.1016/j.rasd.2012.05.006

Hermans, H., van der Pas, F. H., & Evenhuis, H. M. (2011). Instruments assessing anxiety in adults with intellectual disabilities: A systematic review. *Research in Developmental Disabilities, 32(3)*, 861–870. https://doi.org/10.1016/j.ridd.2011.01.034

Hermans, H., Wieland, J., Jelluma, N., Van der Pas, F., & Evenhuis, H. (2013). Reliability and validity of the Dutch version of the Glasgow Anxiety Scale for people with an Intellectual Disability (GAS-ID). *Journal of Intellectual Disability Research, 57*(8), 728–736. https://doi.org/10.1111/j.1365-2788.2012.01632.x

Herr, K., Coyne, P. J., McCaffery, M., Manworren, R., & Merkel, S. (2011). Pain assessment in the patient unable to self-report: Position statement with clinical practice recommendations. *Pain Management Nursing, 12*(4), 230–250. https://doi.org/10.1016/j.pmn.2011.10.002

Hoch, J., Symons, F., & Sng, S. (2013). Sequential analysis of autonomic arousal and self-injurious behavior. *American Journal on Intellectual and Developmental Disabilities, 118*(6), 435–446. https://doi.org/10.1352/1944.7558-118.6.435

Hoffmann, A. N., Sellers, T. P., Halversen, H., & Bloom, S. E. (2018). Implementation of interventions informed by precursor functional analyses with young children: A replication. *Journal of Applied Behavior Analysis, 51*(4), 879–889. https://doi.org/10.1002/jaba.502

Hollins, S., & Esterhuyzen, A. (1997). Bereavement and grief in adults with learning disabilities. *British Journal of Psychiatry, 170*(6), 497–501. https://doi.org/10.1192/bjp.170.6.497

Horner, R. H., Day, H. M., & Day, J. R. (1997). Using neutralizing routines to reduce problem behaviors. *Journal of Applied Behavior Analysis, 30*(4), 601–614. https://doi.org/10.1901/jaba.1997.30-601

Hulbert-Williams, L., Hastings, R., Owen, D. M., Burns, L., Day, J., Mulligan, J., & Noone, S. J. (2014). Exposure to life events as a risk factor for psychological problems in adults with intellectual disabilities: A longitudinal design. *Journal of Intellectual Disability Research, 58*(1), 48–60. https://doi.org/10.1111/jir.12050

Hulbert-Williams, L., & Hastings, R. P. (2008). Life events as a risk factor for psychological problems in individuals with intellectual disabilities: A critical review. *Journal of Intellectual Disability Research, 52*(11), 883–895. https://doi.org/10.1111/j.1365-2788.2008.01110.x

Hunt, A., Goldman, A., Seers, K., Crichton, N., Mastroyannopoulou, K., Moffat, V., … Brady, M. (2004). Clinical validation of the Paediatric Pain Profile. *Developmental Medicine and Child Neurology, 46*(1), 9–18. https://doi.org/10.1017/S0012162204000039

Hunt, A., Wisbeach, A., Seers, K., Goldman, A., Crichton, N., Perry, L., & Mastroyannopoulou, K. (2007). Development of the Paediatric Pain Profile: Role of video analysis and saliva cortisol in validating a tool to assess pain in children with severe neurological disability. *Journal of Pain and Symptom Management, 33*(3), 276–289. https://doi.org/10.1016/j.jpainsymman.2006.08.011

Hyman, P., Oliver, C., & Hall, S. (2002). Self-injurious behavior, self-restraint, and compulsive behaviors in Cornelia de Lange syndrome. *American Journal on Mental Retardation, 107*(2), 146–154+156-157. https://doi.org/10.1352/0895-8017(2002)107<0146:SIBSRA>2.0.CO;2

Iwata, B. A., Deleon, I. G., & Roscoe, E. M. (2013). Reliability and validity of the functional analysis screening tool. *Journal of Applied Behavior Analysis, 46*(1), 271–284. https://doi.org/10.1002/jaba.31

Iwata, B. A., Dorsey, M. F., Slifer, K. J., Bauman, K. E., & Richman, G. S. (1982). Toward a functional analysis of self-injury. *Analysis and Intervention in Developmental Disabilities, 2*, 3–20. https://doi.org/10.1016/0270-4684(82)90003-9

Iwata, B. A., Pace, G. M., Dorsey, M. F., Zarcone, J. R., Vollmer, T. R., Smith, R. G., … Willis, K. D. (1994). The functions of self-injurious behavior: An experimental-epidemiological analysis. *Journal of Applied Behavior Analysis, 27*(2), 215–240. https://doi.org/10.1901/jaba.1994.27-215

Jennett, H., Hagopian, L. P., & Beaulieu, L. (2011). Analysis of heart rate and self-injury with and without restraint in an individual with autism. *Research in Autism Spectrum Disorders, 5*(3), 1110–1118. https://doi.org/10.1016/j.rasd.2010.12.007

Jessel, J., Ingvarsson, E. T., Metras, R., Kirk, H., & Whipple, R. (2018). Achieving socially significant reductions in problem behavior following the interview-informed synthesized contingency analysis: A summary of 25 outpatient applications. *Journal of Applied Behavior Analysis, 51*(1), 130–157. https://doi.org/10.1002/jaba.436

Kahng, S., Hausman, N. L., Fisher, A. B., Donaldson, J. M., Cox, J. R., Lugo, M., & Wiskow, K. M. (2015). The safety of functional analyses of self-injurious behavior. *Journal of Applied Behavior Analysis, 48*(1), 107–114. https://doi.org/10.1002/jaba.168

Kahng, S., Iwata, B. A., Fischer, S. M., Page, T. J., Treadwell, K. R., Williams, D. E., & Smith, R. G. (1998). Temporal distributions of problem behavior based on scatter plot analysis. *Journal of Applied Behavior Analysis, 31*(4), 593–604. https://doi.org/10.1901/jaba.1998.31-593

Kahng, S., Iwata, B. A., Thompson, R. H., & Hanley, G. P. (2000). A method for identifying satiation versus extinction effects under noncontingent reinforcement schedules. *Journal of Applied Behavior Analysis, 33*(4), 419–432. https://doi.org/10.1901/jaba.2000.33-419

Kearney, C. A., Cook, L. C., Chapman, G., & Bensaheb, A. (2006). Exploratory and confirmatory factor analyses of the motivation assessment scale and resident choice assessment scale. *Journal of Developmental and Physical Disabilities, 18*(1), 1–11. https://doi.org/10.1007/s10882-006-9000-1

Kern, L., Sokol, N. G., & Dunlap, G. (2006). Assessment of antecedent influences on challenging behavior. In J. K. Luiselli (Ed.), *Antecedent assessment & intervention* (pp. 53–71). Baltimore, MD: Paul H. Brookes.

Kettering, T. L., Fisher, W. W., Kelley, M. E., & LaRue, R. H. (2018). Sound attenuation and preferred music in the treatment of problem behavior maintained by escape from noise. *Journal of Applied Behavior Analysis, 51*(3), 687–693. https://doi.org/10.1002/jaba.475

Kirkpatrick, B., Louw, J. S., & Leader, G. (2019). Efficacy of parent training incorporated in behavioral sleep interventions for children with autism spectrum disorder and/or intellectual disabilities: A systematic review. *Sleep Medicine, 53*, 141–152. https://doi.org/10.1016/j.sleep.2018.08.034

Kochman, A., Howell, J., Sheridan, M., Kou, M., Ryan, E. E. S., Lee, S., … Yoder, L. (2017). Reliability of the faces, legs, activity, cry, and consolability scale in assessing acute pain in the pediatric emergency department. *Pediatric Emergency Care, 33*(1), 14–17. https://doi.org/10.1097/PEC.0000000000000995

Koegel, R. L., Openden, D., & Koegel, L. K. (2004). A systematic desensitization paradigm to treat hypersensitivity to auditory stimuli in children with autism in family contexts. *Research and Practice for Persons with Severe Disabilities, 29*(2), 122–134. https://doi.org/10.2511/rpsd.29.2.122

Kooij, J. J. S., Bijlenga, D., Salerno, L., Jaeschke, R., Bitter, I., Balázs, J., … Asherson, P. (2019). Updated European consensus statement on diagnosis and treatment of adult ADHD. *European Psychiatry, 56*, 14–34. https://doi.org/10.1016/j.eurpsy.2018.11.001

Koritsas, S., & Iacono, T. (2013). Psychometric comparison of the Motivation Assessment Scale (MAS) and the Questions About Behavioral Function (QABF). *Journal of Intellectual Disability Research, 57*(8), 747–757. https://doi.org/10.1111/jir.12022

Kurtz, P. F., Chin, M. D., Huete, J. M., Tarbox, R. S. F., O'Connor, J. T., Paclawskyj, T. R., & Rush, K. S. (2003). Functional analysis and treatment of self-injurious behavior in young children: A summary of 30 cases. *Journal of Applied Behavior Analysis, 36*(2), 205–219. https://doi.org/10.1901/jaba.2003.36-205

Lamy, M., & Erickson, C. A. (2018). Pharmacological management of behavioral disturbances in children and adolescents with autism spectrum disorders. *Current Problems in Pediatric and Adolescent Health Care, 48*(10), 250–264. https://doi.org/10.1016/j.cppeds.2018.08.015

Lanovaz, M. J., Argumedes, M., Roy, D., Duquette, J. R., & Watkins, N. (2013). Using ABC narrative recording to identify the function of problem behavior: A pilot study. *Research in Developmental Disabilities, 34*(9), 2734–2742. https://doi.org/10.1016/j.ridd.2013.05.038

LaRue, R. H., Lenard, K., Weiss, M. J., Bamond, M., Palmieri, M., & Kelley, M. E. (2010). Comparison of traditional and trial-based methodologies for conducting functional analyses. *Research in Developmental Disabilities, 31*(2), 480–487. https://doi.org/10.1016/j.ridd.2009.10.020

Lecavalier, L., Wood, J. J., Halladay, A. K., Jones, N. E., Aman, M. G., Cook, E. H., … Scahill, L. (2014). Measuring anxiety as a treatment endpoint in youth with autism spectrum disorder. *Journal of Autism and Developmental Disorders, 44*(5), 1128–1143. https://doi.org/10.1007/s10803-013-1974-9

Lerman, D. C., & Iwata, B. A. (1993). Descriptive and experimental analyses of variables maintaining self-injurious behavior. *Journal of Applied Behavior Analysis, 26*(3), 293–319. https://doi.org/10.1901/jaba.1993.26-293

Lewis, T. J., Scott, T. M., & Sugai, G. (1994). The Problem Behavior Questionnaire: A teacher-based instrument to develop functional hypotheses of problem behavior in general education classrooms. *Diagnostique, 19*(2-3), 103–115. https://doi.org/10.1177/073724779401900207

Lotan, M., Ljunggren, E. A., Johnsen, T. B., Defrin, R., Pick, C. G., & Strand, L. I. (2009). A modified version of the Non-Communicating Children Pain Checklist-revised, adapted to adults with intellectual and developmental disabilities: Sensitivity to pain and internal consistency. *The Journal of Pain, 10*(4), 398–407. https://doi.org/10.1016/j.jpain.2008.09.006

Lotan, M., Moe-Nilssen, R., Ljunggren, A. E., & Strand, L. I. (2010). Measurement properties of the Non-Communicating Adult Pain Checklist (NCAPC): A pain scale for adults with intellectual and developmental disabilities, scored in a clinical setting. *Research in Developmental Disabilities, 31*(2), 367–375. https://doi.org/10.1016/j.ridd.2009.10.008

Luiselli, J. K., Cochran, M. L., & Huber, S. A. (2005). Effects of otitis media on a child with autism receiving behavioral intervention for self-injury. *Child and Family Behavior Therapy, 27*(2), 51–56. https://doi.org/10.1300/J019v27n02_05

Lydon, S., Healy, O., & Dwyer, M. (2013). An examination of heart rate during challenging behavior in autism spectrum disorder. *Journal of Developmental and Physical Disabilities, 25*(1), 149–170. https://doi.org/10.1007/s10882-012-9324-y

Malviya, S., Voepel-Lewis, T., Burke, C., Merkel, S., & Tait, A. R. (2006). The revised FLACC observational pain tool: Improved reliability and validity for pain assessment in children with cognitive impairment. *Paediatric Anaesthesia, 16*(3), 258–265. https://doi.org/10.1111/j.1460-9592.2005.01773.x

Manworren, R. C. B., & Stinson, J. (2016). Pediatric pain measurement, assessment, and evaluation. *Seminars in Pediatric Neurology, 23*(3), 189–200. https://doi.org/10.1016/j.spen.2016.10.001

Matson, J. L., Bamburg, J. W., Cherry, K. E., & Paclawskyj, T. R. (1999). A validity study on the Questions About Behavioral Function (QABF) scale: Predicting treatment success for self-injury, aggression, and stereotypies. *Research in Developmental Disabilities, 20*(2), 163–175. https://doi.org/10.1016/S0891-4222(98)00039-0

Matson, J. L., Kuhn, D. E., Dixon, D. R., Mayville, S. B., Laud, R. B., Cooper, C. L., … Matson, M. L. (2003). The development and factor structure of the Functional Assessment for multiple CausaliTy (FACT). *Research in Developmental Disabilities, 24*(6), 485–495. https://doi.org/10.1016/j.ridd.2003.07.001

May, M. E., Sheng, Y., Chitiyo, M., Brandt, R. C., & Howe, A. P. (2014). Internal consistency and inter-rater reliability of the Questions About Behavioral Function (QABF) rating scale when used by teachers and paraprofessionals. *Education and Treatment of Children, 37*(2), 347–364. https://doi.org/10.1353/etc.2014.0013

McAtee, M., Carr, E. G., & Schulte, C. (2004). A contextual assessment inventory for problem behavior: Initial development. *Journal of Positive Behavior Interventions, 6*(3), 148–165. https://doi.org/10.1177/10983007040060030301

Miltenberger, R. G. (2001). *Behavior modification: principles and procedures* (2nd ed.). Belmont, CA: Wadsworth/Thomson Learning.

Moskowitz, L. J., Mulder, E., Walsh, C. E., McLaughlin, D. M., Zarcone, J. R., Proudfit, G. H., & Carr, E. G. (2013). A multimethod assessment of anxiety and problem behavior in children with autism spectrum disorders and intellectual disability. *American Journal on Intellectual and Developmental Disabilities, 118*(6), 419–434. https://doi.org/10.1352/1944.7558.118.6.419

Muething, C. S., Call, N. A., Lomas Mevers, J., Zangrillo, A. N., Clark, S. B., & Reavis, A. R. (2017). Correspondence between the results of functional analyses and brief functional analyses. *Developmental Neurorehabilitation, 20*(8), 549–559. https://doi.org/10.1080/17518423.2017.1338776

Neef, N. A., & Peterson, S. M. (2007). Functional behavior assessment. In J. O. Cooper, T. E. Heron, & W. L. Heward (Eds.), *Applied behavior analysis* (2nd ed., pp. 500–524). Upper Saddle River, NJ: Pearson.

Newton, J. T., & Sturmey, P. (1991). The Motivation Assessment Scale: Inter-rater reliability and internal consistency in a British sample. *Journal of Mental Deficiency Research, 35*(5), 472–474. https://doi.org/10.1111/j.1365-2788.1991.tb00429.x

Nicholson, J., Konstantinidi, E., & Furniss, F. (2006). On some psychometric properties of the Questions About Behavioral Function (QABF) scale. *Research in Developmental Disabilities, 27*(3), 337–352. https://doi.org/10.1016/j.ridd.2005.04.001

Nuske, H. J., Finkel, E., Hedley, D., Parma, V., Tomczuk, L., Pellecchia, M., ... Dissanayake, C. (2019). Heart rate increase predicts challenging behavior episodes in preschoolers with autism. *Stress, 22*(3), 303–311. https://doi.org/10.1080/10253890.2019.1572744

O'Dwyer, C., McCallion, P., Burke, É., Carroll, R., O'Dwyer, M., & McCarron, M. (2018). Prevalence and associated factors of challenging behaviours among older adults with intellectual disabilities in Ireland. *Research in Developmental Disabilities, 80*, 192–204. https://doi.org/10.1016/j.ridd.2018.05.007

O'Neill, R. E., Albin, R. W., Storey, K., Horner, R. H., & Sprague, J. R. (2015). *Functional assessment and program development for problem behavior: a practical handbook* (3rd ed.). Stamford, CT: Cengage Learning.

O'Reilly, M. F. (1995). Functional analysis and treatment of escape-maintained aggression correlated with sleep deprivation. *Journal of Applied Behavior Analysis, 28*(2), 225–226. https://doi.org/10.1901/jaba.1995.28-225

O'Reilly, M. F. (1997). Functional analysis of episodic self-injury correlated with recurrent otitis media. *Journal of Applied Behavior Analysis, 30*(1), 165–167. https://doi.org/10.1901/jaba.1997.30-165

Owen, D. M., Hastings, R. P., Noone, S. J., Chinn, J., Harman, K., Roberts, J., & Taylor, K. (2004). Life events as correlates of problem behavior and mental health in a residential population of adults with developmental disabilities. *Research in Developmental Disabilities, 25*(4), 309–320. https://doi.org/10.1016/j.ridd.2004.01.003

Paclawskyj, T. R., Matson, J. L., Rush, K. S., Smalls, Y., & Vollmer, T. R. (2000). Questions About Behavioral Function (QABF): A behavioral checklist for functional assessment of aberrant behavior. *Research in Developmental Disabilities, 21*(3), 223–229. https://doi.org/10.1016/S0891-4222(00)00036-6

Paclawskyj, T. R., Matson, J. L., Rush, K. S., Smalls, Y., & Vollmer, T. R. (2001). Assessment of the convergent validity of the Questions About Behavioral Function scale with analogue functional analysis and the Motivation Assessment Scale. *Journal of Intellectual Disability Research, 45*(6), 484–494. https://doi.org/10.1046/j.1365-2788.2001.00364.x

Pary, R. J., & Khan, S. (2002). Cyclic behaviors in persons with developmental disabilities: Are cluster and migraine headaches being overlooked? *Mental Health Aspects of Developmental Disabilities, 5*(4), 125–129. Retrieved from https://www.mh-idd.com/journal

Petty, J. L., Bacarese-Hamilton, M., Davies, L. E., & Oliver, C. (2014). Correlates of self-injurious, aggressive and destructive behaviour in children under five who are at risk of developmental delay. *Research in Developmental Disabilities, 35*(1), 36–45. https://doi.org/10.1016/j.ridd.2013.10.019

Posey, D. J., Erickson, C. A., Stigler, K. A., & McDougle, C. J. (2006). The use of selective serotonin reuptake inhibitors in autism and related disorders. *Journal of Child and Adolescent Psychopharmacology, 16*(1-2), 181–186. https://doi.org/10.1089/cap.2006.16.181

Reese, R. M., Richman, D. M., Belmont, J. M., & Morse, P. (2005). Functional characteristics of disruptive behavior in developmentally disabled children with and without autism. *Journal of Autism and Developmental Disorders, 35*(4), 419–428. https://doi.org/10.1007/s10803-005-5032-0

Richman, D. M., Barnard-Brak, L., Grubb, L., Bosch, A., & Abby, L. (2015). Meta-analysis of noncontingent reinforcement effects on problem behavior. *Journal of Applied Behavior Analysis, 48*(1), 131–152. https://doi.org/10.1002/jaba.189

Richman, D. M., & Hagopian, L. P. (1999). On the effects of "quality" of attention in the functional analysis of destructive behavior. *Research in Developmental Disabilities, 20*(1), 51–62. https://doi.org/10.1016/S0891-4222(98)00031-6

Ringdahl, J. E., & Sellers, J. A. (2000). The effects of different adults as therapists during functional analyses. *Journal of Applied Behavior Analysis, 33*(2), 247–250. https://doi.org/10.1901/jaba.2000.33-247

Ringdahl, J. E., Vollmer, T. R., Marcus, B. A., & Roane, H. S. (1997). An analogue evaluation of environmental enrichment: The role of stimulus preference. *Journal of Applied Behavior Analysis, 30*(2), 203–216. https://doi.org/10.1901/jaba.1997.30-203

Roane, H. S., Vollmer, T. R., Ringdahl, J. E., & Marcus, B. A. (1998). Evaluation of a brief stimulus preference assessment. *Journal of Applied Behavior Analysis, 31*(4), 605–620. https://doi.org/10.1901/jaba.1998.31-605

Rojahn, J., Schroeder, S. R., & Hoch, T. A. (2008). *Self-injurious behavior in intellectual disabilities*. Amsterdam: Elsevier.

Roscoe, E. M., Iwata, B. A., & Rand, M. S. (2003). Effects of reinforcer consumption and magnitude on response rates during noncontingent reinforcement. *Journal of Applied Behavior Analysis, 36*(4), 525–539. https://doi.org/10.1901/jaba.2003.36-525

Roscoe, E. M., Schlichenmeyer, K. J., & Dube, W. V. (2015). Functional analysis of problem behavior: A systematic approach for identifying idiosyncratic variables. *Journal of Applied Behavior Analysis, 48*(2), 289–314. https://doi.org/10.1002/jaba.201

Sanberg, S. A., Kuhn, B. R., & Kennedy, A. E. (2018). Outcomes of a behavioral intervention for sleep disturbances in children with autism spectrum disorder. *Journal of Autism and Developmental Disorders, 48*(12), 4250–4277. https://doi.org/10.1007/s10803-018-3644-4

Sequeira, H., Howlin, P., & Hollins, S. (2003). Psychological disturbance associated with sexual abuse in people with learning disabilities. *British Journal of Psychiatry, 183*(5), 451–456. https://doi.org/10.1192/bjp.183.5.451

Shabani, D. B., Carr, J. E., Pabico, R. S., Sala, A. P., Lam, W. Y., & Oberg, T. L. (2013). The effects of functional analysis test sessions on subsequent rates of problem behavior in the natural environment. *Behavioral Interventions, 28*(1), 40–47. https://doi.org/10.1002/bin.1352

Shanahan, P. J., Palod, S., Smith, K. J., Fife-Schaw, C., & Mirza, N. (2019). Interventions for sleep difficulties in adults with an intellectual disability: A systematic review. *Journal of Intellectual Disability Research, 63*(5), 372–385. https://doi.org/10.1111/jir.12587

Shogren, K. A., & Rojahn, J. (2003). Convergent reliability and validity of the Questions About Behavioral Function and the Motivation Assessment Scale: A replication study. *Journal of Developmental and Physical Disabilities, 15*(4), 367–375. https://doi.org/10.1023/A:1026314316977

Shore, B. A., Iwata, B. A., DeLeon, I. G., Kahng, S. W., & Smith, R. G. (1997). An analysis of reinforcer substitutability using object manipulation and self-injury as competing responses. *Journal of Applied Behavior Analysis, 30*(1), 21–41. https://doi.org/10.1901/jaba.1997.30-21

Sigafoos, J., Kerr, M., & Roberts, D. (1994). Interrater reliability of the Motivation Assessment Scale: Failure to replicate with aggressive behavior. *Research in Developmental Disabilities, 15*(5), 333–342. https://doi.org/10.1016/0891-4222(94)90020-5

Simó-Pinatella, D., Alomar-Kurz, E., Font-Roura, J., Giné, C., Matson, J. L., & Cifre, I. (2013). Questions About Behavioral Function (QABF): Adaptation and validation of the Spanish version. *Research in Developmental Disabilities, 34*(4), 1248–1255. https://doi.org/10.1016/j.ridd.2013.01.015

Simpson, N., Mizen, L., & Cooper, S.-A. (2016). Intellectual disabilities. *Medicine (United Kingdom), 44*(11), 679–682. https://doi.org/10.1016/j.mpmed.2016.08.008

Singh, A. N., Matson, J. L., Mouttapa, M., Pella, R. D., Hill, B. D., & Thorson, R. (2009). A critical item analysis of the QABF: Development of a short form assessment instrument. *Research in Developmental Disabilities, 30*(4), 782–792. https://doi.org/10.1016/j.ridd.2008.11.001

Smiley, E., Cooper, S., Finlayson, J., Jackson, A., Allan, L., Mantry, D., … Morrison, J. (2007). Incidence and predictors of mental ill-health in adults with intellectual disabilities. Prospective study. *British Journal of Psychiatry, 191*(4), 313–319. https://doi.org/10.1192/bjp.bp.106.031104

Smith, C. E., Carr, E. G., & Moskowitz, L. J. (2016). Fatigue as a biological setting event for severe problem behavior in autism spectrum disorder. *Research in Autism Spectrum Disorders, 23*, 131–144. https://doi.org/10.1016/j.rasd.2015.12.003

Smith, C. M., Smith, R. G., Dracobly, J. D., & Pace, A. P. (2012). Multiple-respondent anecdotal assessments: An analysis of interrater agreement and correspondence with analogue assessment outcomes. *Journal of Applied Behavior Analysis, 45*(4), 779–795. https://doi.org/10.1901/jaba.2012.45-779

Spreat, S., & Connelly, L. (1996). Reliability analysis of the Motivation Assessment Scale. *American Journal on Mental Retardation, 100*(5), 528–532.

Symons, F. J., Byiers, B., Tervo, R. C., & Beisang, A. (2013). Parent-reported pain in Rett syndrome. *Clinical Journal of Pain, 29*(8), 744–746. https://doi.org/10.1097/AJP.0b013e318274b6bd

Tarbox, J., Wilke, A. E., Najdowski, A. C., Findel-Pyles, R. S., Balasanyan, S., Caveney, A. C., … Tia, B. (2009). Comparing indirect, descriptive, and experimental functional assessments of challenging behavior in children with autism. *Journal of Developmental and Physical Disabilities, 21*(6), 493–514. https://doi.org/10.1007/s10882-009-9154-8

Taylor, L., Oliver, C., & Murphy, G. (2011). The chronicity of self-injurious behaviour: A long-term follow-up of a total population study. *Journal of Applied Research in Intellectual Disabilities, 24*(2), 105–117. https://doi.org/10.1111/j.1468-3148.2010.00579.x

Thompson, R. H., & Iwata, B. A. (2007). A comparison of outcomes from descriptive and functional analyses of problem behavior. *Journal of Applied Behavior Analysis, 40*(2), 333–338. https://doi.org/10.1901/jaba.2007.56-06

Tomlin, M., & Reed, P. (2012). Effects of fixed-time reinforcement delivered by teachers for reducing problem behavior in special education classrooms. *Journal of Behavioral Education, 21*(2), 150–162. https://doi.org/10.1007/s10864-012-9147-z

Toogood, S., & Timlin, K. (1996). The functional assessment of challenging behaviour: A comparison of informant-based, experimental and descriptive methods. *Journal of Applied Research in Intellectual Disabilities, 9*(3), 206–222. https://doi.org/10.1111/j.1468-3148.1996.tb00110.x

Touchette, P. E., MacDonald, R. F., & Langer, S. N. (1985). A scatter plot for identifying stimulus control of problem behavior. *Journal of Applied Behavior Analysis, 18*(4), 343–351. https://doi.org/10.1901/jaba.1985.18-343

Van de Wouw, E., Evenhuis, H. M., & Echteld, M. A. (2012). Prevalence, associated factors and treatment of sleep problems in adults with intellectual disability: A systematic review. *Research in Developmental Disabilities, 33*(4), 1310–1332. https://doi.org/10.1016/j.ridd.2012.03.003

Vervoort-Schel, J., Mercera, G., Wissink, I., Mink, E., van der Helm, P., Lindauer, R., & Moonen, X. (2018). Adverse childhood experiences in children with intellectual disabilities: An exploratory case-file study in Dutch residential care. *International Journal of Environmental Research and Public Health, 15*(10), E2136. https://doi.org/10.3390/ijerph15102136

Vessells, J., Sy, J. R., Wilson, A., & Green, L. (2018). Effects of delay fading and signals on self-control choices by children. *Journal of Applied Behavior Analysis, 51*(2), 374–381. https://doi.org/10.1002/jaba.454

Vigneau, F., & Cormier, S. (2008). The factor structure of the State-Trait Anxiety Inventory: An alternative view. *Journal of Personality Assessment, 90*(3), 280–285. https://doi.org/10.1080/00223890701885027

Virues-Ortega, J., Segui-Duran, D., Descalzo-Quero, A., Carnerero, J. J., & Martin, N. (2011). Caregivers' agreement and validity of indirect functional analysis: A cross cultural evaluation across multiple problem behavior topographies. *Journal of Autism and Developmental Disorders, 41*(1), 82–91. https://doi.org/10.1007/s10803-010-1022-y

Vollmer, T. R., Marcus, B. A., & Ringdahl, J. E. (1995). Noncontingent escape as treatment for self-injurious behavior maintained by negative reinforcement. *Journal of Applied Behavior Analysis, 28*(1), 15–26. https://doi.org/10.1901/jaba.1995.28-15

Vollmer, T. R., & Matson, J. L. (1995). *User's guide: Questions about behavioral function (QABF)*. Baton Rouge, LA: Scientific Publishers.

Vollmer, T. R., & Smith, R. G. (1996). Some current themes in functional analysis research. *Research in Developmental Disabilities, 17*(3), 229–249. https://doi.org/10.1016/0891-4222(96)00006-6

Wacker, D. P., Berg, W. K., Cooper, L. J., Derby, K. M., Steege, M. W., Northup, J., & Sasso, G. (1994). The impact of functional analysis methodology on outpatient clinic services. *Journal of Applied Behavior Analysis, 27*(2), 405–407. https://doi.org/10.1901/jaba.1994.27-405

Wallace, M. D., Vega, C. M., & Hernandez, A. (2015). Translating the QABF to Spanish with an eye toward reliability and validity. *Behavioral Interventions, 30*(1), 65–72. https://doi.org/10.1002/bin.1397

Weeden, M., Mahoney, A., & Poling, A. (2010). Self-injurious behavior and functional analysis: Where are the descriptions of participant protections? *Research in Developmental Disabilities, 31*(2), 299–303. https://doi.org/10.1016/j.ridd.2009.09.016

Zaja, R. H., Moore, L., Van Ingen, D. J., & Rojahn, J. (2011). Psychometric comparison of the functional assessment instruments QABF, FACT and FAST for self-injurious, stereotypic and aggressive/destructive behaviour. *Journal of Applied Research in Intellectual Disabilities, 24*(1), 18–28. https://doi.org/10.1111/j.1468-3148.2010.00569.x

Zarcone, J. R., Rodgers, T. A., Iwata, B. A., Rourke, D. A., & Dorsey, M. F. (1991). Reliability analysis of the Motivation Assessment Scale: A failure to replicate. *Research in Developmental Disabilities, 12*(4), 349–360. https://doi.org/10.1016/0891-4222(91)90031-M

Chapter 6
Intervention with Self-Injurious Behavior

6.1 Individualizing Intervention for Self-Injurious Behavior

Despite the fact that longitudinal studies, especially in childhood, suggest that substantial proportions of people who engage in self-injurious behavior (SIB) have ceased to do so at a later time (see Chap. 2), the literature on interventions for SIB suggests that for any individual, the probability of an intervention succeeding is difficult to predict. There is general agreement that the limitations of our current understanding of the biological processes involved in SIB, together with the relative paucity of relevant randomized controlled trials, severely limit the possibility of rational pharmacological therapy for both children and adults with intellectual disabilities (IDs) and/or autism spectrum conditions (ASCs) (Farmer & Aman, 2013; Gormez, Rana, & Varghese, 2014; McQuire, Hassiotis, Harrison, & Pilling, 2015, 2016; Sawyer, Lake, Lunsky, Liu, & Desarkar, 2014). Behavioral interventions are often reported to be highly effective when used under controlled conditions, but with little data regarding generalization and maintenance of effects (Chezan, Gable, McWhorter, & White, 2017; Gregori, Rispoli, Gerow, & Lory, 2018). Additionally, it is often asserted that for a substantial minority of people who engage in SIB, behavioral interventions are of limited or no benefit (Rojahn, Schroeder, & Hoch, 2008). Recommended algorithms and pathways for intervention with people engaging in SIB often suggest beginning with a functional behavioral assessment, proceeding to behavioral intervention based on such assessment, and considering pharmacological intervention only if behavioral intervention proves to be minimally effective or ineffective (Minshawi, Hurwitz, Morriss, & McDougle, 2015). Further, there is a perception that psychotropic medications are overused with people with IDs and ASCs, and policy initiatives are underway to ensure that such medications are used only where appropriate (Royal College of Psychiatrists Faculty of Psychiatry of Intellectual Disability, n.d.; Mehta & Glover, 2019). There is also acceptance however that in clinical practice, behavioral and pharmacological

F. Furniss, A. B. Biswas, *Self-Injurious Behavior in Individuals with Neurodevelopmental Conditions*, Autism and Child Psychopathology Series,
https://doi.org/10.1007/978-3-030-36016-0_6

interventions are often implemented with relatively limited communication between the professionals involved (Minshawi et al., 2015).

Undoubtedly, one factor contributing to this situation is the lack of data on personal characteristics associated with differential outcomes in response to currently available interventions. Research into behavioral interventions has perhaps particularly neglected this topic, possibly because it has been assumed that a careful functional analysis provides a sufficient basis for individualizing treatment to the needs of the individual engaging in SIB. This situation possibly parallels that seen in general medicine, in which the concept of "personalized medicine," which emphasized the tailoring of treatments to the needs of individualized patients, was seen by some as a simple restatement of good clinical practice and has now been superseded by the framework of "precision medicine" (König, Fuchs, Hansen, von Mutius, & Kopp, 2017). Although precision medicine has been variously defined, it is generally conceptualized as using the integration of clinical and other data to enable "stratification" of individuals on the basis of genetic, biomarker, phenotypic, or psychosocial characteristics to predict differential individual risk of disease and probability of response to treatment among people who present with apparently similar clinical problems (König et al., 2017). To date, few attempts have been made to take such a "precision medicine" approach to intervention with SIB. In one pioneering attempt, Mace and Mauk (1995) suggested that SIB could be differentiated into operant SIB and four subtypes of "possibly biologic" SIB, distinguishable by clinical presentation, and hypothesized to be related to impairments in specific neurotransmitter systems and hence potentially treatable using different pharmacological agents. Mace and Mauk (1995) suggested that severe self-inflicted tissue damage suggested possible disturbance of the opioid system, with naltrexone a possible candidate for initial pharmacological intervention, while repetitive or stereotypic SIB suggested dysfunction in dopaminergic pathways, with a trial of low-dose atypical antipsychotics a logical first step in psychopharmacological intervention. Mace and Mauk (1995) suggested two further "biologic" subtypes of SIB, "high rate with agitation when interrupted" and "SIB co-occurring with agitation," for which they proposed use of selective serotonin reuptake inhibitors (SSRIs) and propranolol or mood stabilizers, respectively. Despite the face validity of Mace and Mauk's subtyping of "biologic" SIB, there are however no well-controlled studies demonstrating selective impact of specific agents on specific subtypes of SIB, and improved methods for stratification of cases involving SIB remain an important goal for research (Thompson & Symons, 1999). Despite the paucity of relevant evidence, several researchers have however suggested that each of four types of characteristic (genetic, biomarker, phenotypic, or psychosocial) may be related to differential responses to interventions for people engaging in SIB. As was noted in Chap. 3, people with Lesch-Nyhan syndrome have been reported to show "paradoxical" worsening of SIB in response to attempts to reduce the behavior using contingent electric shock punishment (Olson & Houlihan, 2000), although no mechanism has been proposed as underpinning this phenomenon. With respect to biomarkers, signs of dysregulation of the hypothalamic-pituitary-adrenal stress system have been proposed as a possible biomarker for positive response to treatment with naltrexone, with recent interest in the pro-opiomelanocortin (POMC) system (Sandman & Kemp, 2011). The POMC molecule, which in humans is produced mainly in the anterior pituitary, undergoes enzyme cleavage producing a number of biologically active products including the opioid peptide β-endorphin and the peptide hormone adrenocorticotrophin (ACTH). These products of POMC are normally released together by the pituitary in response to stress, and in adults plasma levels of the two products are normally highly correlated. Studies have suggested however that this normal "coupling" of β-endorphin and ACTH is reduced following episodes of SIB in adults with developmental disabilities (Sandman, Touchette, Lenjavi, Marion, & Chicz-DeMet, 2003), with levels of β-endorphin elevated with respect to levels of ACTH. Elevation of β-endorphin levels relative to ACTH in measurements taken in the morning (not directly related to an episode of SIB) is also related to the extent to which occurrence of SIB shows a "contagious" pattern in which SIB is strongly predicted by previous SIB events (Sandman, Touchette, Marion, & Chicz-Demet, 2008; Sandman, Touchette, Marion, Lenjavi, & Chicz-Demet, 2002). Subsequent studies of response to naltrexone revealed a complex pattern of results in which higher basal levels of β-endorphin relative to ACTH and elevation of β-endorphin levels following episodes of SIB were associated with different patterns of response to treatment with naltrexone. Elevation of β-endorphin levels following episodes of SIB was associated with greater disruption of "contagious" SIB following naltrexone treatment, i.e., reduced probability that one episode of SIB would lead to another. Higher basal levels of β-endorphin were not directly associated with this effect of naltrexone, but did strengthen the relationship between post-SIB elevation of β-endorphin and response to naltrexone (Sandman et al., 2008). Further study of the long-term effects of naltrexone treatment however suggested that higher basal levels of β-endorphin relative to ACTH might indeed predict better response to longer-term treatment with low doses of naltrexone (Sandman & Kemp, 2011).

With regard to phenotypic predictors of response to treatment, the distinction between "impulsive" and "compulsive" types of SIB has been supported by factor analytic studies (Bodfish & Lewis, 2002), and Aman, Buitelaar, De Smedt, Wapenaar, and Binder (2005) suggested that risperidone may be useful primarily in treatment of "impulsive" rather than "compulsive" forms of SIB. Finally, with regard to "stratification" on the basis of psychosocial characteristics, Hagopian, Rooker, and Yenokyan (2018) have proposed that patterns of responding in experimental functional analyses (EFAs: see Chap. 5) can be used as "predictive behavioral markers," with high levels of SIB in the "alone" condition of an EFA relative to the "play" condition predictive of positive response, and high and variable levels of SIB across all EFA conditions predictive of negative response, to purely reinforcement-based interventions.

Although the evidence for each of these suggestions is currently limited, it is apparent that there are points of convergence between these proposals regarding stratification of cases of SIB, summarized in Table 6.1 together with the stages/subtypes of SIB outlined in Chaps. 3 and 5 of this volume.

Consistent with the proposal that these subtypes represent stages in the development of SIB, the points of divergence between these proposals mainly concern their

Table 6.1 Convergence of proposals for stratification of cases of SIB

Mace and Mauk (1995)	Aman et al. (2005)	Hagopian et al. (2018)	Present proposal
			Emergent SIB
Operant SIB		Socially reinforced SIB and automatically reinforced SIB Subtype 1	Operant (goal-directed) SIB
	Impulsive SIB		Habitual/ impulsive (S-R) SIB
		Automatically reinforced SIB Subtype 2	Generalized impulsive SIB
Stereotyped SIB			Stereotyped SIB
High rate SIB with agitation when interrupted	Compulsive SIB	Automatically reinforced SIB Subtype 3	Compulsive SIB
SIB co-occurring with agitation			

range (e.g., Aman et al., 2005, were concerned only with possible subtypes of response to risperidone) and the number of subtypes proposed together with the boundaries between them. Each of these proposals however suggests that specific phenotypic characters and/or predictive behavioral markers can be used to guide the initial approach to intervention. Consideration of the subtypes as stages in the development of SIB implies however that interventions indicated for more than one "subtype" may be indicated for some individuals. In the remainder of this chapter, we will review the evidence base for interventions within the framework described in Chap. 3 together with its associated terminology.

6.2 Intervention with "Emergent" Self-Injurious Behavior

The early age at which SIB emerges, together with the relatively early age at which operant functions are acquired in many cases (see Chap. 2), makes it rather unlikely that specialist clinicians will see many children presenting with "emergent" SIB which has yet to acquire operant functions. Such cases may however be seen among children diagnosed at a very young age with one of the neurodevelopmental conditions (NDCs) known to be associated with particularly high risk for SIB. No study on the persistence of SIB in very young children has yet differentiated outcomes for those whose SIB does and does not appear to be operant in nature. It is however known that approximately 40–50% of young children with IDs and/or ASCs who do engage in SIB will later cease to do so (Baghdadli et al., 2008; Chadwick, Kusel, Cuddy, & Taylor, 2005; Davies & Oliver, 2016; Dimian et al., 2017). Whether SIB in such cases has already acquired operant functions or has yet to do so, energetic intervention with young children who engage in SIB therefore has a high probability of success.

Where SIB has acquired operant functions, intervention using the approaches described in Sect. 6.3 below is obviously indicated, and behavioral methods of intervention for challenging behaviors have been widely and successfully used (Durand & Moskowitz, 2015; Lang et al., 2013). If however assessment suggests that behaviors have yet to acquire operant functions, functional assessment will still identify contexts and specific situations (e.g., transitions) and stimuli which elicit SIB. Further assessment should have also evaluated the child's communication, self-help, and coping skills relevant to overcoming the frustrations which they are experiencing in these situations. Behavioral intervention in such cases will focus on helping the child to develop and apply the necessary skills. In many cases these will be communication skills required, for example, to request adult assistance or indicate disagreement with adult requests, and in such cases interventions such as functional communication training (FCT: see Sect. 6.3.4 below) will be applicable. Such interventions will simultaneously provide the child with a constructive means of dealing with difficult situations and minimize the probability of SIB acquiring operant functions. In some situations however, developing the child's independent self-help skills may be preferable to teaching them to request adult assistance. Children may engage in SIB when they are passively washed, dressed, or have their teeth cleaned or hair brushed, by adults. Behavioral skill-teaching methods, such as prompting and physical guidance, prompt fading, and reinforcement contingent on completion of self-care task steps, can be used to build independence skills and reduce SIB and other challenging behaviors (Roberts, Mace, & Daggett, 1995).

Particularly for children with ASCs, there is now a considerable body of research documenting the effects of both early intensive behavioral intervention (EIBI) and a variety of parent-training interventions, on children's development in various developmental domains. Recent meta-analyses suggest that EIBI is moderately to very effective in improving various aspects of communication skills, moderately effective in improving socialization skills, and of low effectiveness in improving daily living skills (Makrygianni, Gena, Katoudi, & Galanis, 2018). Parent training interventions on the other hand have a small positive effect on socialization skills and a statistically significant but very small effect in improving communication skills (Nevill, Lecavalier, & Stratis, 2018). Despite substantial interest in the potential for behavioral interventions to prevent the development of SIB and other behavioral difficulties (e.g., McGill, 1999), there is however very little empirical work investigating the effects of such intervention. Luczynski and Hanley (2013) provided a potential model for such research in a study involving young children (without NDCs) who were considered to be at risk for development of challenging behaviors. Two groups of six children (one with mean age 4.8 years and one with mean age 3.4 years) were each split into two groups of three, matched on teachers' levels of concern regarding their behavior and communication. One older and one younger group of three children participated in activity sessions in class of 15–30-min duration, four or five times a week, in which they were taught skills for requesting adult attention, requesting materials, and tolerating situations in which adults denied or delayed responding to their requests. Sessions were continued until the children reached preset criteria for demonstrating acquisition of these skills, with the younger group participating in over 80 training sessions. The other two groups also participated in sessions, but in these strenuous attempts were made to ensure that the children had access to adult attention and play/activity materials at all times. Before and after the intervention, both groups were tested in situations in which access to materials was periodically limited, adult attention diverted, and requests from the children either denied or responded to in delayed fashion; in these sessions adults responded to both challenging behaviors (including aggression) and appropriate communicative requests. Pre-intervention, the six children who later participated in communication training engaged in challenging behavior on significantly more trials than the control group. Post-intervention however the group who had learned communication and delay tolerance skills never engaged in challenging behavior, whereas children from the control group engaged in challenging behavior on a much higher proportion of trials than originally.

A possible model for parent training interventions was provided by Fodstad, Kirsch, Faidley, and Bauer (2018), who evaluated such an intervention with the families of 11 children with IDs, who were 1–5 years of age and had engaged in SIB for at least 2 months at the time of initial evaluation. The training comprised 11 individual sessions of 60–90 min, with direct instruction, use of video examples, practice exercises, role-play with feedback, and collaborative development of function-based interventions for the child's SIB which parents implemented as "homework." Topics covered included antecedent interventions, use of reinforcement and extinction, functional communication skills, communicating clear expectations and encouraging cooperation with parental requests, skill development, and strategies for generalization. Although the purpose of Fodstad et al.'s (2018) study was primarily to evaluate the feasibility and acceptability to parents of the intervention, and no control group was employed, significant pre- to post-training reductions were found on parent-rated severity of SIB and in child challenging behavior (including but not limited to SIB) during brief observations.

Intervention with emergent SIB and the long-term effects of such intervention are clearly issues requiring much more attention. The studies of Luczynski and Hanley (2013) and Fodstad et al. (2018) however provide hope that both structured therapist-led intervention in educational settings and parent training interventions in outpatient settings may be able to produce meaningful change at this critical early stage in the evolution of SIB.

6.3 Intervention with Operant/Goal-Directed Self-Injurious Behavior

6.3.1 Basic Principles of Behavioral Intervention

In Chaps. 3 and 5, we defined operant or goal-directed SIB as being characterized either by the identification of an external source of reinforcement for the behavior through an experimental functional analysis (EFA: see Chap. 5) or by responsiveness of the behavior to a trial of "noncontingent reinforcement" (NCR: see Chap. 5) using a reinforcer hypothesized to maintain SIB following a functional assessment of the behavior. Intervention using the methods of applied behavior analysis is clearly the appropriate intervention in such cases (Hagopian et al., 2018; Mace & Mauk, 1995). Historically, behavioral interventions such as that described in the pioneering study of Wolf, Risley, and Mees (1963), described in Chap. 1, proceeded from the assumption that some form of reinforcement, probably socially mediated, must be maintaining SIB and that making "time-out" from all possible sources of socially mediated reinforcement contingent on the behavior should reduce it. Concerns that such interventions reduced SIB without developing more appropriate behaviors however led to a rapid shift in emphasis toward intervention procedures aimed primarily at strengthening socially valued behaviors in the hope that these would effectively compete with and reduce SIB. Such differential reinforcement approaches included differential reinforcement of other behavior (DRO), in which reinforcement is provided contingent on the absence or omission of SIB; differential reinforcement of alternative behavior (DRA), in which reinforcement is delivered contingent on the occurrence of a specified alternative behavior to SIB; and differential reinforcement of incompatible behavior (DRI) in which reinforcement is delivered contingent on the occurrence of a behavior which is physically incompatible with the person's SIB (e.g., playing with a toy or performing a task requiring simultaneous use of both hands for SIB comprising head-hitting). Early applications of differential reinforcement approaches used reinforcers chosen empirically without reference to the consequences presumed to be maintaining the challenging behavior. Differential reinforcement treatments continue to have a role in behavioral intervention with SIB, and their use will be discussed further in the section on intervention with habitual/impulsive SIB below. Behavioral approaches to intervention with SIB were however dramatically influenced by a seminal paper by Carr (1977), who reviewed evidence suggesting that SIB could be maintained by a variety of consequences in different individuals and argued that treatment should therefore be individualized with respect to the function of the behavior. The EFA method first described by Iwata, Dorsey, Slifer, Bauman, and Richman (1982) provided the foundation for the widespread application of this principle. In a review of a case series involving use of EFA in 152 cases of SIB in persons with developmental disabilities, Iwata et al. (1994) reported that social-negative reinforcement (e.g., escape from task demands) maintained SIB in 38.1% of the sample, social-positive reinforcement (e.g., securing attention from carers) maintained SIB for 26.3%, automatic (sensory) reinforcement accounted for 25.7%, and for 5.3% of cases SIB was found to be maintained by multiple controlling variables.

There are two principal methods of behavioral intervention in cases involving operant SIB. The first is modification of motivating operations (MOs: Michael, 2000) in order to devalue the reinforcing value of the events which have previously reinforced SIB and/or reduce their ability to evoke SIB. The second is teaching (and/or increasing the density of reinforcement for) alternative more adaptive behaviors which compete with SIB for the reinforcer(s) which have previously maintained the SIB. Success with the second type of intervention often also requires increasing the effort involved in SIB and/or reducing or eliminating reinforcement of the behavior in order to ensure that the alternative prosocial behavior is more efficient than SIB in obtaining reinforcement (Iwata, Roscoe, Zarcone, & Richman, 2002). Each of these intervention methods has been applied with people whose SIB has been maintained by each of the sources of reinforcement (social-positive, social-negative, and automatic) identified as commonly maintaining SIB by Iwata et al. (1994). In the following sections of this chapter, we illustrate by examples how each broad intervention strategy has been applied in cases where SIB has been identified as maintained by each type of reinforcement and then discuss some of the difficulties and potential adverse side effects of these interventions and how these may be minimized.

6.3.2 Reducing Operant Self-Injurious Behavior by Modifying Motivating Operations and/or People's Exposure to Those Operations

Two types of socially mediated positive reinforcement have frequently been reported to be involved in maintenance of SIB in people with NDCs: attention from/interaction with carers (Love, Carr, & LeBlanc, 2009) and delivery of tangible items (e.g., food, toys), access to which is controlled or mediated by caregivers (O'Reilly et al., 2010). Rojahn et al. (2008) have pointed out that in cases where socially mediated tangible reinforcement has been identified as maintaining SIB, it may be the delivery of the tangible, social interaction involved in the delivery of the tangible, or both, which reinforces the SIB. Since in many cases it will be impossible to separate delivery of the tangible and social interaction, careful assessment of which is the primary source of reinforcement will be necessary. Where an EFA has been carried out, comparison of levels of SIB in conditions where social interaction alone, and social interaction plus tangible delivery, is made contingent on SIB should clarify the issue. If no EFA has been completed, but contingent access to a tangible has been suggested as the reinforcer by functional assessment, it will in most cases be clinically appropriate to proceed with an intervention in which both the putative tangible reinforcer and the social interaction involved in its delivery are targeted.

Since reinforcement is defined as an increase in the strength of a behavior when an event is contingent on that behavior, the term "noncontingent reinforcement" (NCR) has been criticized as conceptually incoherent. Nevertheless, it was the term first employed to describe the delivery of a reinforcer assessed as maintaining SIB on a schedule largely independent of the occurrence of the behavior and continues to be widely used. Vollmer, Iwata, Zarcone, Smith, and Mazaleski (1993) provided the first demonstration of the application of NCR in intervention with SIB. They treated long-established SIB (headbanging and hitting, body hitting, or hand-mouthing) engaged in by three women with severe/profound IDs, which had been shown by EFA to be reinforced by contingent carer attention, by providing attention on a fixed-time (FT) schedule. Attention was initially provided continuously, then progressively reduced to 10 s of attention in each 5 min, with steps in the reduction in the amount of attention provided dependent on low rates of SIB in the previous session. Rigid FT schedules might be difficult to sustain in everyday settings, but the potential for clinical application of NCR was increased when Van Camp, Lerman, Kelley, Contrucci, and Vorndran (2000) subsequently showed that variable-time (VT) schedules in which inter-reinforcement intervals varied randomly around a mean value were as effective as corresponding fixed-time schedules, suggesting the applicability of this approach for applied settings provided that such VT schedules could at least be approximated. Kahng, Iwata, DeLeon, and Wallace (2000) further demonstrated that the reduction in frequency with which reinforcers were delivered could be achieved more rapidly than using the fixed-step approach of Vollmer et al. (1993), and without reducing the effectiveness of the intervention, by a procedure in which the interval between reinforcer delivery was adjusted based on the mean interval between participants' self-injurious behaviors. Where a person engages in frequent SIB, both FT and VT schedules risk maintaining the behavior through adventitious reinforcement when SIB occurs immediately before a scheduled reinforcer delivery. This problem can however be avoided by briefly postponing reinforcement when a scheduled delivery is immediately preceded by SIB (Carr & LeBlanc, 2006). NCR has been used to reduce SIB maintained by contingent social interaction but also socially mediated tangible reinforcement (e.g., access to food) (Ingvarsson, Kahng, & Hausman, 2008).

Time-based schedules have also been used to reduce SIB maintained by socially mediated negative reinforcement. The negative reinforcement process which has received most attention is escape from or avoidance of task demands, although escape from or avoidance of a variety of other aversive events, and from people or situations which have been associated with such events, is also frequently implicated in maintenance of SIB (Reese, Richman, Belmont, & Morse, 2005). Vollmer, Marcus, and Ringdahl (1995) treated the SIB of two young males with developmental disabilities for whom EFA had suggested that SIB was maintained by contingent escape from instructional activities. Provision of brief breaks from instructional activities on fixed-time schedules, with the interval between breaks progressively increased to 10 min for one participant and 2.5 min for the second, substantially reduced rates of SIB for both. Time-based schedules have additionally been used with "automatically reinforced SIB Subtype 1" (Hagopian et al., 2018). These applications are discussed in Sect. 6.5 below.

Overall, NCR is a highly effective approach to reducing operant SIB. Richman, Barnard-Brak, Grubb, Bosch, and Abby (2015) conducted a meta-analysis of data from 55 single-case design studies in which NCR was used as an intervention for challenging behaviors engaged in by 91 people. Self-injury was the most frequently occurring behavior of concern for over 25% of the people concerned. Overall, use of NCR, using a reinforcer identified as the effective reinforcer of the challenging behavior or an alternative reinforcer, produced substantial reductions in challenging behavior (Cohen's d equivalent = −1.58, 95% confidence interval −1.44 to −1.71).

Interventions using reinforcers identified as maintaining the target behavior were associated with significantly, but not greatly, higher effectiveness than others (e.g., when the reinforcer used was identified by a preference assessment). In studies in which it was possible to compare the effects of NCR during initial implementation with effects during schedule thinning, the therapeutic effect of NCR was only slightly reduced by schedule thinning. Further analysis of this data together with additional data from 15 studies involving 43 participants showed that the effect of NCR on SIB was as great as that on other forms of challenging behavior (aggression to others or property destruction). Although NCR was effective overall in reducing both socially and automatically reinforced challenging behaviors, its effect on automatically reinforced behaviors was smaller (but also less variable) than its effect on socially reinforced behaviors (Ritter, Barnard-Brak, Richman, & Grubb, 2018). A similar conclusion was drawn from a case series comprising 27 consecutive applications of NCR to treat a variety of challenging behaviors, including SIB in many cases, presented by 21 children and young adults with intellectual and developmental disabilities (Phillips, Iannaccone, Rooker, & Hagopian, 2017). Effective treatment was defined as achieving at least an 80% reduction in levels of challenging behavior compared to the rate of behavior seen in the relevant condition of the EFA (e.g., the "social disapproval"/contingent attention condition if it was concluded that the behavior was reinforced by attention). Using this criterion, NCR was an effective treatment for 14 of the 15 applications in which it was used as an intervention for socially reinforced challenging behavior, but for only 4 of 9 applications in which it was used to treat automatically reinforced behavior (in the other 3 applications, the behavior was either assessed as controlled by multiple sources of reinforcement or functional analysis had been inconclusive). Further analysis of five cases in which automatically reinforced SIB could be identified as Hagopian et al.'s "Subtype 1" or "Subtype 2" showed that NCR was effective with two of the three cases of "Subtype 1" SIB, but neither of the 2 cases of "Subtype 2" SIB (Phillips et al., 2017).

Successful use of NCR to reduce disruptive behaviors engaged in by people with developmental disabilities in everyday settings such as classrooms has been reported (e.g., Tomlin & Reed, 2012). In considering the use of NCR as a treatment for SIB, it should also be considered however that a review of 24 studies of NCR treatments found that although 13 had included thinning of the NCR schedule, the mean terminal inter-reinforcement time was just under 5 min, with a range from 45 s to 12 min (Carr, Severtson, & Lepper, 2009). Maintaining this level of NCR over a person's whole waking day (or even a full school day) on a long-term basis would clearly be a challenge in many settings. Intervention using NCR for operant SIB (especially for socially reinforced SIB) may therefore best be viewed as a valuable option which can reliably and rapidly reduce SIB and stabilize situations so that additional treatment options can be developed and introduced.

6.3.3 *Difficulties and Potential Adverse Side Effects of, and Alternatives to, Noncontingent Reinforcement*

NCR may be effective in reducing SIB by reducing motivation to engage in SIB through making the reinforcer freely available, by extinction (removing the contingency between the behavior and the reinforcer), and by increasing tolerance of delay to reinforcement through the schedule thinning process (Vollmer et al., 1998). Alternatively, the effects of NCR may be interpreted as a reallocation of responding from SIB maintained by gaining access to the reinforcer to the behaviors involved in engaging with the reinforcer (Hagopian, Crockett, van Stone, DeLeon, & Bowman, 2000). Interventions using NCR often start by providing the reinforcer on a dense schedule. Such schedules often rapidly produce substantial reductions in SIB but will in many situations also interfere substantially with the person's engagement in planned activities. As noted in several of the examples given above, NCR reinforcement schedules are therefore often thinned (i.e., the reinforcer is progressively provided less frequently) to reduce the impact of the intervention on the person's other activities. Such schedule thinning is often accompanied however by temporary increases in levels of the targeted challenging behavior (e.g., Kahng et al., 2000; Vollmer et al., 1998). Such effects are often interpreted as extinction bursts (i.e., temporary increases in the rate and intensity of a behavior, commonly seen on transition from reinforcement to extinction of operant behavior), suggesting that at this point in the intervention, the primary effect of NCR has shifted from reducing motivation for challenging behavior to extinction of the response-reinforcer contingency (Wallace, Iwata, Hanley, Thompson, & Roscoe, 2012). For some people, maintaining low rates of challenging behavior through the schedule thinning process will require an explicit extinction contingency, i.e., a procedure to ensure that the reinforcer is not provided contingent on the challenging behavior (Hagopian et al., 2000; Wallace et al., 2012). In situations where extinction would be impractical or ethically problematic (e.g., in the case of seriously harmful SIB), SIB may initially be reduced using a dense NCR schedule. Teaching the person involved to request the reinforcer using a more adaptive response (i.e., functional communication training; see below) before initiating thinning of the NCR schedule may then enable subsequent thinning to proceed without extinction while maintaining a low rate of SIB (Fritz, Jackson, Stiefler, Wimberly, & Richardson, 2017).

Combining NCR with functional communication training may however be complicated by a further possible adverse side effect of NCR. Dense schedules of NCR which devalue the reinforcer maintaining SIB can also reduce the effectiveness of that reinforcer in teaching and/or maintaining communicative or other adaptive behaviors (Goh, Iwata, & DeLeon, 2000; Kelley, Nadler, Rey, Cowie, & Podlesnik, 2017). Acquisition of such positive responses is facilitated when the NCR schedule is thinned (Goh et al., 2000; Marcus & Vollmer, 1996), so decisions on the speed with which NCR schedules are thinned must balance the reductions in SIB which can be achieved by dense schedules against the impediment which they place on learning of more adaptive responses. Successful thinning of NCR schedules may also be aided by using a visual signal to help the person discriminate periods of time in which the reinforcer will not be provided and also by providing access to preferred activities and stimuli other than those which maintain the SIB during periods when the reinforcer for SIB is not available (Slocum, Grauerholz-Fisher, Peters, & Vollmer, 2018).

With negatively reinforced SIB, especially SIB reinforced by escape from task demands, modifying the demand characteristics of the situation may provide an alternative to enabling the person to leave the situation on a time-based schedule. Pace, Iwata, Cowdery, Andree, and McIntyre (1993) reduced levels of SIB presented by three young people with IDs by initially completely withdrawing demands and then gradually increasing these over sessions to pre-intervention levels, while also preventing escape from activities contingent on SIB. This extinction component to the intervention appears to be necessary if reduction of SIB is to be maintained as demand levels are increased (Zarcone, Iwata, Smith, Mazaleski, & Lerman, 1994). Alternatively, particularly in educational or training settings where providing frequent opportunities for a person to leave the setting might be disruptive to their progress, other characteristics of the demand environment may be modified on a long-term basis. Options may include identifying specific tasks which elicit SIB and then interspersing requests to complete these among other tasks less likely to elicit SIB (Horner, Day, Sprague, O'Brien, & Heathfield, 1991), increasing levels of reinforcement for task engagement (Hoch, McComas, Thompson, & Paone, 2002; Lalli et al., 1999), preceding demands which elicit SIB by a sequence of demands with which the person typically cooperates while preventing escape from the demand contingent on SIB (Zarcone, Iwata, Mazaleski, & Smith, 1994), increasing levels of assistance with tasks, embedding task demands in reinforcing activities, increasing the predictability of demands, and increasing choice of activity (Miltenberger, 2006). Attending to patterns of activity across the whole day may reveal other options for reducing SIB. O'Reilly, Sigafoos, Lancioni, Edrisinha, and Andrews (2005) found that the SIB of a 12-year-old boy with an ASC, which was normally high in the task demand condition of an EFA, did not occur when the task demand condition was preceded successively by no interaction and play conditions. Introduction of a similar structure (a repeating schedule of 5 min each of no interaction, play, and task demand) into the classroom situation produced substantial reductions of SIB in the classroom which were maintained at 5-month follow-up.

Where MOs cannot be directly modified, it may be possible to increase the person's tolerance of them. McCord, Iwata, Galensky, Ellingson, and Thomson (2001), for example, treated challenging behaviors (including SIB) maintained by escape from noise by progressively exposing people to increasing noise levels accompanied by extinction (challenging behavior did not lead to noise termination). In one case, differential reinforcement for absence of challenging behavior in the presence of noise was added to the intervention. It may also be possible to disrupt the long-term effects of some MOs. Horner, Day, and Day (1997) discovered that the escape-maintained aggression and SIB of two children with severe IDs occurred in response to error correction, but only when this experience followed earlier delay or postponement of planned, preferred activities. Implementation of individually developed calming routines (e.g., formally rescheduling the activity and reviewing pictures from the past) following such events reduced levels of challenging behavior in later instructional sessions.

6.3.4 Reducing Self-Injurious Behavior by Teaching and Reinforcing Competing Prosocial Responses

Although interventions which help people to better tolerate MOs may result in long-term reductions in SIB, those which are based on modifying the MO, or reducing the person's exposure to the MO, will only be expected to reduce levels of SIB as long as they remain in effect. Maintaining such interventions, especially when a person is living in their local community, moving between different environments, and interacting with members of the public as well as their families and professional staff will present many challenges. Alternative interventions which may avoid such difficulties are those which develop people's abilities to obtain the reinforcement maintaining their SIB by more prosocial behaviors, usually alternative skills which serve a specifically communicative function. Such "functional communication training" (FCT) interventions aim to replace SIB by communicative behaviors which can serve the same social function as the person's SIB (Carr & Durand, 1985).

In their initial demonstration of the effectiveness of this approach, Carr and Durand (1985) reduced the challenging behaviors (including aggression, tantrums, and self-injury) of four children with developmental disabilities, who presented challenging behaviors maintained by socially mediated positive or negative (escape from difficult tasks) reinforcement, by teaching them to verbally request attention and/or assistance from adults. Carr and Durand (1985) further showed that the effectiveness of FCT depended on teaching the child to verbally solicit the reinforcer maintaining the challenging behavior. Importantly, they also showed that the positive effects of FCT on the children's challenging behaviors occurred with carers naïve with respect to the purposes of the study and suggested that this aspect of FCT might constitute an important advantage for FCT by comparison with other intervention approaches in which carers have to be trained in how to respond to different behaviors. SIB may of course have several behavioral functions. Day, Horner, and O'Neill (1994) demonstrated that the SIB (or aggression) of three individuals with autism or severe IDs was in each case maintained both by escape from tasks and by access to preferred items and showed that establishing a communicative response appropriate to each function was necessary to reduce challenging behavior across both contexts in which it was displayed. Helping people with multiply controlled SIB by using interventions such as NCR can require carers to dynamically assess the current importance of different sources of reinforcement to the maintenance of the behavior. FCT may offer particular advantages in such cases by enabling the client to indicate which source of reinforcement is most important to them on a moment-by-moment basis.

FCT has been shown to be effective in reducing a variety of challenging behaviors, including SIB, which are maintained by socially mediated positive reinforcement including social interaction and tangibles, and socially mediated negative reinforcement including escape from task demands and other contexts with characteristics which some people find aversive, such as noise or social interaction (Durand & Moskowitz, 2015; Kurtz, Boelter, Jarmolowicz, Chin, & Hagopian, 2011; Tiger, Hanley, & Bruzek, 2008). FCT has also been successfully used in combination with augmentative and alternative communication devices and systems to reduce SIB and other challenging behaviors engaged in by people who had very limited communicative abilities prior to intervention (Durand, 1999; Mirenda, 1997; Walker & Snell, 2013). It might be thought that by definition, FCT would not be applicable in situations where SIB was maintained by automatic reinforcement. For some people with ASCs however, SIB may be reinforced by access to opportunities to engage in stereotyped behaviors (STBs) or more complex repetitive and restrictive behaviors, in situations where other people attempt to restrict such access, and in these situations FCT may give the person an alternative means to request this access. Hausman, Kahng, Farrell, and Mongeon (2009), for example, reduced the SIB and other challenging behaviors of a 9-year-old girl with an ASC and moderate ID by teaching her to use a picture card and the phrase "My way, please" to request the opportunity to position the room door as she preferred it. Working with three preschool children with ASCs, Rispoli, Camargo, Machalicek, Lang, and Sigafoos (2014) used FCT to reduce their challenging behaviors (including, in one case, SIB) which were reinforced by continued access to restricted and repetitive behaviors (e.g., rapidly turning book pages or lining up toy trains) in the face of attempts by carers to interrupt or redirect the children away from these activities. The children were taught to use a verbal phrase ("I don't want that"), or to give the carer a symbol card, which resulted in carers allowing them to continue with their preferred behaviors for 30 s. In some cases, SIB may be maintained by consequences, apparently intrinsically important to the person engaging in SIB, which involve the physical placement of other people. Torres-Viso, Strohmeier, and Zarcone (2018), for example, used FCT to reduce levels of challenging behaviors (including SIB) which were reinforced (in part) by the parents of a 12-year-old girl with Smith-Magenis syndrome adopting particular bodily postures or positions.

6.3.5 Difficulties, Potential Adverse Side Effects, and Further Developments of Functional Communication Training

Acquisition of a communicative functional equivalent to SIB, even if that response is consistently reinforced, will not necessarily reduce the level of SIB. If both behaviors elicit qualitatively similar responses from carers, the proportion of responses which are prosocial and self-injurious will be determined by the effort (and other costs) associated with each response (Richman, Wacker, & Winborn,

2001), the magnitude of the reinforcer, and the latency and schedule (reliability) with which reinforcement is delivered (Symons, Hoch, Dahl, & McComas, 2003). In most studies which have shown a positive effect of FCT, the SIB or other challenging behavior has been placed on extinction (i.e., is no longer followed by the reinforcer) simultaneously with the communicative response being reinforced (Kurtz et al., 2011). Several studies have found that FCT reduced challenging behaviors only when extinction or time-out contingencies were in effect for those behaviors in addition to positive reinforcement of the communicative response (e.g., Shirley, Iwata, Kahng, Mazaleski, & Lerman, 1997; Wacker et al., 1990). Even if a communicative response is well-established while SIB is on extinction, SIB may increase to pre-treatment levels if it is once again reinforced (Shirley et al., 1997). Worsdell, Iwata, Hanley, Thompson, and Kahng (2000), treating the SIB of five adults with profound IDs, showed that for one person, FCT (with every prosocial communication reinforced) reduced rates of SIB even when SIB was also continuously reinforced. For the other 4 people however, meaningful reductions in SIB were achieved only when the appropriate communication was continuously reinforced and rate of reinforcement of SIB was reduced, in 2 cases to 1 reinforcement per 20 responses. Since with even the highest level of training and support for families and other carers SIB may continue to be at least intermittently reinforced (e.g., by members of the public), successful long-term use of FCT may require an ongoing dense schedule of reinforcement for the communicative response.

There are additional reasons for eliminating or minimizing reinforcement of SIB during FCT interventions. If reinforcement of SIB continues, then functionally the communicative response and the person's SIB may become members of the same functional class, and reinforcement of the communicative response may strengthen the entire functional class, including SIB, in terms of rate of occurrence and resistance to extinction (Derby, Fisher, Piazza, Wilke, & Johnson, 1998). Consideration also needs to be given to these issues in situations where a person already has in their repertoire a potentially appropriate communicative response for use in FCT. For example, a person may sometimes engage in SIB, and sometimes use a manual sign for "finished," when they wish to end an activity. Although using the manual sign as the communicative response in FCT avoids the need for the person to learn a new response, the sign also has a history of membership of the same functional class as SIB. It may be preferable therefore to teach the person a novel communicative response which has no history of membership of the same functional class as SIB (Tiger et al., 2008; Winborn, Wacker, Richman, Asmus, & Geier, 2002).

A problem commonly encountered in implementing FCT interventions is that the person uses the alternative communicative response so frequently that to reinforce every occurrence is impracticable in the long term (Fisher et al., 1993; Lalli, Casey, & Kates, 1995). In the early stages of FCT intervention, it is generally recommended that a communicative response which requires little effort is used, to increase the probability that the person will use that response rather than their presumably more effortful SIB (Horner & Day, 1991; Tiger et al., 2008). As a consequence of this reduced effort however, the person may use the communicative response much more frequently than they previously engaged in SIB, possibly to the extent that continuous reinforcement of the response on an ongoing basis would result in, for example, health-damaging levels of consumption of tangibles or continuous avoidance of educational activities. On the other hand, in everyday settings it may not be practicable to reinforce every communicative response, leading to a risk of resurgence of the SIB (Fisher, Thompson, Hagopian, Bowman, & Krug, 2000). Several strategies for addressing this problem have been evaluated. One is to attempt to progressively delay the reinforcement of the communicative response (Fisher et al., 2000). The probability of success using this approach can be increased by additionally providing the person with preferred items or activities during the period in which they are waiting for reinforcement, especially if these have been demonstrated to be associated with reduced levels of challenging behavior (e.g., Austin & Tiger, 2015; Hagopian, Kuhn, Long, & Rush, 2005). The second strategy is to commence FCT using continuous reinforcement of the communicative response but then to introduce progressively increasing periods during which neither SIB nor the communicative response is reinforced, i.e., a "multiple schedule" with fixed-ratio 1 (FR1) and extinction (EXT) components. Hanley, Iwata, and Thompson (2001), for example, initiated FCT treatment of the SIB and aggression of three adults with profound IDs by establishing the communicative response using continuous reinforcement and then introduced and progressively lengthened periods of (signalled) extinction in which an S^{Δ} (a colored card) indicated that the communicative response would not be reinforced. Other strategies with more limited applicability have also been used. The strategy of "demand fading," or chained schedules, has been used when SIB or other challenging behaviors are reinforced by escape from task demands and involves the communicative response being reinforced only once the person has completed a predetermined amount of the task involved, with the amount progressively increased over sessions. Hagopian, Boelter, and Jarmolowicz (2011) provide a detailed practice-focused review of options for thinning reinforcement schedules in FCT together with guidance on selecting a strategy appropriate to the individual case.

Even when these strategies are used however, resurgence of SIB may well occur at some stage in the process of thinning reinforcement of the communicative response. In a review of 24 applications of FCT in which a multiple-schedule approach to thinning the reinforcement of the communicative response was used, Saini, Miller, and Fisher (2016) noted resurgence of challenging behavior at some stage of the process in over half of the cases. Greer, Fisher, Saini, Owen, and Jones (2016) reported a case series of 25 applications of FCT to reduce challenging behaviors in children and a young adult, including 3 targeting SIB, in which various strategies were used to thin the reinforcement schedule following initial FCT. In 88% of cases, it was possible to thin the schedule of reinforcement for FCT to the point where reinforcement of the communicative response was not provided for a period of 4 min out of 5, while still maintaining low rates of challenging behavior. In two of the three cases involving SIB however, these reductions were only achieved by also using NCR or response blocking. Further, in a supplementary analysis of the data from Greer et al.'s (2016) study, Briggs, Fisher, Greer, and Kimball (2018) reported that resurgence of challenging behavior during the thinning process occurred in the course of 76% of applications of reinforcement thinning following FCT, and in over 40% of individual schedule-thinning steps, with levels of challenging behavior sometimes exceeding mean baseline levels. Briggs et al. (2018) observed that although resurgence of challenging behavior had been successfully managed in all cases by the professional staff involved in the research study, families or other unqualified carers faced with such sudden resurgence of challenging behavior might well have responded by reinforcing that behavior.

Recent research has continued to investigate methods to improve the effectiveness and efficiency of FCT, including methods for manipulating motivating operations to minimize levels of challenging behavior during FCT (Fisher et al., 2018), choosing an initial communicative response to use in FCT (Kunnavatana, Wolfe, & Aguilar, 2018), selecting the initial duration of non-reinforcement periods during schedule thinning (Call et al., 2018), and shaping increasingly complex communicative responses during FCT (Ghaemmaghami, Hanley, Jessel, & Landa, 2018). However, the resurgence of SIB if the functionally equivalent communicative response is not reliably reinforced remains a major issue in using FCT in everyday settings, and there is only limited research on the use of FCT by non-specialists and into the generalization of treatment effects. In a review of studies using FCT to reduce challenging behaviors of children and adults with IDs, Kurtz et al. (2011) reported that although teachers or parents had implemented the intervention in 25% of cases, in 60% it was professional therapists or behavior analysts who had done so. A review of behavioral interventions including FCT used to treat SIB in children with ASCs and published between 2000 and 2016 similarly reported that in 75% of studies, the researcher or a therapist (in this case meaning a researcher, graduate student, or practitioner) had implemented the intervention (Chezan et al., 2017). In a review of 37 studies of FCT which reported data on generalization and/or maintenance of treatment effects, Neely, Garcia, Bankston, and Green (2018) reported that 24 (65%) reported data on 1 or more aspects of generalization of treatment effects (across people, settings, tasks, etc.), and 19 (51%) presented data on maintenance of treatment effects, although 3 of these used only a single maintenance probe. However, of those 19 studies, 11 collected maintenance data immediately after the intervention phase of the study, with only 6 collecting maintenance data more than 3 months after completion of the intervention phase. One study (Bailey, McComas, Benavides, & Lovascz, 2002) collected follow-up data 2 years after the initial stage of the study and found that the "aggressive behaviors" (which included SIB) of a man with a profound ID living in a group home were reduced in frequency from a mean of 21.2 episodes per month before initial assessment to 1.4 episodes per month in the first 4 months of intervention and remained at 3.8 episodes per month 2 years later.

Although the effectiveness of FCT in short-term applications by trained therapists is therefore well-established, there is still relatively little evidence on sustainability of effects in everyday settings. Research has however begun to investigate conditions affecting the probability of re-emergence of challenging behavior following FCT and related interventions, and this issue is discussed further in Sect. 6.8 below.

Many early behavioral interventions used with SIB engaged in by persons with NDCs used differential reinforcement approaches (e.g., Cowdery, Iwata, & Pace, 1990). These include DRO, DRA, and DRI (see Sect. 6.3.1 above). In the early stages of implementation of DRA/DRI procedures, the individual concerned may be assisted to engage in the alternative responses by prompting or physical guidance. Differential reinforcement procedures have, for example, been used to replace SIB and other challenging behaviors with self-care skills (Roberts et al., 1995). FCT itself is a differential reinforcement approach, and since its development, other types of differential reinforcement interventions targeting noncommunicative behaviors, and using reinforcers not assessed as maintaining the challenging behavior, have been relatively less used (Petscher, Rey, & Bailey, 2009). Such approaches however continue to be relevant in cases where SIB is not maintained by socially mediated reinforcement, and they are discussed further in Sect. 6.4.2.

6.3.6 Reducing or Eliminating Reinforcement of Self-Injurious Behavior

Most applications of FCT involve eliminating or reducing the reinforcement maintaining SIB in addition to teaching and reinforcing the communicative response. Extinction alone however is rarely used to treat SIB. Aside from the ethical issue that extinction used alone denies the person access to an outcome which presumably is important to her/him without providing an alternative means for the person to access that outcome, extinction used alone is likely to produce adverse side effects. Lerman, Iwata, and Wallace (1999) found evidence for extinction bursts in 62% of 41 datasets for children and adults with moderate to profound IDs whose SIB was treated by extinction alone, versus 15% of cases in which antecedent change and/or reinforcement procedures were used in combination with extinction. Aggression was also more commonly observed when extinction was used alone than when it was used in combination with other procedures (Lerman et al., 1999). Extinction bursts may lead to carers reinstating reinforcement of SIB and hence contribute to shaping of progressively more severe forms of the behavior (Oliver & Head, 1990).

6.4 Intervention with Habitual/Impulsive (Stimulus-Response Controlled) Self-Injurious Behavior

6.4.1 Short-Term Management of Habitual/Impulsive (Stimulus-Response Controlled) Self-Injurious Behavior

As was discussed in Chap. 5, if SIB occurs in specific situations, or is reliably evoked by specific stimuli, but the behavior is not responsive to NCR, it is probable that the behavior is habitual/impulsive SIB in which operant processes have become less influential and stimulus-response (S-R) processes are predominant. Nevertheless, the behavioral interventions described above for treatment of operant SIB continue to have some relevance. In the short term, NCR providing very frequent positive reinforcement, or complete avoidance of aversive situations, may enable serious SIB to be safely managed. FCT may also be helpful in enabling the person to achieve the same outcomes. In some cases, it may be possible to successfully manage a person's SIB for long periods of time using such strategies. In the case of habitual/impulsive SIB, the behavior is likely, however, to continue to occur when the person is challenged by deprivation (however brief) of positive reinforcement or by exposure to an aversive situation, and further active intervention may be necessary.

6.4.2 Behavioral Intervention with Habitual/Impulsive (Stimulus-Response Controlled) Self-Injurious Behavior

In cases of habitual/impulsive SIB, behavioral assessment may have identified specific situations or stimuli which evoke SIB and/or identified eliciting processes which may occur in a variety of situations (e.g., high-pitched noise, having to wait, supporting persons being present but interacting with each other rather than the person engaging in SIB). The fundamental component of behavioral intervention in such cases is progressively increasing exposure to the eliciting situation using a hierarchy of steps. The hierarchy may be developed as a series of task steps or along dimensions such as the severity of eliciting stimuli, the person's proximity to the stimulus or situation, or the amount of time they are exposed to the stimulus. For example, in the case of a person who engages in SIB at mealtimes in school, the hierarchy may involve the series of task steps involved (entering the school dining room, collecting a tray, indicating meal choices, etc.), or it may involve how crowded and noisy the dining room is, or where the person sits (perhaps starting in an adjoining room before moving progressively closer to the dining room), or how long the person remains in the room. Appropriate hierarchy construction requires careful assessment of the specific aspects of the situation which elicit SIB, and in many cases the treatment hierarchy will combine elements from several approaches to hierarchy construction. For example, the hierarchy may begin with a series of steps involving proximity of approach to the dining room, followed by a series of task-related steps, followed by a series of steps involving progressively increasing time in the dining room.

Progression to each step of the hierarchy is generally arranged dependent on the person concerned successfully completing the previous step without engaging in SIB for a predetermined number of trials. Schmidt, Luiselli, Rue, and Whalley (2013), for example, developed an intervention for a teenager with severe ID and an ASC who engaged in SIB (and other challenging behaviors) when he was asked to enter the music room, gymnasium, or gross-motor exercise room at his school. The initial series of hierarchy steps involved the young man progressively approaching closer to the rooms concerned. Baseline measures were taken of the distance which he walked from his classroom toward the rooms concerned until he began to engage in challenging behaviors. The first step in the intervention hierarchy involved him walking from his classroom to a point which was 30% of the distance he managed without engaging in challenging behavior during baseline assessment. The distance he was asked to walk was increased by 20% each time he successfully achieved the previous criterion distance on two successive occasions without engaging in SIB or other challenging behaviors. When the teenager successfully reached the threshold of each room, the hierarchy was modified to one comprising a series of steps involving spending progressively longer periods of time in the room without engaging in SIB or other challenging behavior.

Although progression through the hierarchy is the central element in behavioral treatment, successful intervention will generally require use of additional techniques. Most important is differential positive reinforcement, preferably using stimuli which have been assessed as highly preferred by the person involved using a systematic stimulus preference assessment (see Chap. 5). Reinforcement is provided for completing a hierarchy step successfully, contingent either on the person actively completing a task step without engaging in SIB or contingent on the person facing progressively more challenging situations without engaging in SIB (Jennett & Hagopian, 2008). For example, once he had entered the activity room concerned, Schmidt et al. (2013) gave the teenager with whom they worked a small amount of a preferred edible for engaging in each step of an activity, while Shabani and Fisher (2006) provided a young adult with ID and an ASC with access to preferred items if he kept his arm still, without engaging in SIB or other challenging behavior, as a lancet (to be used to take a small blood sample) was moved to a criterion distance from his fingertip. Other supplementary techniques which may be helpful are verbal prompting and/or physical guidance to help a person to engage in hierarchy steps or social modelling (e.g., another person completing the hierarchy step and gaining access to reinforcement for doing so).

Reviews of the use of graduated exposure with reinforcement and other techniques, not only with SIB, by Jennett and Hagopian (2008) and Rosen, Connell, and Kerns (2016) support their effectiveness with people with IDs and ASCs. Pharmacological intervention is sometimes regarded as the only intervention option for habitual/impulsive SIB showing little sensitivity to social contingencies. Where this type of SIB is elicited by specific situations or stimuli however, progressive exposure with reinforcement is a viable behavioral treatment option with roots shared with differential reinforcement interventions (e.g., Roberts et al., 1995).

6.4.3 Pharmacological Intervention with Habitual/Impulsive (Stimulus-Response Controlled) Self-Injurious Behavior

6.4.3.1 Overview of Research into Pharmacological Therapy for Challenging Behaviors

In their authoritative text on SIB in people with IDs, Rojahn et al. (2008) described several difficulties in interpreting the research base for pharmacological interventions for SIB in that population. Aside from the logistical and ethical difficulties of conducting randomized, placebo-controlled trials of medication with double-blind evaluation of outcomes, which have led to a relative paucity of such studies, they noted several other issues, two of which remain prominent. The first was that most of the rating scales used to assess outcomes in pharmacological intervention studies were not constructed to measure change in specific classes of behavior such as SIB. A Cochrane systematic review (Gormez et al., 2014) concerned with pharmacological treatments in adults with IDs, which specified measurement of frequency, intensity, or duration of SIB as a criterion for inclusion of studies, could, for example, find only five randomized controlled trials, one of clomipramine and four of naltrexone. The second issue was that much research had been conducted with groups of people with IDs of unknown and probably heterogeneous origins, leading to the probability of high variability in response to any one treatment. Aman and his colleagues (Aman, Arnold, & Armstrong, 1999; Aman & Madrid, 1999; Farmer & Aman, 2013) have periodically presented authoritative reviews of the effects of antipsychotic, serotonergic, and other medications commonly used in treatment of challenging behaviors in people with intellectual and developmental disabilities, while other reviews have focused on children with IDs (e.g., McQuire et al., 2015, 2016), children with ASCs (e.g., Fallah et al., 2019; Lamy & Erickson, 2018; Siegel & Beaulieu, 2012), children and adults with ASCs (e.g., Politte & McDougle, 2014), and adults with ASCs and IDs (e.g., Sawyer et al., 2014). Farmer and Aman (2013) noted that between 2001 and 2010, research in this field had concentrated very largely on the use of second-generation antipsychotics with people (many of them children) with ASCs and that the outcome measures used often made it difficult to determine the impact of treatments on specific types of behavior such as SIB. They also characterized the "pool" of research as "wide and shallow" (Farmer & Aman, 2013, p. 315), with many different drugs evaluated, but often in a small number of methodologically limited studies, a situation which necessarily leads to inconclusive results regarding efficacy. In this chapter we shall therefore focus only on those medications for which there is robust evidence of efficacy and/or a specific rationale for their use in treatment of specific subtypes of SIB. Firstly however we briefly describe three rating scales which have been used to measure change in many of the relevant studies.

The Aberrant Behavior Checklist (ABC; Aman, Singh, Stewart, & Field, 1985a), a generalized behavior rating scale with five subscales (irritability, lethargy, stereotypy, hyperactivity, and inappropriate speech), has been widely used in evaluating the effectiveness of pharmacological interventions. Psychometric studies have generally found that the scale has a factor structure corresponding to its subscale structure (e.g., Aman, Burrow, & Wolford, 1995; Bihm & Poindexter, 1991; Marshburn & Aman, 1992), adequate to very good criterion validity (Aman, Singh, Stewart, & Field, 1985b; Rojahn & Helsel, 1991), very good internal consistency and test-retest reliability (Aman et al., 1985b), and moderate interrater reliability (Aman, Singh, & Turbott, 1987). The "irritability" subscale of the ABC has three items referring to (topographically non-specified) SIB. The Nisonger Child Behavior Rating Form (NCBRF; Aman, Tassé, Rojahn, & Hammer, 1996; Tassé, Aman, Hammer, & Rojahn, 1996), another third-party rating scale with good psychometric properties, has also been widely used. The NCBRF has a 66-item "Problem Behaviors" section with 6 subscales, 1 of which (self-injurious behavior/stereotypic) includes 6 items describing SIB, with some level of differentiation in terms of topography. The Behavior Problems Inventory (BPI; Rojahn, Matson, Lott, Esbensen, & Smalls, 2001) is a more focused behavior rating scale. The BPI was originally a 32-item rating scale containing only items relating to self-injurious behavior and stereotypies (Rojahn, 1984, 1986) but has been developed over time, with the addition of an aggressive/destructive behavior subscale and the replacement of the original stereotypies subscale with the independently developed "stereotyped behavior scale" (Rojahn, Matlock, & Tassé, 2000; Rojahn, Tassé, & Sturmey, 1997). The current version of the scale (BPI-01; Rojahn et al., 2001) is a 49-item scale with a 14-item self-injurious behavior subscale, a 24-item stereotypic behavior subscale, and an 11-item aggressive/destructive behavior subscale. Each item is scored on a five-point frequency of occurrence scale and a four-point severity scale, provided that the behavior has occurred in the 2 months prior to scale completion. Rojahn et al. (2001) performed a confirmatory factor analysis on data from 432 individuals with IDs, assuming 3 oblique factors corresponding to the BPI subscales, and found a reasonable fit with this a priori model, with mean factor loadings of 0.34 for the SIB, 0.38 for the stereotypic behavior, and 0.54 for the aggression/destruction subscales. Subsequent confirmatory factor analyses have generally replicated these finding (González et al., 2009; Lundqvist, 2011), although Rojahn et al. (2010) found a less adequate fit in a study involving school students (children, adolescents, and young adults) with IDs. Rojahn et al. (2001) found the internal consistencies of all three BPI subscales to be adequate or better, with the self-injurious behavior showing the lowest internal consistency (Cronbach's alpha = 0.61). González et al. (2009) also found the internal consistencies of the aggressive/destructive behavior and stereotyped behavior subscales to be good to excellent (for both frequency and severity ratings) but that the self-injurious behavior subscale had lower internal consistency (Cronbach's alpha between 0.40 and 0.48). The relatively poor internal consistency of the self-injurious behavior subscale has been repeatedly replicated (Lundqvist, 2011; Rojahn et al., 2010; van Ingen, Moore, Zaja, & Rojahn, 2010) and may be due to the fact that some items on the SIB subscale (e.g., those concerning air-swallowing and excessive drinking) are relatively infrequently endorsed, but also may relate to the limited coherence of conceptualizations of SIB which include such items (Rojahn et al., 2008). Interrater and test-retest reliabilities for BPI-01 subscale scores have however consistently been found to be adequate to excellent (González et al., 2009; Rojahn et al., 2001, 2010; van Ingen et al., 2010), with the exception of interrater agreement between teachers and parents (Rojahn et al., 2010).

Changes in scores on the ABC "irritability" subscale or the NCBRF "self-injurious behavior/stereotypic" subscale are therefore suggestive (although not necessarily indicative) of changes in SIB, while changes in BPI-01 self-injurious behavior subscale scores are a specific measure of changes in the frequency and/or severity of SIB.

6.4.3.2 Second-Generation Antipsychotics

The suggestion that supersensitivity of the D_1 dopamine receptor subtype may be implicated in the self-injury observed in the neonatally 6-hydroxydopamine-lesioned rat model of SIB (Breese et al., 2005) has led to particular interest in the potential therapeutic value of dopamine receptor antagonists. Although no specific D_1 receptor antagonist is currently available for clinical use, the "second-generation" antipsychotics typically have a complex pattern of action at multiple receptor subtypes including D_1, D_2, and other receptors and therefore are of specific interest as potential treatments for SIB.

6.4.3.2.1 Risperidone

Risperidone primarily blocks D_2, serotonergic, and adrenergic receptors (Aman & Madrid, 1999). An 8-week, double-blind, placebo-controlled study (McCracken et al., 2002) examined the effect of risperidone (in doses between 0.5 and 3.5 mg/day at the end of the study) on the behavior of 49 children and teenagers with ASCs (the majority of whom also had IDs) compared with 52 children receiving placebo. Participants were reported to engage in tantrums, aggression, SIB, or multiple challenging behaviors, with high parent-rated scores (≥ 18) on the ABC irritability subscale. Repeated assessment on that subscale showed a significant group by time interaction, with a mean 57% decrease in irritability score in the risperidone-treated group compared with a 14% decrease in the placebo group. ABC stereotypy and hyperactivity subscales scores also showed significantly greater reductions for the risperidone than the placebo group. Reports of increased appetite, fatigue, and drowsiness were significantly associated with risperidone treatment, with parental reports of tremor and tachycardia also associated (at a $p = 0.06$ level) with risperidone use. Weight gain was significantly greater in the children taking risperidone. A 16-week open-label follow-up (Research Units on Paediatric Psychopharmacology Autism Network, 2005) of 63 children who either had received risperidone in the double-blind trial, or were given 8 weeks of open-label treatment following placebo, found significant (but small) increases in ABC irritability subscale score, with the mean score remaining well below the baseline level of the double-blind phase. The participants experienced a mean 6-month weight increase of 5.1 kg. An 8-week double-blind placebo-substitution phase showed relapse rates of 13% with ongoing risperidone and 63% with placebo substitution. Anderson et al. (2007) showed that approximately one-third of participants had prolactin levels above the normal range at 22 months of treatment. Shea et al. (2004) reported results from an 8-week, double-blind, placebo-controlled trial involving 79 children, aged between 5 and 12, all with ASCs, 69% having diagnoses of autistic disorder, with the majority also having mild to severe IDs. All subscales of the ABC showed significantly greater decreases for the risperidone group than for the placebo group, as did the conduct problem, hyperactive, insecure/anxious, and overly sensitive subscales of the NCBRF. There were no significant differences between groups in change on the NCBRF self-isolated/ritualistic or self-injurious/stereotypic subscales. Somnolence was reported for over 70% of the risperidone group but was reported to resolve in most cases (usually following dose rescheduling or reduction). Increases in weight, pulse rate, and systolic blood pressure at study endpoint were all significantly greater for the risperidone than for the placebo group.

These studies therefore have produced limited and mixed evidence specifically relevant to the impact of risperidone on SIB, with improvements in ABC irritability, but not NCBRF self-injurious/stereotypic subscales, greater with risperidone than placebo. Arnold et al. (2003) however asked parents of 87 children participating in McCracken et al.'s (2002) study to identify their two greatest concerns regarding their child's behavior. SIB was selected as a primary concern by parents of 11 children receiving placebo and 8 receiving risperidone. After 4 and 8 weeks, descriptions of the child's current status with respect to these problems were rated for degree of change by a panel of clinical judges blind to treatment group. The mean improvement rating for SIB was significantly higher for the children receiving risperidone, showing the greatest effect size of all target symptoms.

The effects of risperidone in children with IDs, but without ASCs, have also been evaluated. Table 6.2 summarizes the results of two large placebo-controlled double-blind evaluations of risperidone with children aged 5–12, with IQs between 36 and 84, and presenting severely disruptive behaviors, together with results from the subsequent open-label follow-ups. It can be seen that the BPI-01 and NCBRF were used as outcome measures in addition to the ABC, increasing the probability that SIB-specific outcomes could be evaluated. Taken together, these studies provided convincing evidence of a positive effect of risperidone on behavioral difficulties in young children with moderate, mild, or borderline levels of ID. Specific measures of SIB and STBs however frequently showed either no significant change, or changes of less significance than those shown for externally directed aggression, during risperidone treatment. A post hoc analysis (LeBlanc et al., 2005) of data from 163 participants in the Aman et al. (2002) and Snyder et al. (2002) studies confirmed that risperidone-treated participants showed significantly greater decreases than placebo-treated participants on an "aggression score" derived from six core aggression items on the NCBRF, but no analysis was presented on change in a similarly derived "self-harm score." Aman et al. (2005), examining pooled data from these studies, showed that only one item from the NCBRF self-injury/stereotypic subscale showed improvement with risperidone.

Table 6.2 Evaluations of risperidone for behavioral difficulties in young children with moderate-borderline IDs

Study	Participants (in parentheses: number completing study)	Design (in parentheses: dose range in double-blind phase if any)	General outcome measures	Specific SIB measures	Selected side effects reported
Aman et al. (2002)	115 (87) children, ages 5–12, IQ 36–84, with severely disruptive behaviors	6-week double-blind parallel placebo-controlled (0.02–0.06 mg/kg/day)	NCBRF conduct problem and all other subscales, ABC irritability, lethargy and hyperactivity subscales, BPI aggressive/destructive behavior subscale: greater improvement with risperidone vs. placebo	1. BPI self-injurious behavior subscale: no difference in change between groups 2. NCBRF self-injury/stereotypic subscale: greater improvement with risperidone vs. placebo	Weight and (boys only) prolactin levels increased with risperidone vs. placebo; transient heart rate increase also noted. Somnolence, headaches, vomiting, dyspepsia in 15% or more with risperidone. No between group difference in extrapyramidal symptoms
Snyder et al. (2002)	110 (85) children, ages 5–12, IQ 36–84, with severely disruptive behaviors	6-week double-blind parallel placebo-controlled (0.02–0.06 mg/kg/day)	NCBRF conduct problem and most other subscales, all ABC subscales, BPI aggressive/destructive behavior subscale: greater improvement with risperidone vs. placebo	1. BPI self-injurious behavior subscale: no difference in change between groups 2. NCBRF self-injury/stereotypic subscale: greater improvement with risperidone vs. placebo	Weight and prolactin levels increased with risperidone vs. placebo. Somnolence, headaches, dyspepsia in 15% or more with risperidone. No between-group difference in extrapyramidal symptoms
Findling, Aman, Eerdekens, Derivan, and Lyons (2004)	107 participants from Aman et al. (2002) study	48-week open-label follow-up to Aman et al. (2002)	Both for children receiving risperidone in double-blind phase and those receiving placebo in that phase, all NCBRF subscales improved from baseline of double-blind phase to study endpoint	NCBRF self-injury/stereotypic subscale: for children receiving risperidone in double-blind baseline, showed smallest improvement of all NCBRF subscales from double-blind baseline to study endpoint	91% reported adverse events including somnolence (33%), headache (33%), rhinitis (28%), and weight increase (21%). Eleven withdrew from trial after adverse events including weight gain ($N = 4$), depression ($N = 3$), suicide attempt ($N = 2$). Prolactin increased but within normal limits by end

(continued)

Table 6.2 (continued)

Study	Participants (in parentheses: number completing study)	Design (in parentheses: dose range in double-blind phase if any)	General outcome measures	Specific SIB measures	Selected side effects reported
Turgay, Binder, Snyder, and Fisman (2002)	77 children from Snyder et al. (2002) study	48-week open-label follow-up to Snyder et al. (2002)	Children receiving risperidone in double-blind phase: all subscales of NCBRF improved by comparison with double-blind baseline. Children receiving placebo in double-blind phase: all subscales of NCBRF except self-injury/stereotyped and self-isolated/ritualistic subscales improved from follow-up baseline to endpoint	NCBRF self-injury/stereotypic subscale: improved for children receiving risperidone during double-blind from double-blind baseline to endpoint; not improved for children receiving placebo in double-blind from open-label baseline to endpoint	Somnolence (over 50%), headache (over 35%). Prolactin levels increased, but levels at endpoint within or just above normal range. Mean weight increase 8.5 kg from baseline of 30.7 kg, half attributed to normal growth. Mild-moderate extrapyramidal symptoms in 26%

NCBRF Nisonger Child Behavior Rating Form (Aman et al., 1996), *ABC* Aberrant Behavior Checklist (Aman et al., 1985a), *BPI* Behavior Problems Inventory (BPI-01) (Rojahn et al., 2001). (Reprinted/adapted by permission from Springer Nature: Springer Science + Business Media LLC, *Treating Childhood Psychopathology and Developmental Disabilities* by Johnny L. Matson, Frank Andrasik and Michael L. Matson (Editors), © Springer Science + Business Media LLC, 2009)

Evidence regarding the effectiveness of risperidone for treating adults with ASCs is substantially less than that available for children. McDougle et al. (1998) reported data from 30 adults with ASCs and a mean age of 28 years randomized to treatment with either risperidone (mean dose 2.0 mg/day) or placebo over a period of 12 weeks. Risperidone treatment was associated with greater improvement than placebo on Clinical Global Impression, repetitive behavior as assessed by a modified form of the Yale-Brown Obsessive-Compulsive Scale (Y-BOCS; Goodman et al., 1989), and the Self-Injurious Behaviour Questionnaire (SIB-Q). The latter however, despite its name, includes only five items relating to SIB, the others being concerned with other behavioral, attentional, and emotional difficulties (Rojahn et al., 2008). Hellings et al. (2006) investigated the effects of risperidone in a study involving 19 adults together with 21 children and adolescents. All had at least mild ID, and 36 had an ASC. In the initial double-blind period of the study, participants were randomized to either 3, 4, or 5 weeks of placebo, then randomized to 4 weeks of either a low (1.0 mg/day for children; 2.0 mg/day for adults) or high (0.05 mg/kg/day: mean actual doses 2.0 mg/day for children; 3.6 mg/day for adults), and then crossed over to the alternate dose of risperidone, followed by another 3, 4, or 5 weeks of placebo. Two weeks of dose tapering took place between each phase. At this stage of the study, the treating clinicians were released from blinding, and participants were offered a further 24 weeks of treatment with dose optimized for each individual in terms of balancing therapeutic effect and side effects (excluding weight gain). Mean ABC irritability subscale scores, using mean scores from the first placebo phase as covariates, were significantly lower during both drug phases than during the second placebo phase, but not significantly different between high- and low-dose phases. Acute side effects including sedation and gastrointestinal disturbance were however more common with the higher doses of risperidone. Of the 40 participants in the trial, 31 engaged in both SIB and aggression to others, and 5 engaged in SIB without aggression. Hellings et al. (2006) did not report SIB-specific outcomes. However, in an earlier preliminary report on 9 adult and 11 child/teenager participants, Zarcone et al. (2001) also presented scores on the NCBRF (for children/adolescents) and SIB-Q (for adults), completed (as for the ABC) by caregivers. Although no statistical analyses were completed, and substantial variability between participants was noted, mean scores for the NCBRF self-injury/stereotypic subscale for the young people were lower during both drug phases than both placebo phases. For the adults however, mean scores for the SIB-related items of the scale showed little difference between pre-study baseline, both drug phases, the second placebo phase, and the open-label maintenance phase of the study, although they were highest during the first placebo phase. Direct observation of challenging behaviors in their everyday environment was undertaken for 30 min approximately three times a week for five participants. The behaviors observed included SIB but also aggression toward persons and property and disruptive behaviors. Two participants showed lower frequencies of challenging behavior during drug than in placebo phases, two showed inconclusive results, and one showed higher frequency behavior with risperidone than in both placebo phases. Zarcone et al. (2004) further reported on direct observation of challenging behaviors (including aggression, SIB, and disruption) during approximately weekly EFAs conducted with eight children and five adults with ASCs and other developmental disabilities who participated in the Zarcone et al. (2001) study. Zarcone et al. (2004) presented data on mean rates per minute of all "destructive responses" combined for each acute study phase, concluding that for 10 individuals, rates of destructive behavior were reduced with at least 1 dose level of risperidone when compared with the first placebo phase. Their data also show however that for two of these "responders," rates of challenging behavior were lower during the second placebo phase than under either risperidone dose, and in two further cases, there was little difference between rates of behavior in the second placebo phase and in the drug phase with the lowest rate of behavior (no second placebo phase data were available for one participant).

The above studies clearly indicate a beneficial effect of risperidone on behavioral difficulties of children and adolescents with IDs and with ASCs, and there is some evidence for a therapeutic effect of risperidone in adults with IDs and ASCs. The evidence for a positive effect of risperidone specifically on SIB however is much less compelling. The one study which has used clinician ratings of change in specifically described challenging behaviors (Arnold et al., 2003) reported a larger effect size for risperidone treatment related to SIB than for any other challenging behavior considered. However, this figure relates to only 8 children treated with risperidone and 11 given placebo. Findings regarding changes on the NCBRF self-injury/stereotypic subscale have been generally positive but mixed (Shea et al., 2004), no study has found an effect using the BPI self-injurious behavior subscale, and Zarcone et al. (2001) reported little change between risperidone and the final placebo phase of their study using the SIB-Q. When SIB has been a specific focus, direct observation during blinded trials of medication for individual cases has suggested both a specific beneficial effect of risperidone on SIB greater than that on aggression (Crosland et al., 2003) and both positive and negative effects (Zarcone et al., 2004), across different individuals.

6.4.3.2.2 Aripiprazole

Aripiprazole has a complex pattern of activity; in addition to antagonism at dopamine receptors, it is a partial D_2 agonist. It acts in complex fashion also at serotonin (5-HT) receptors, acting as a partial 5-HT_{1A} agonist as well as a 5-HT_{2A} antagonist (Posey, Stigler, Erickson, & McDougle, 2008). Two randomized, placebo-controlled, double-blind, parallel-group studies have evaluated the impact of aripiprazole on challenging behaviors presented by young people with ASCs. In a fixed-dose study, Marcus et al. (2009) randomized 218 young people with ASCs and challenging behaviors including SIB, 178 of whom completed the study, to 8 weeks of treatment with placebo or 1 of 3 fixed-dose levels of aripiprazole (5, 10, or 15 mg/day). All three doses of aripiprazole produced significantly greater reductions from baseline to week 8 in ABC irritability, stereotypy, and hyperactivity subscale scores than did placebo, and all three groups receiving aripiprazole demonstrated greater ABC irritability subscale score reduction than the placebo group by week 2 of treatment (at which time all three groups were receiving 5 mg/day). In another 8-week study, Owen et al. (2009) randomized 98 young people (age 6–17 years) with autistic disorder and challenging behaviors such as tantrums, aggression, and SIB to treatment with either placebo or flexibly dosed aripiprazole (starting dose 2 mg/day, maximum dose 15 mg/day). Mean improvement on the ABC irritability subscale was significantly greater for the aripiprazole group than the placebo group throughout treatment, commencing at week 1 when all aripiprazole doses were 2 mg/day, and at week 8 aripiprazole treatment was also associated with greater improvement than placebo on the ABC hyperactivity, stereotypy, and inappropriate speech subscales. Participants from both of the above studies, together with additional participants, were further evaluated in a 52-week open-label extension study (Marcus et al., 2011a). By the end of the study, the mean decrease from baseline in ABC irritability subscale scores was 8 in newly recruited participants and 6.1 in those who had received placebo in the double-blind studies. These results were largely replicated by another double-blind randomized placebo-controlled study (Ichikawa et al., 2017) with open-label follow-up (Ichikawa et al., 2018). However, Aman et al. (2010), examining changes in individual ABC items in the studies of Marcus et al. (2009) and Owen et al. (2009), reported that items referring to SIB had low baseline values and showed only nonsignificant improvement in both studies. In a further evaluation of the long-term effects of aripiprazole, Findling et al. (2014) randomized 85 children with ASCs (aged 6–17 years), whose challenging behaviors had shown a positive response to aripiprazole treatment for 12 consecutive weeks, to maintenance with aripiprazole or placebo, for up to 16 weeks or until their behavior relapsed. Relapse rates by week 16 were 35% for aripiprazole and 52% for placebo, with no significant between-group difference in time to relapse.

6.4.3.2.3 Other Second-Generation Antipsychotics

A variety of other second-generation antipsychotics have been evaluated as possible treatments for irritability and challenging behaviors in children and adults with ASCs and IDs, but there is no evidence that any are more effective than risperidone and aripiprazole (see reviews by Farmer & Aman, 2013; Goel, Hong, Findling, & Ji, 2018; Howes et al., 2018), and risperidone and aripiprazole remain the only two medications approved by the US Food and Drug Administration for treatment of irritability (in children with ASCs).

6.4.3.2.4 Difficulties and Potential Adverse Side Effects of Treatment with Risperidone and Aripiprazole

Weight gain, increased appetite, raised prolactin levels, and somnolence/sedation are frequently reported adverse events associated with risperidone treatment (Goel et al., 2018; Howes et al., 2018), and extrapyramidal symptoms have been reported in up to 26% of participants in 1-year follow-ups of children using risperidone

(Turgay, Binder, Snyder, & Fisman, 2002). Safety data from trials of aripiprazole have been reported by Marcus et al. (2011b) and Robb et al. (2011). Commonly experienced adverse events in the short-term studies of aripiprazole by Marcus et al. (2009) and Owen et al. (2009) have included sedation, fatigue, somnolence, vomiting, increased appetite, tremor, and nasopharyngitis. One participant taking aripiprazole experienced presyncope, and one demonstrated aggression 1 day after discontinuing aripiprazole owing to increased agitation. In the long-term study (Marcus et al., 2011a), pyrexia, upper respiratory tract infection, and insomnia were also reported as adverse events, and nine participants experienced serious adverse events, aggression being the most frequently reported. Almost 15% of participants experienced extrapyramidal symptoms including tremor, psychomotor hyperactivity, akathisia, and (non-tardive) dyskinesia. In both short-term studies, groups taking aripiprazole (at all doses) gained significantly more weight over the course of the study than placebo participants, and 23% of participants in the long-term study had significant weight gain. Aripiprazole treatment was however associated with significant reductions in serum prolactin over the course of the study, in contrast to the increase in serum prolactin often observed in people taking risperidone and other second-generation antipsychotics.

In 2004 a joint statement from the American Psychiatric Society, American Association of Clinical Endocrinologists, American Diabetes Association, and North American Association for the Study of Obesity recommended extensive metabolic screening and monitoring for all patients taking antipsychotic medications, irrespective of age and psychiatric diagnosis (see Table 6.3), although research suggests that these guidelines have not been consistently followed in clinical practice (Lamy & Erickson, 2018). Monitoring for other less frequent adverse events such as neuroleptic malignant syndrome also remains important with second-generation antipsychotics.

6.4.3.3 Treatment of Habitual/Impulsive Self-Injurious Behavior with Other Medications

Since overactivity and impulsivity are associated with SIB in general, and presumably more specifically with impulsive SIB, it might be expected that medications used to treat overactivity and impulsivity might also assist in treatment of impulsive SIB. Relevant studies have focused almost entirely on children, mostly with ASCs, and most have measured outcomes primarily in terms of overactivity and inattention (for reviews and meta-analyses, see Farmer & Aman, 2013; Patra, Nebhinani, Viswanathan, & Kirubakaran, 2019; Reichow, Volkmar, & Bloch, 2013; Tarrant et al., 2018). The great majority of studies have examined the effects of immediate-release or extended-release methylphenidate or the norepinephrine reuptake inhibitor atomoxetine, with the alpha-2 adrenergic agonist guanfacine also receiving some attention. With regard to methylphenidate, placebo-controlled trials show positive effects on overactivity and impulsivity, with sleeping difficulties, reduced appetite and weight loss being commonly reported adverse effects, and increased irritability,

Table 6.3 Recommended medical monitoring for patients prescribed antipsychotic medications

Parameter	Baseline	Time after medication initiation			Ongoing frequency of monitoring
		1 month/ 4 weeks	2 months/ 8 weeks	3 months/ 12 weeks	
Height	X				
Weight	X	X	X	X	Every 3 months with routine visits
Waist circumference	X				
Blood pressure	X			X	Once a year
Fasting plasma glucose	X			X	Once a year
Fasting lipid profile	X			X	5 years if profile normal, more frequent if clinically indicated
Personal/family medical history[a]	X				

Reproduced with permission of Elsevier from Lamy, M., & Erickson, C. A. (2018). Pharmacological management of behavioral disturbances in children and adolescents with autism spectrum disorders. *Current Problems in Pediatric and Adolescent Health Care, 48*(10), 250–264. © Elsevier 2018

[a]Personal or family history of the following: obesity, diabetes, dyslipidemia, hypertension, or cardiovascular disease

social withdrawal, and increased motor activity also reported in some cases. Several studies have suggested that the probability of positive response is reduced, and the probability of adverse effects increased, in children with ASCs and/or IDs by comparison with children without these conditions but with symptoms of ADHD (Farmer & Aman, 2013; Reichow et al., 2013; Tarrant et al., 2018). The more limited evidence from controlled trials of atomoxetine also suggests an overall positive effect on overactivity/impulsivity, with negative side effects again including sleep difficulties, reduced appetite, nausea and vomiting, and in some cases increased irritability (Farmer & Aman, 2013; Patra et al., 2019; Reichow et al., 2013). However, there is almost no evidence to suggest any effect of these medications on SIB (which has rarely been a focus for the relevant studies). This lack of evidence for a therapeutic effect of methylphenidate and atomoxetine on SIB may of course partly be due to participants in trials of these medications having been selected because of their overactivity/impulsivity rather than engagement in SIB, limiting potential for any therapeutic impact. Nevertheless, some studies have reported change in other challenging behaviors, without effect on potentially SIB-relevant measures. Pearson et al. (2003), for example, reported improvements in teacher-reported aggressive behavior with methylphenidate, but this was not accompanied by any improvement in parent ratings on the ABC irritability subscale. Arnold et al. (2006), using a measurement scale with some items focusing specifically on SIB, found no effect of atomoxetine on scores on the SIB-related group of items.

6.4.3.4 Pharmacological Treatment of Habitual/Impulsive Self-Injurious Behavior: Conclusions

There is some limited specific evidence for a positive effect of risperidone in treatment of SIB. In the case of aripiprazole, the equally limited amount of information available suggests that it may not have any positive effect on SIB (Aman et al., 2010). Its positive effect on irritability (as measured by the ABC irritability subscale) suggests however that it might be tried in cases where the possibility of hyperprolactinemia is of particular concern. Use of both of these medications is frequently accompanied by increased appetite and weight gain, with potential to cause serious long-term health problems. Careful monitoring of weight and key metabolic indicators and periodic attempts to reduce daily dosage or discontinue use of the medication are recommended (Howes et al., 2018). A number of small placebo-controlled double-blind trials involving children and adults with IDs have shown that in many cases, it is possible to reduce or withdraw risperidone after substantial periods of use without significant deterioration in challenging behavior (McNamara et al., 2017; Ramerman et al., 2019). A recent systematic review of the available evidence on reduction or discontinuation of antipsychotics in adults with IDs taking the medication because of challenging behavior concluded however that although the relevant evidence was limited in scope and quality, withdrawal of medication led to behavioral deterioration for some people, with no evident personal characteristics distinguishing the group who experienced these adverse effects (Sheehan & Hassiotis, 2017). A person's ongoing need for pharmacological treatment should be therefore be subject to regular interdisciplinary review on an individual basis (Sheehan & Hassiotis, 2017).

6.4.4 Intervention with "Generalized Habitual" Self-Injurious Behavior

As outlined in Chap. 5, for some people who regularly engage in SIB for extended periods and across many environments, who cannot readily be diverted from engaging in SIB by competing positive stimulation, and who immediately recommence SIB if they are briefly interrupted, this pattern of SIB may have developed from habitual/impulsive (S-R) SIB through a process in which Pavlovian conditioning has led to a wide range of stimuli acquiring the power to elicit SIB. The basic dynamics of such a situation closely resemble those seen with habitual/impulsive SIB evoked in specific situations. The behavioral and pharmacological interventions appropriate to the latter accordingly remain appropriate in cases where the person concerned engages in generalized habitual SIB. The practicalities of behavioral intervention with a person engaging in generalized habitual SIB however will necessarily differ from those in which SIB is evoked by specific environmental challenges. As described earlier, the cornerstone of behavioral intervention where this type of habitual/impulsive SIB is elicited by specific situations or stimuli is progressive exposure with reinforcement. In cases of generalized habitual SIB, however, the ability to evoke SIB may have become generalized by means of perceptual similarity of stimuli, but also by associative, categorical, and semantic processes (Dymond, Dunsmoor, Vervliet, Roche, & Hermans, 2015), and it may be extremely difficult or impossible to determine the nature of the contexts which originally elicited SIB. If a good history of the development of the behavior can be obtained, however, it may be possible to develop a reasonable hypothesis regarding the relevant characteristics of the contexts in which the behavior developed. It is likely that the originating situations involved aversive experiences, and situations associated with physical discomfort or pain, restraint being used to enable personal care to be provided, task demands, aversive sensory experiences, traumatic experiences (including, but not limited to, abuse), and a variety of other aversive experiences may have been the originating context. Behavioral intervention will require the initial establishment of a "safe situation," as distinct as possible from other contexts in which the person engages in SIB. The logistics of such intervention may involve finding a particular space which the person has not previously encountered, providing support from therapeutic staff who the person has not previously met in SIB-eliciting contexts, gradually developing interactions through preferred activities, and encouraging the person to engage with those activities through differential reinforcement. If this initial phase of intervention is successful in terms of establishing a situation in which the person does not engage in SIB (or does so with reduced frequency or intensity), the safe situation may be used to establish by association a "safety signal" (e.g., a distinctive piece of "uniform" worn by supporting persons) to encourage the person to progressively enter other situations and engage in other activities. The logistical challenges involved in developing and maintaining such interventions are obvious, and there will always be a risk that progress will be disrupted by the person encountering a person or situation with some physical or conceptual similarity with the originally eliciting contexts. The situation will be further complicated in cases where there is a need for the person to continue to engage with activities or contexts which elicit SIB, such as personal care routines. Such situations provide ongoing opportunities for novel stimuli to become associated with SIB-eliciting stimuli and thereby potentially evoke SIB even in the presence of a previously established effective safety signal.

6.4.5 Intervention with Habitual/Impulsive Self-Injurious Behavior: Summary and Conclusions

With people whose SIB shows limited sensitivity to social contingencies and appears to be habitual/impulsive in nature, if the behavior is nevertheless evoked by specific situations, behavioral intervention using graduated exposure with reinforcement and other techniques should be the first choice of intervention. Further, the behavioral interventions described above as relevant for intervention with operant SIB, and FCT in particular, should also continue to be used. Progression from operant (goal-directed) control to habitual/impulsive (S-R) control of SIB is a progressive, and in principle reversible, developmental path, and the development of a complex repertoire of goal-directed behaviors is potentially an important therapeutic process in reversing the dominance of S-R processes. Encouraging and developing communicative skills therefore has an importance beyond attempts to directly replace SIB with a functionally equivalent communicative response. Pharmacological intervention may also be of value in treating habitual/impulsive SIB. There is however only limited evidence for the utility of such intervention, with specific evidence of effectiveness only for risperidone, use of which is frequently accompanied by increased appetite and weight gain. Although therefore there may be a role for pharmacological intervention, with close specialist supervision, in tandem with behavioral intervention for habitual/impulsive SIB, its likely effectiveness should not be overestimated. In a study of referrals to a specialist (tertiary) treatment center for children and adults with ASCs, many of whom also had IDs, Adler et al. (2015) reported that in over half of those referred because of concerns about aggression, SIB, and "severe tantrums," these behaviors were "drug-refractory" in the sense that they were not adequately controlled by drug treatment, either by trials of risperidone and aripiprazole or by trials of one of these drugs plus trials of at least two other medications. Although the participants in this study may have experienced particularly severe difficulties, these findings are a useful reminder of the limitations of current treatment options.

6.5 Intervention with Stereotyped Self-Injurious Behavior ("Automatically Reinforced Self-Injurious Behavior Subtype 1")

If assessment suggests that SIB is "stereotyped," i.e., the person engages in SIB continuously or almost continuously for extended periods, but can readily be diverted from SIB if they are offered a stimulating alternative activity, or meets Hagopian et al.'s (2018) criteria for "automatically reinforced SIB Subtype 1," i.e., high levels of SIB in the "alone" condition of an EFA relative to the "play" condition, the principal challenge for behavioral intervention is identification of effective alternative sources of reinforcement of sufficient variety to compete effectively with engagement in SIB over extended periods of time. In some cases, further assessment may give some indication as to the effective reinforcer. Goh et al. (1995), for example, searching for sources of stimulation to reduce hand-mouthing, provided objects to manipulate to four adults with profound IDs and showed that for all four hand-object contact was more extensive than mouth-object contact, suggesting that hand stimulation was the reinforcer maintaining hand-mouthing. However, in cases involving putative automatic reinforcement, the nature of the reinforcement involved can rarely be specified with any confidence. In the absence of this information, NCR interventions typically provide noncontingent access to sensory and other stimuli selected using structured preference assessments (see Chap. 5). The most straightforward method of intervention is then to provide the person with noncontingent access to, and encouragement to engage with, these activities. Vollmer, Marcus, and LeBlanc (1994) showed that noncontingent access to preferred items reduced levels of SIB in three young children with developmental disabilities, although additional procedures, including brief (5 s) restraint of one child's hands, were necessary to achieve acceptable reductions in SIB for two of the children. Vollmer et al. (1994) noted that treatment effectiveness might reduce owing to satiation if such treatments were used over extended time periods. Subsequent studies have however reported that where necessary, providing access to a variety of sources of stimulation and/or rotating the objects provided can produce long-term reductions in extent of SIB (DeLeon, Anders, Rodriguez-Catter, & Neidert, 2000; Lindberg, Iwata, Roscoe, Worsdell, & Hanley, 2003). Van Camp, Vollmer, and Daniel (2001), working with a boy diagnosed with autism whose SIB involved placing harmful substances into his eyes, showed that increasing the effort involved in SIB relative to that involved in accessing a preferred item (keyboard), by ensuring that items required to engage in SIB were further away from him than the keyboard, produced greater reduction in SIB than providing the keyboard alone. In treatment of stereotyped SIB, noncontingent presentation of competing stimulation has been more widely used than attempts to use the stimulation to reinforce behaviors alternative to and/or incompatible with SIB. Early attempts to use differential reinforcement to intervene with SIB had suggested that even where competing stimuli could be identified, attempts to use them in differential reinforcement interventions were ineffective (Shore, Iwata, DeLeon, Kahng, & Smith, 1997). Shore et al. suggested that this failure was a consequence of the increased response effort required to gain stimulation in DRA by comparison with SIB. Reducing the response effort required to produce the alternative stimulation, e.g., by use of microswitches, may therefore increase the effectiveness of DRA intervention. Steege, Wacker, Berg, Cigrand, and Cooper (1989) reduced the damaging hand-mouthing of a child with severe multiple disabilities by teaching him to use a microswitch to activate reinforcing stimuli (a radio or a fan). However, providing access to stimulation noncontingently is more effective than DRO or DRA when these are used without additional interventions (Rooker, Bonner, Dillon, & Zarcone, 2018). Perhaps unsurprisingly, Rooker et al. (2018) also found that interventions using competing stimuli selected on the basis of direct observation of their effectiveness in reducing SIB were more effective than those using stimuli selected from stimulus preference assessments.

6.6 Intervention with "Compulsive" Self-Injurious Behavior

Within the model we propose for the development of SIB, compulsive SIB presenting with elevated levels of arousal, anxiety, and agitation, particularly if these levels increase further if attempts are made to persuade the person to stop engaging in SIB, or SIB presenting with self-restraint (SR), with agitation if SR is interrupted, represents one of the final possible stages in the development of SIB. People who engage in compulsive SIB usually do so in response to particular environmental events (e.g., being asked to wait for something) or the interruption of SR. If other people then attempt to remedy the person's problem (e.g., by giving them the desired item or allowing them to resume SR), the person's SIB and agitation, rather than abating, is however likely to continue or even escalate further.

It seems likely therefore that the initiation of compulsive SIB is under S-R control, and the behavioral interventions described above in discussion of intervention with habitual/impulsive SIB can in principle also be used in the treatment of compulsive SIB. In cases involving compulsive SIB however, systematic progress through a desensitization hierarchy is often very difficult or impossible because the point in the hierarchy at which SIB occurs will often vary dramatically from day to day depending on the anxiety and arousal levels of the person concerned. For any progress to be made, therefore, it will usually be necessary to make attempts to help the person to reduce her/his levels of anxiety and agitation before beginning attempts at desensitization. For some people, it may be possible to achieve this through behavioral relaxation training (Lindsay, Richardson, & Michie, 1989). In other cases, pharmacological intervention may be tried. Two classes of agent, anticonvulsants (used for their potential mood-stabilizing properties) and beta-adrenergic receptor blockers, have been investigated for use in the treatment of irritability, including SIB. Two randomized controlled trials of anticonvulsants with children with ASCs have reported significant positive effects on ABC irritability subscale scores. Rezaei et al. (2010) reported a significant effect for topiramate (in combination with risperidone) versus topiramate plus placebo, while Hollander et al. (2010) reported a positive effect of divalproex sodium. However, Hollander et al. (2010) found no effect of divalproex sodium on scores on the Overt Aggression Scale-Modified, a scale which includes a subsection of items relevant to SIB, and a further placebo-controlled study of valproate in young people with ASCs found no effect on aggressive behaviors (Hellings et al., 2005). Prospective open-label and other studies of topiramate, valproate, and other anticonvulsants for the treatment of challenging behavior in people with ASCs and/or IDs have produced mixed results (Farmer & Aman, 2013; Lamy & Erickson, 2018). Beta-adrenergic receptor blockers (beta-blockers) such as propranolol are competitive antagonists of noradrenaline and adrenaline at beta-adrenergic receptor sites in the peripheral and central nervous system (Ward, Tharian, Roy, Deb, & Unwin, 2013) and have been used in the treatment of generalized anxiety and acute stress in people without NDCs, particularly when physical symptoms such as tachycardia are prominent in the person's experience of anxiety. In their systematic review of studies on the use of beta-blockers with children and adults with IDs (including those with ASCs), Ward et al. (2013) identified 5 studies, involving a total of 11 participants, in which effects on SIB were reported. Positive effects were reported in all cases, although the quality of evidence available from the studies (case reports, retrospective casenote review, and open clinical trial) was low. Hypotension and bradycardia, followed by gastrointestinal and respiratory disturbance, were the most commonly reported adverse events. Ward et al. (2013) noted that in the absence of clear dosing guidelines, particularly careful clinical monitoring is essential if beta-blockers are used with people with limited ability to communicate symptoms. It should also be noted that beta-blockers can inhibit the release of insulin, an issue of particular concern for people at risk for adverse metabolic effects of antipsychotics, and are not generally recommended for treatment of anxiety in people without NDCs. Close specialist psychiatric supervision is therefore required if their use is considered with people engaging in SIB.

The use of selective serotonin reuptake inhibitors (SSRIs) such as citalopram, fluoxetine, fluvoxamine, and sertraline in the treatment of obsessive-compulsive disorder in people without NDCs has encouraged some interest in their possible use in treating compulsive SIB. A retrospective case review study of 38 adults with IDs living in institutional care, most of whom had additional psychiatric diagnoses and were taking other medications, reported significant improvement in global ratings of SIB (on a seven-point scale) made by the researchers from clinical records following the addition of an SSRI (most often paroxetine), or for 2 participants clomipramine, to their medication regime (Janowsky, Shetty, Barnhill, Elamir, & Davis, 2005). However, a large, 12-week, randomized controlled trial of the effectiveness of citalopram for treatment of repetitive behaviors (including SIB) in children and teenagers with ASCs (King et al., 2009) showed no advantage for citalopram over placebo in reducing SIB. Citalopram treatment was however associated with significantly higher rates of a range of adverse effects including increased energy levels, impulsivity, hyperactivity, attentional difficulties, stereotypy, gastrointestinal problems, insomnia, and dry skin. Two children (one with a previous history of seizures) experienced seizures during the trial. Additional retrospective review, open-label trial, and case report studies of the effects of SSRIs on challenging behaviors in children and adults with ASCs have yielded variable results (Farmer & Aman, 2013; Lamy & Erickson, 2018). A retrospective review of 22 young people with ASCs treated with an SSRI following a clinically unsuccessful trial of a previous SSRI reported that over two-thirds showed activation side effects with the second SSRI (Henry et al., 2009). For children with ASCs therefore lack of evidence of effectiveness, frequent occurrence of adverse reactions and uncertainties regarding appropriate dosage (Lamy & Erickson, 2018; Posey, Erickson, Stigler, & McDougle, 2006) do not support the utility of currently available SSRIs in treatment of SIB. There is much less evidence relevant to the effects of SSRIs on SIB in adults with ASCs and/or IDs, but a retrospective review of the use of SSRIs to treat depression in adults with IDs reported that over 30% of episodes of treatment with SSRIs resulted in behavioral activation side effects similar to those reported for children with ASCs (Biswas, Bhaumik, & Branford, 2001).

6.7 Monitoring the Effects of Intervention with Self-Injurious Behavior

In the applied behavior analytic literature, frequency of SIB, or the proportion of time which a person spends engaging SIB, is often used as the primary outcome measure, whereas in most evaluations of pharmacological treatments, the irritability subscale of the ABC has been the primary outcome measure. Both of these techniques are however of limited utility in outpatient clinical practice. The clinician may rarely actually see the person concerned engaging in SIB, and the person's behavior in the clinical setting may differ substantially from that in their everyday environment. Even if the clinician arranges to regularly observe the person in their everyday environment, the rate of SIB observed will often differ markedly between sessions, and substantial amounts of observation may be required in order to derive meaningful estimates of the rate of SIB before and during intervention. On the other hand, a wide-ranging behavioral measure such as the ABC includes only a small number of items specifically relevant to SIB and will be relatively insensitive to incremental changes which may be expected during intervention.

In clinical practice therefore, the most practical way of evaluating progress (or its absence) during intervention will be to regularly complete a focused rating scale with input from the person engaging in SIB and/or people supporting her/him. There are two obvious choices of rating scale for this purpose. The first is the BPI-01 described in Sect. 6.4.3.1 above. Rojahn and his colleagues have developed a short (30-item) form derived from the BPI-01, the BPI-S, with 8 items assessing SIB, 10 assessing aggressive/destructive behavior, and 12 assessing stereotyped behavior. Each item is rated on a five-point frequency scale and a four-point severity scale, based on the person's behavior in the 6 months prior to rating. For the SIB (and aggressive/destructive behavior) subscales, multiplication of the frequency and severity score for each item and addition of the resulting scores can be used to generate an overall subscale score. The BPI-S has adequate to good internal consistency (Mascitelli et al., 2015; Rojahn et al., 2012a) and interrater and test-retest reliability (Mascitelli et al., 2015). Confirmatory factor analysis has demonstrated adequate fit of derived factors with the three BPI-S subscales (Mascitelli et al., 2015), and Rojahn et al. (2012a, 2012b) have presented evidence for the confirmatory and discriminant validity of the BPI-S. Bowring, Totsika, Hastings, and Toogood (2018) have provided normative data from a total population sample of adults with IDs in the UK, enabling a clinician to determine what percentage of individuals with IDs in the normative sample achieved each level of severity and frequency rating for each BPI-S item. Bowring et al. (2018) also provide "cutoff" scores for each BPI-S subscale which are proposed to indicate the boundary between population subgroups with and without clinically significant challenging behaviors and "reliable change" scores which indicate change scores which are unlikely to arise simply owing to the limitations on the reliability of the BPI-S.

All items of the SIB subscale of the BPI-S, and all but two of the items on the aggressive/destructive behavior scale, refer to simple physical (nonvocal) behaviors (e.g., self-biting, head-hitting, pushing others). Clinicians working with more verbally able people may however also be interested in verbal aggression directed toward the self or others, together with more sophisticated types of SIB such as self-cutting or self-burning. Staff of the New York State Institute for Basic Research in Developmental Disabilities (IBR) developed the IBR Modified Overt Aggression Scale (IBR-MOAS; Cohen et al., 2010), a wide-ranging instrument which includes a section on aggressive behaviors covering verbal aggressive behaviors directed toward the self and others in addition to more physical behaviors. This section (which we refer to hereafter as the IBR-MOAS Aggression Scale to differentiate it from the wider questionnaire) has five domains (verbal aggression toward others, verbal aggression toward self, physical aggression against other people, physical aggression against objects, physical aggression against self). The four items within each domain describe behaviors with increasing levels of severity, with each item rated on a four-point frequency scale ranging from "never" to "often," with the latter operationally defined as once or more per day on average. Data on the scale are available from a large population-based sample very largely comprising adults with IDs. Cohen et al. (2010) reported internal consistencies of the IBR-MOAS Aggression Scale domains ranging from fair to good, with levels of interrater reliability ranging from good to excellent, and test-retest reliability excellent for all domains. Principal components analysis of data from a subgroup of participants who were identified as engaging in significant aggression toward themselves, others, or property identified two factors, the first factor with high loadings from items from the verbal aggression toward others, physical aggression against other people, and physical aggression against objects domains. The second factor showed high loadings from the physical aggression against self-domain, while items from the verbal aggression toward self-domain loaded on both factors. The IBR-MOAS Aggression Scale therefore offers an alternative to the BPI-01 or BPI-S for clinicians wishing to monitor SIB engaged in by more able people.

Clinicians working with people engaging in SIB will normally want to know whether any changes in frequency or severity of the behavior are being accompanied by changes in the range of opportunities open to them. The Guernsey Community Participation and Leisure Assessment (GCPLA; Baker, 2000) is a useful tool in monitoring such change. The GCPLA is a checklist of six categories of community contact and activity (contact with health and law enforcement staff, use of public transport, indoor leisure activities, out-of-home leisure, sporting, and recreational activities, social activities, and use of facilities and amenities such as shops and post offices). The 6 categories list a total of 49 types of activity (e.g., going to the cinema), each of which are rated on a 5-point scale of frequency of occurrence ranging from less than once every 3 months to once or more daily. For each type of contact, information is also collected on whether the person engaged in the activity alone, with peers, accompanied by carers but not directly supervised, or directly supervised by carers. The GCPLA is intended to be completed on the basis of a semi-structured interview with the person concerned or a carer regarding the last 6 months, but the ratings can be used to generate numerical scores such as a range score (the number of activities which are engaged in at least once every 3 months). Preliminary studies of interrater reliability when care staff complete the GCPLA, and test-retest reliabilities for completion of the GCPLA by staff and by interview of service users, suggest that these are acceptable. The GCPLA has been used to assess changes in levels of community participation following behavioral intervention for challenging behavior (Hassiotis et al., 2012) and provides a convenient method of monitoring changes in community access associated with behavioral changes in intervention with SIB.

6.8 Preventing and Responding to Relapse of Self-Injurious Behavior Following Successful Intervention

Cooper et al. (2009) suggested that SIB could usefully be thought of as a remitting-relapsing disorder, and certainly any clinician who has worked with individuals engaging in SIB over substantial time periods will have witnessed situations in which a person who has successfully controlled their SIB for varying periods of time then experiences a further increase in the rate and/or severity of the behavior. Such relapses can usefully be divided into two groups. The first group comprises relapses which occur during or shortly after apparently successful intervention. The second group comprises those situations in which a person who has refrained from SIB, or maintained the behavior at a very low level, for months or even years, begins again to engage in SIB of substantial severity.

The first type of relapse is often seen with behavioral interventions, and in some cases the cause is simply that carers have ceased to implement a previously effective intervention. In educational or residential care settings, this may occur because not all staff have been sufficiently trained in implementing the intervention, or because of turnover in the staff members working with the person concerned. In these situations further training, or improving the availability of written behavior support plans, may be sufficient to remedy the situation, and proactive planning to train new staff members in details of the person's support plan may be sufficient to avoid further relapses. In other cases, staff may have ceased to implement an intervention because of a change in the topography of SIB. Particularly if the intervention includes a component of extinction of the SIB, another topography of SIB which is a member of the same operant class may become more salient. Intervention may, for example, have involved carers reinforcing adaptive communicative responses with breaks from task demands while not responding to head-hitting which has been assessed as being maintained by such access. In these circumstances an alternative topography of SIB (e.g., the person kicking herself) may increase in frequency, and alarmed carers may reinforce this topography by providing breaks from task demands contingent on its occurrence. In these situations, supporting carers to recognize that the intervention plan requires the planned response contingent on both topographies of SIB should be sufficient to restore the effectiveness of the intervention.

Other than these situations when interventions have temporarily completely broken down, there will of course be many others where behavioral interventions are implemented inconsistently. Even if carers working with the person implement the plan with complete fidelity, the person engaging in SIB will meet with other people who may respond to their behavior in ways inconsistent with the planned intervention. In many situations however, when caregivers are attempting to implement an intervention while simultaneously meeting the other needs of the person concerned for social interaction, intellectual stimulation, and personal care, even the most committed and skilled carers are unlikely to implement interventions with perfect fidelity (Bloom & Lambert, 2015). With FCT (and other DRA interventions), fidelity may be compromised in two ways. Carers may not consistently reinforce the adaptive communicative (or other) response (omission errors), or they may occasionally reinforce SIB (commission errors). In general, commission errors result in higher levels of challenging behavior than omission errors. Achieving a high level of fidelity during initial intervention appears to have an important effect on the consequences of later failures in treatment integrity. Following initial high-fidelity DRA treatment, inconsistent maintenance with both adaptive replacement and challenging behaviors reinforced on 50% of occurrences results in a situation where both behaviors will occur with similar frequencies; if however DRA treatment is implemented from the outset with a similar limited degree of fidelity, the person is likely to continue to engage in challenging behavior with little use of the prosocial alternative response (Pipkin, Vollmer, & Sloman, 2010). Since some degree of deterioration in fidelity of implementation is likely with behavioral interventions, an initial phase of intervention in which treatment is implemented with high fidelity is therefore important in reducing the probability of relapse.

Some degree of re-emergence of SIB if the behavior is occasionally reinforced following successful FCT or DRA intervention with extinction of SIB would of course be predicted by a straightforward behavioral account. Just short of two decades ago, Layng, Andronis, and Goldiamond (1999) showed in an animal model that previously extinguished headbanging recurred, even without any reinstatement of reinforcement, and with alternative behavior continuing to be reinforced, as schedules of reinforcement of the alternative behavior changed and thinned. This re-emergence of a previously reinforced but then extinguished behavior (such as SIB) when a second behavior (such as communication) which has been reinforced simultaneously with the extinction of the first, but is then itself placed on extinction or reinforced sparsely, is generally referred to as resurgence. As mentioned in the discussion on FCT in Sect. 6.3.5 above, Briggs et al. (2018) reported resurgence of challenging behavior during schedule thinning in 76% of applications of reinforcement thinning following FCT. In principle, resurgence can be readily managed by re-instating a higher level of reinforcement for the communicative (or other alternative) behavior. If family members or other carers are insufficiently supported in maintaining the intervention however, resurgence of SIB might well result in loss of confidence in the intervention and reinforcement of SIB being reinstated (Bloom & Lambert, 2015). Resurgence of SIB might also occur if the communicative or other alternative response is unavailable (rather than available but unreinforced), as when a person's augmentative or alternative communicative system is unavailable to them (Kimball, Kelley, Podlesnik, Forton, & Hinkle, 2018). Research interest has therefore recently turned to modelling the effects of factors which influence the probability of resurgence of a challenging behavior if reinforcement of an alternative behavior is discontinued or thinned, with a view to modifying interventions so as to reduce the probability of such resurgence (Fisher et al., 2018). Most attention has been focused on FCT/DRA interventions, although resurgence may also occur if delivery of noncontingent reinforcement is discontinued or thinned in NCR interventions (Liggett, Nastri, & Podlesnik, 2018). Much of the relevant research to date, even when it has involved participants with NDCs, has modelled resurgence processes using arbitrary responses such as button-pressing as the "target" response, so caution must be exercised in generalizing results to interventions for SIB (or other challenging behaviors). To date, however, it appears that interventions (FCT or NCR) in which the target response is placed on extinction may result in lower rates of resurgence (Fisher, Greer, Craig, et al., 2018; Saini, Fisher, & Pisman, 2017). A further method of reducing the risk of resurgence of challenging behavior if the communicative response faces periods of extinction following FCT may be to thin reinforcement of the communicative response using a multiple schedule, in which the communicative response is reinforced in the presence of an S^D (e.g., a green card) and not reinforced in the presence of an S^Δ (e.g., a red card) and the proportion of time in which the S^Δ is present is progressively increased. Fuhrman, Fisher, and Greer (2016) showed that following such training, resurgence of challenging behavior during subsequent extinction (with the S^Δ present) was reduced by comparison with that following a "traditional" FCT sequence without the multiple-schedule process. An alternative strategy for reducing risk of resurgence following FCT is to sequentially train and extinguish a series of different communicative responses, in the expectation that if the last trained response is faced with extinction, previously trained alternative communicative responses will resurge rather than (or at least prior to) challenging behavior. Although resurgence of previously trained communicative responses has been demonstrated in controlled situations, (e.g., Hoffman & Falcomata, 2014; Lambert, Bloom, Samaha, Dayton, & Rodewald, 2015), when this strategy is applied in FCT treatment of established challenging behaviors, resurgence of previously trained communicative responses may not always occur, and the challenging behavior may resurge to a greater degree than any of the trained communicative responses (Lambert, Bloom, Samaha, & Dayton, 2017).

Relapse following successful behavioral intervention may also occur through a process generally termed renewal (Podlesnik, Kelley, Jimenez-Gomez, & Bouton, 2017). Extinction is an active learning process, and following successful FCT, both the newly learned communicative response and the SIB or other challenging behavior which have been extinguished may have come under stimulus control of aspects of the context in which FCT was implemented. If the treatment context (e.g., an inpatient setting) is different from the context in which challenging behavior was originally reinforced (e.g., the person's home), then on return home the person may fail to use the communicative response learned in FCT and recommence engaging challenging behavior (Saini, Sullivan, Baxter, DeRosa, & Roane, 2018). Treatment effects may similarly fail to transfer to a third context (e.g., work or school). The most effective way to avoid minimizing such effects is to implement intervention in the person's everyday environment and with the people who normally support them. Even when this is done however, renewal may be seen when the person visits other environments. Fortunately however a number of strategies to avoid or minimize renewal effects have long been recognized (Stokes & Baer, 1977). If intervention is implemented in multiple settings, during multiple activities, and involving many different individuals as therapists ("training sufficient exemplars"), intervention effects should eventually generalize to novel settings. Training sufficient exemplars may obviously be a lengthy process. An alternative strategy which is less labor-intensive is to "program common stimuli." This approach aims to bring the responding established during intervention under the control of a portable discriminative stimulus which can then be transported to other settings. Fisher, Greer, Fuhrman, and Querim (2015) used FCT to reduce challenging behaviors of two children with ASCs and then used a distinctive stimulus (a yellow wristband worn by the person acting as "therapist") to signal periods when use of the communicative response would be followed by reinforcement. Once the children had learned to use the communicative response only when the therapist wore the wristband, Fisher et al. (2015) showed that their use of the communicative response (and low rates of challenging behavior) rapidly and reliably generalized across new settings and therapists (provided that the latter were wearing the wristband). Fisher et al.'s (2015) procedure offers a possible method for rapid generalization of treatment effects across settings. However, generalization was demonstrated only in different rooms and with different personnel within the broader treatment setting. Establishing the robustness of this approach when treatment is extended to the situation in which challenging behavior had originally been reinforced will require further research. In addition, it remains to be investigated whether this method assists or inhibits generalization of the communicative response to such natural situations during the eventual withdrawal of the discriminative stimulus (e.g., wristband).

Although renewal has been primarily investigated in relation to maintenance of the effects of FCT, renewal may also be seen following successful behavioral intervention with habitual/impulsive SIB using progressive exposure with reinforcement, and similar approaches may be used to minimize such renewal effects. Research into relapse prevention is a major focus of current research in behavioral interventions, and we return to this issue in Chap. 9.

The second type of relapse, in which a person who has refrained from SIB, or maintained the behavior at a low level, for a substantial period of time, recommences engaging in SIB, has received much less research attention than relapse shortly following treatment. In individual cases, such relapse may be seen in connection with stressful experiences such as illness or with major life events such as changes in living situation. Changes which simultaneously change or disrupt a person's physical environment, significant relationships, and overall patterns of activity, in addition to specific support plans or treatment programs, are likely to cause substantial stress and impact broadly on the person's behavior. In such situations, it may be helpful to attempt to mitigate the effects of the overall change, e.g., by facilitating ongoing contact with friends with whom contact might otherwise be lost following a change in residence. Sometimes it will be necessary to formally reinstate interventions (e.g., FCT) which may have previously been helpful in reducing SIB but which may have become more informally and irregularly used as the person engaged less in SIB.

In other cases however a person may recommence engaging in SIB, sometimes of considerable frequency and severity, after a lengthy period of "remission," without any obvious precipitating event. Such relapses may bear some resemblance to the "return of fear" sometimes experienced by people who have successfully participated in behavioral intervention for phobic anxiety. Such relapses are believed to result from people encountering stimuli which have acquired the ability to evoke anxiety through association with other stimuli (Dymond et al., 2015), but which have not been included in the hierarchy used in progressive exposure therapy. Relapse for a person whose SIB was evoked by stimuli associated with mealtimes may for example occur when they hear the theme music of a TV or radio program (perhaps long since withdrawn from the schedules) which was often playing just before one of their main meals of the day. Once SIB has been re-evoked, other stimuli newly associated with the eliciting stimuli can rapidly acquire the ability to evoke the behavior. Often therefore, whether or not the stimulus which initiated relapse can be identified, it will be necessary to completely re-assess the person's SIB and intervene according to the current, rather than the historic, dynamics of the situation.

6.9 Intervention with Self-Injurious Behavior: Summary and Conclusions

In this chapter we have suggested that conceptualizing the development of SIB through a series of stages (emergent, operant, habitual/impulsive, stereotyped, and compulsive) provides a useful foundation on which to base choice of initial intervention. We emphasize once again that progress along this proposed developmental path involves changes in the relative influences of diverse processes rather than abrupt changes in sources of control. Further, progress through the stages is a process which can be inhibited or reversed by environmental influences. Our intention is that the framework proposed can be used to understand the processes currently predominant in causing the SIB of each particular person at any one time and provide a starting point for consideration of intervention. The proposed model clearly suggests that for some individuals whose SIB can be thought of as emergent, operant, or stereotyped, behavioral interventions should be the first choice of intervention, and there is little rationale for pharmacological treatment. In situations however where a person's SIB presents as habitual/impulsive (including cases where such behavior is widely generalized), or where the behavior appears compulsive, non-operant behavioral interventions such as progressive exposure with reinforcement are also viable intervention options but can in some cases rationally be combined with pharmacological intervention.

For socially reinforced operant SIB, and stereotyped (or "automatically reinforced Type 1") SIB, behavioral interventions when implemented with fidelity can clearly produce significant reductions in SIB in most cases. Significant challenges however remain in maintaining these interventions over long periods in people's everyday environments. Fortunately, the attention of researchers and behavioral clinicians is increasingly turning to methods for effective maintenance, and we shall briefly outline some of the work currently being undertaken in Chap. 9.

With regard to pharmacological interventions, the only convincing evidence for specific effectiveness in treatment for SIB concerns the atypical antipsychotics and specifically risperidone. The effectiveness of these medications might be expected to be restricted by their limited ability to block dopamine D_1 receptors. Other medications such as beta-blockers may be helpful adjuncts to behavioral intervention in cases involving compulsive SIB. However, all possibly effective pharmacological interventions are accompanied by significant risk of side effects and require specialist psychiatric supervision for their use.

In clinical practice, members of different professions may work with one individual with varying levels of communication between each other and with varying levels of coordination of their inputs. A distinction between "operant" and "biological" SIB is often still made in considering choice of intervention. The model proposed in this and preceding chapters will we hope contribute to the development of a more integrated and effective basis for multidisciplinary intervention.

6.10 Case Studies

Ayanna B

Although Ayanna continued to use her "I want to leave" symbol to ask to be excused from group activities, and rarely engaged in SIB, as the weather improved with the approach of summer, her teacher noticed a change in her behavior. She started to use the "I want to leave" symbol at the very beginning of group activities and also started to use the symbol at other times. Being concerned about the activities that Ayanna was missing, and about the amount of time the teaching assistant was having to spend with her, the teacher decided that Ayanna's requests to leave an activity would only be agreed to during specific group activities. Having obtained the consent of Ayanna's mother to make this change, the teacher explained it to Ayanna with the aid of a symbol timetable with which Ayanna was familiar. Since Ayanna had learned to use the "leave" symbol so rapidly, the teacher was confident that she would understand the restriction being placed on its use. Ayanna appeared to understand, and assent to, the proposed limitation on her use of the symbol.

Ayanna's teacher was therefore surprised and disappointed to see Ayanna's reaction on the first occasion when she used the "leave" symbol and was told that she could not leave the classroom at that moment. Ayanna started to cry and slap her face as she used to do before. Although on the first occasion that this happened the teacher insisted that Ayanna should remain in the activity, on subsequent similar occasions Ayanna became so distressed and self-injurious that her teacher felt obliged to let her leave the activity for the sake of the other students. After 2 weeks, there was no sign that Ayanna was becoming more accepting of the limitation placed on her ability to leave the classroom on request. Her teacher became seriously worried following an episode in which Ayanna requested to leave an activity, was told she could not immediately do so, and then not only started to cry and slap herself but also tore the "leave" symbol into pieces.

Ayanna's teacher sought an urgent consultation with the speech and language therapist, and after a discussion with Ayanna's parents in which they consented to the plan, the teacher removed the "leave" symbol from the wallet in which Ayanna stored her symbols for a period of 2 weeks. During this period there were occasions when Ayanna became distressed and started to slap her face during group activities, and she was allowed to leave these activities as in the past. During other activities however she seemed accepting of the fact that there was no option to leave except at scheduled breaks. Following the 2-week period, the teacher reintroduced the "leave" symbol. The symbol was however made twice as large as Ayanna's other symbols and set on a differently colored background. Also, Ayanna was not given the symbol to keep with her at all times. Instead, she was given the symbol at the beginning of group activities and asked to hand it back to the teacher at the end. Ayanna again started to use the symbol to ask to leave group activities almost as soon as they had begun, but also continued to participate in other classroom activities, while episodes of SIB were again rapidly reduced in frequency.

Darren C

Although the Educational Psychologist had mentioned the possibility of conducting a stimulus preference assessment to identify a reinforcer to use in conjunction with a progressive exposure intervention, Darren's teacher saw little need for a formal assessment in order to identify a probable effective reinforcer. Like many other students at the school, Darren loved playing simple games and watching videos on a tablet computer. As a matter of general policy, the school limited students' access to these devices (other than for educational purposes) to strictly defined periods at the end of breaks and mealtimes, but the headteacher was happy to endorse a temporary arrangement for Darren to have additional tablet time as a consequence of participating in the program.

In consultation with the Educational Psychologist, Darren's teacher worked out a sequence of program steps which initially involved Darren walking progressively further from his classroom toward the dining room, then involved him entering the dining room and spending progressively longer periods of time sitting at a table, and finally involved him going progressively further through the sequence of steps involved in selecting and consuming his meal. Understanding that there might be a risk that Darren might engage in SIB during the intervention, the teacher arranged a meeting to explain the plan to Darren's parents and obtain their consent to its implementation before putting it into practice. At each step until the program was completed, Darren returned to his classroom to actually eat his meal. Progression through the series of steps was decided on the basis of Darren's behavior, with progression to the next stage provided that he had successfully completed the previous step without engaging in SIB on two consecutive days. Each time Darren completed a step without engaging SIB, he was given a voucher which he could exchange for 5 min extra time with his tablet computer.

Darren completed the first five steps of the program, which involved walking progressively further toward the dining room, in 2 weeks, engaging in no SIB at all. On the Monday of the next week, he entered the dining room without engaging in

SIB, but on the Tuesday he appeared to become a little distressed on entering the dining room and started to bite his hand. He was asked to return to his classroom and was disappointed not to receive a voucher. The next day he successfully entered the dining room without engaging in SIB, and for the remainder of that week and the next, he spent progressively increasing lengths of time in the dining room, until he was successfully remaining there for 20 min. His teacher anticipated that there might be difficulties when Darren was asked to start going through the series of steps to actually collect a meal. Darren however received a tremendous reception from the school's catering staff, who were delighted to see him back in the dining room, and he completed the remaining steps of the program without any further SIB.

Arshad D

The clinical psychologist who had assessed Arshad's SIB wrote a brief report, including her recommendations for intervention, which included her conclusion that to be effective, a noncontingent reinforcement program would need to commence with a mean inter-reinforcement interval of no more than 60 s. At a further meeting between school staff, Arshad's mother, his social worker, and the clinical psychologist, there was an extended discussion on the options available both to reduce Arshad's SIB and to improve his independent toileting skills. His social worker pointed out that given Arshad's age and lack of capacity to make his own decisions on the issues, it was necessary to decide which course of action would be in Arshad's best interests and pointed out the possible negative consequences should his SIB deteriorate when he left school. His mother reiterated her view that improving Arshad's independent toileting should be a priority and suggested that improving his skills in this area would improve his quality of life by widening the range of social situations his family would be confident to take him into. The school's head teacher, although agreeing that decisions should be taken in Arshad's best interests, observed that implementing the NCR program recommended by the psychologist together with an intensive program to teach him to use the toilet independently would require assigning a teaching assistant to work full time with Arshad, which would limit opportunities for other students. After a lengthy discussion, it was agreed to trial a noncontingent reinforcement program for a period of 1 h in each school day in order to evaluate its effectiveness and determine how rapidly reinforcement schedule thinning could be achieved, while also introducing a highly structured prompt fading program to teach Arshad to go to the toilet independently.

Sarah E

The experimental functional analysis (EFA) sessions in which Sarah had participated had identified escape from task demands as the primary reinforcer of Sarah's SIB. The BCBA therefore discussed with the residential service manager the possibility of piloting a noncontingent reinforcement intervention, starting from a position of completely withdrawing any requests for Sarah to participate in any activity other than essential personal care. There was naturally some concern regarding the possible impact of such a proposal on Sarah's quality of life. Following extensive consultations with staff of the residential service, Sarah's parents, and Sarah's consultant psychiatrist, who had been closely involved in her care for several years, the BCBA and the manager of the residential service agreed that a time-limited trial of such an approach would be in Sarah's best interests. It was however considered that it would also be in Sarah's best interests to closely monitor the effects of the intervention on Sarah's SIB, and in addition to support staff keeping records, the BCBA undertook to carry out 1 h of structured observation on each day for 2 weeks before the intervention started and then on each of the 14 days of the proposed period of intervention.

The results of the intervention were disappointing. Neither the support workers' records nor the results of the BCBA's observations suggested any meaningful change in the amount of time that Sarah spent engaging in SIB when compared with the 2 weeks prior to the intervention starting. Anecdotal reports from the staff supporting Sarah suggested that although they had refrained from any attempts to engage her in all but absolutely essential activities, even the minimal requests which they had to make of Sarah in the course of providing basic personal care sometimes resulted in her head-hitting or headbanging. Sarah's support workers also mentioned that on these occasions, they sometimes temporarily withdrew requests, e.g., for Sarah to brush her hair (or cooperate with a support worker brushing it) but that even then she would continue to hit her head. When the support workers asked Sarah to brush her hair, they showed her a particular bright red hairbrush as a visual signal to support the request, but even when they took this away and told Sarah that she could do her hair later, she was sometimes continuing to hit her head. The support workers said that it was as though Sarah was becoming so agitated that she was hardly aware of what was happening in her environment.

The BCBA wondered whether the occasional postponements of attempts to persuade Sarah to engage in these activities such as hairbrushing were continuing to reinforce her self-injury. In the course of an informal discussion with the BCBA, Sarah's psychiatrist however mentioned that she had by chance witnessed an incident when Sarah had started to self-injure in response to a suggestion that she should brush her hair. The psychiatrist described Sarah as becoming extremely agitated and self-injurious in response to the request, almost as is she were having a panic attack.

Reflecting on this discussion later, the BCBA considered the possibility that although Sarah's self-injury might have developed through negative reinforcement processes, it could later have become a habitual response to requests to engage in activities and stimuli associated with such requests. Being familiar with the literature on behavioral treatments of phobias in people with severe intellectual disabilities, the BCBA considered the possibility of an intervention using progressive exposure with reinforcement. She discussed this possibility with Sarah's parents, support staff, and Sarah's psychiatrist. There was general agreement that a trial of such an intervention would be in Sarah's best interests. The manager of the residential service suggested that the intervention should initially focus on Sarah's response to suggestions that she should brush her hair, since staff were frequently having to postpone attempts to persuade her to do so because of the severity of the self-injury with which she sometimes responded. The irregularity with which Sarah brushed her hair (or cooperated with someone else doing so) had an obvious effect on her appearance. In addition, if Sarah avoided having her hair brushed, it could become tangled, increasing the difficulty and potential aversiveness of the experience when it was eventually done.

Sarah's support workers thought that in general, it was easier to persuade Sarah to brush her own hair than to allow someone else to do it. Through discussion with Sarah's staff, the BCBA worked out a hierarchy of task steps which Sarah would go through in brushing her hair, starting with holding the brush and then progressing to raising it to her head, brushing her fringe, brushing the ends of her hair (which were generally tangle-free), and then progressing to brushing the full length of her hair, one area at a time. It was initially planned to progress to the next step in the hierarchy after Sarah completed the previous step for two consecutive sessions without self-injury.

Two members of Sarah's staff who had good working relationships with her agreed to model the behaviors involved, including cooperating with light physical prompts. A stimulus preference assessment identified a number of particular songs from films Sarah particularly liked, and it was planned to play these quietly during the intervention sessions and to offer Sarah a small coconut macaroon biscuit (a particular favorite of hers) if she completed the target task step(s) for each session without engaging in self-injury. Of course, it was also necessary for support workers to continue to ask Sarah to brush her hair at other times. It was arranged however to make the context of the intervention sessions obviously different from the daily routine. Sessions were held in a room used by therapists of various professions who visited the residential service, a hairbrush of a different color to Sarah's own brush was purchased, and the BCBA and the residential service manager acted as "therapists." Two sessions each day were arranged for an initial period of 5 days to evaluate Sarah's initial response to the intervention.

It proved necessary to add preliminary steps of entering the room and sitting on a chair to the task hierarchy. Sarah entered the room with one of her support workers with no difficulty, but did hit her head on the first occasion when she was asked to sit down. After six sessions however, she was entering the room and sitting without difficulty. She seemed to be aware that it was an unusual situation and appeared to focus her attention on the support worker who was acting as a model. With the support worker modelling holding a hairbrush, then raising it to her head, and then brushing her own fringe, with the therapist providing light physical guidance, Sarah also completed each of these steps without difficulty. On the first occasion that she was prompted to brush the ends of her hair on the left-hand side, she did so without engaging in SIB. During the second session in which she was asked to do so, she started to hit her head. The session was ended, and it was decided to increase the criterion for progressing through the hierarchy to four consecutive sessions without self-injury. The intervention with Sarah continued for a further 17 sessions, during which she progressed to brushing the ends of her hair on both left- and right-hand sides. The BCBA was slightly apprehensive about progressing to the next step, which would have involved Sarah brushing her hair at the back of her head, owing to the increased physical effort required for this task step. Although Sarah met the criterion for progressing to this step one Friday, the BCBA asked the residential services manager to delay the progression until the following Tuesday when she could be available to lead that session herself.

Unfortunately, on the intervening Saturday, Sarah seriously hurt herself during an episode of headbanging for which there was no obvious precipitating antecedent. She was treated in the Accident and Emergency Department of the local hospital, and an urgently convened multidisciplinary case conference concluded that the residential service was unable to maintain her safety. Most of the professionals present accepted that Sarah had made progress in her sessions with the BCBA and residential services manager. Most considered however that the gradual pace of progress, the number and diversity of activities for which progressive exposure would be required, and the fact that there were no obvious antecedents for many of Sarah's episodes of SIB meant that there was little chance that such intervention had the potential to reduce Sarah's SIB rapidly enough to make it safe for her to remain living where she was. Since Sarah's SIB had previously not responded to a range of pharmacological interventions, and behavioral and psychological support was available to Sarah in her present placement, the Consultant Psychiatrist in Learning Disabilities who attended the case conference was reluctant to arrange for Sarah to be voluntarily admitted to the local Assessment and Treatment Unit (ATU). With Sarah's current placement insisting that they could no longer meet Sarah's needs, and an emergency placement in a residential service some 2 h travelling from the home of Sarah's parents the only immediately available option, the psychiatrist however eventually agreed that a short-term admission to give her social worker time to identify a more suitable residential placement would be in Sarah's best interests.

Nathan F

At Nathan's home, having discussed the procedure with his mother, and having considered capacity and "best interests" issues, the BCBA carried out a single session of experimental functional analysis (EFA) in order to validate (or otherwise) the results of her earlier assessments. The standard EFA conditions of Iwata et al. (1982) were used, except that the "alone" condition was modified to one in which a person was in the room with Nathan but did not interact with him. With coaching from the BCBA, Nathan's mother led the assessment, with the BCBA observing. The results of the assessment were clear; during 5 min in each condition, Nathan hit himself 23 times in the "alone" condition, three times in the "social disapproval" condition, and not at all in the "task demand" and "unstructured play" conditions, suggesting that Nathan's behavior was maintained by automatic reinforcement. Although only a single session of EFA had been completed, it appeared that Nathan's self-injury resembled the "automatically reinforced self-injury Subtype 1" described by Hagopian, Rooker, and Zarcone (2015). Following discussions with Nathan's mother, the BCBA concluded that she would find it difficult to maintain any highly structured intervention program while still meeting Nathan's other needs. The BCBA therefore carried out several sessions of stimulus preference assessments with Nathan in order to identify a number of items, which mostly appeared to provide sensory feedback, with which liked to interact. The BCBA then provided a selection of such items for Nathan to use, continuing to briefly visit Nathan and his mother on a monthly basis to check his progress and rotate the items which were available to him. The results of brief observations made during these meetings concurred with Mrs. E's reports that although Nathan continued to self-injure while at home, he did so with substantially reduced frequency.

References

Adler, B. A., Wink, L. K., Early, M., Shaffer, R., Minshawi, N., McDougle, C. J., & Erickson, C. A. (2015). Drug-refractory aggression, self-injurious behavior, and severe tantrums in autism spectrum disorders: A chart review study. *Autism, 19*(1), 102–106. https://doi.org/10.1177/1362361314524641

Aman, M. G., Arnold, L. E., & Armstrong, S. C. (1999). Review of serotonergic agents and perseverative behavior in patients with developmental disabilities. *Mental Retardation and Developmental Disabilities Research Reviews, 5*(4), 279–289. https://doi.org/10.1002/(SICI)1098-2779(1999)5:4<279::AID-MRDD5>3.0.CO;2-6

Aman, M., Buitelaar, J., De Smedt, G., Wapenaar, R., & Binder, C. (2005). Pharmacotherapy of disruptive behavior and item changes on a standardized rating scale: Pooled analysis of risperidone effects in children with subaverage IQ. *Journal of Child and Adolescent Psychopharmacology, 15*(2), 220–232. https://doi.org/10.1089/cap.2005.15.220

Aman, M. G., Burrow, W. H., & Wolford, P. L. (1995). The Aberrant Behavior Checklist-community: Factor validity and effect of subject variables for adults in group homes. *American Journal on Mental Retardation, 100*(3), 283–292.

Aman, M. G., De Smedt, G., Derivan, A., Lyons, B., Findling, R. L., Hagerman, R., … Swanson, J. (2002). Double-blind, placebo-controlled study of risperidone for the treatment of disruptive behaviors in children with subaverage intelligence. *American Journal of Psychiatry, 159*(8), 1337–1346. https://doi.org/10.1176/appi.ajp.159.8.1337

Aman, M. G., Kasper, W., Manos, G., Mathew, S., Marcus, R., Owen, R., & Mankoski, R. (2010). Line-item analysis of the Aberrant Behavior Checklist: Results from two studies of aripiprazole in the treatment of irritability associated with autistic disorder. *Journal of Child and Adolescent Psychopharmacology, 20*(5), 415–422. https://doi.org/10.1089/cap.2009.0120

Aman, M. G., & Madrid, A. (1999). Atypical antipsychotics in persons with developmental disabilities. *Mental Retardation and Developmental Disabilities Research Reviews, 5*(4), 253–263. https://doi.org/10.1002/(SICI)1098-2779(1999)5:4<253::AID-MRDD2>3.0.CO;2-R

Aman, M. G., Singh, N. N., Stewart, A. W., & Field, C. J. (1985a). The Aberrant Behavior Checklist: A behavior rating scale for the assessment of treatment effects. *American Journal of Mental Deficiency, 89*(5), 485–491.

Aman, M. G., Singh, N. N., Stewart, A. W., & Field, C. J. (1985b). Psychometric characteristics of the Aberrant Behavior Checklist. *American Journal of Mental Deficiency, 89*(5), 492–502.

Aman, M. G., Singh, N. N., & Turbott, S. H. (1987). Reliability of the Aberrant Behavior Checklist and the effect of variations in instructions. *American Journal of Mental Deficiency, 92*(2), 237–240.

Aman, M. G., Tassé, M. J., Rojahn, J., & Hammer, D. (1996). The Nisonger CBRF: A child behavior rating form for children with developmental disabilities. *Research in Developmental Disabilities, 17*(1), 41–57. https://doi.org/10.1016/0891-4222(95)00039-9

Anderson, G. M., Scahill, L., McCracken, J. T., McDougle, C. J., Aman, M. G., Tierney, E., … Vitiello, B. (2007). Effects of short- and long-term risperidone treatment on prolactin levels in children with autism. *Biological Psychiatry, 61*(4), 545–550. https://doi.org/10.1016/j.biopsych.2006.02.032

Arnold, L. E., Aman, M. G., Cook, A. M., Witwer, A. N., Hall, K. L., Thompson, S., & Ramadan, Y. (2006). Atomoxetine for hyperactivity in autism spectrum disorders: Placebo-controlled crossover pilot trial. *Journal of the American Academy of Child and Adolescent Psychiatry, 45*(10), 1196–1205. https://doi.org/10.1097/01.chi.0000231976.28719.2a

Arnold, L. E., Vitiello, B., McDougle, C., Scahill, L., Shah, B., Gonzalez, N. M., … Tierney, E. (2003). Parent-defined target symptoms respond to risperidone in RUPP autism study: Customer approach to clinical trials. *Journal of the American Academy of Child and Adolescent Psychiatry, 42*(12), 1443–1450. https://doi.org/10.1097/00004583-200312000-00011

Austin, J. E., & Tiger, J. H. (2015). Providing alternative reinforcers to facilitate tolerance to delayed reinforcement following functional communication training. *Journal of Applied Behavior Analysis, 48*(3), 663–668. https://doi.org/10.1002/jaba.215

Baghdadli, A., Picot, M. C., Pry, R., Michelon, C., Burzstejn, C., Lazartigues, A., & Aussilloux, C. (2008). What factors are related to a negative outcome of self-injurious behaviour during childhood in pervasive developmental disorders? *Journal of Applied Research in Intellectual Disabilities, 21*(2), 142–149. https://doi.org/10.1111/j.1468-3148.2007.00389.x

Bailey, J., McComas, J. J., Benavides, C., & Lovascz, C. (2002). Functional assessment in a residential setting: Identifying an effective communicative replacement response for aggressive behavior. *Journal of Developmental and Physical Disabilities, 14*(4), 353–369. https://doi.org/10.1023/A:1020382819146

Baker, P. A. (2000). Measurement of community participation and use of leisure by service users with intellectual disabilities: The Guernsey Community Participation and Leisure Assessment (GCPLA). *Journal of Applied Research in Intellectual Disabilities, 13*(3), 169–185. https://doi.org/10.1046/j.1468-3148.2000.00015.x

Bihm, E. M., & Poindexter, A. R. (1991). Cross-validation of the factor structure of the Aberrant Behavior Checklist for persons with mental retardation. *American Journal on Mental Retardation, 96*(2), 209–211.

Biswas, A. B., Bhaumik, S., & Branford, D. (2001). Treatment-emergent behavioural side effects with selective serotonin re-uptake inhibitors in adults with learning disabilities. *Human Psychopharmacology, 16*(2), 133–137. https://doi.org/10.1002/hup.233

Bloom, S. E., & Lambert, J. M. (2015). Implications for practice: Resurgence and differential reinforcement of alternative responding. *Journal of Applied Behavior Analysis, 48*(4), 781–784. https://doi.org/10.1002/jaba.266

Bodfish, J. W., & Lewis, M. H. (2002). Self-injury and comorbid behaviors in developmental, neurological, psychiatric, and genetic disorders. In S. R. Schroeder, M. L. Oster-Granite, & T. Thompson (Eds.), *Self-injurious behavior: Gene-brain-behavior relationships* (pp. 23–39). Washington, DC: American Psychological Association.

Bowring, D. L., Totsika, V., Hastings, R. P., & Toogood, S. (2018). Toward data-based clinical decision making for adults with challenging behavior using the Behavior Problems Inventory-short form (BPI-S). *Tizard Learning Disability Review, 23*(2), 103–110. https://doi.org/10.1108/TLDR-06-2017-0025

Breese, G. R., Knapp, D. J., Criswell, H. E., Moy, S. S., Papadeas, S. T., & Blake, B. L. (2005). The neonate-6-hydroxydopamine-lesioned rat: A model for clinical neuroscience and neurobiological principles. *Brain Research Reviews, 48*(1), 57–73. https://doi.org/10.1016/j.brainresrev.2004.08.004

Briggs, A. M., Fisher, W. W., Greer, B. D., & Kimball, R. T. (2018). Prevalence of resurgence of destructive behavior when thinning reinforcement schedules during functional communication training. *Journal of Applied Behavior Analysis, 51*(3), 620–633. https://doi.org/10.1002/jaba.472

Call, N. A., Clark, S. B., Mevers, J. L., Parks, N. A., Volkert, V. M., & Scheithauer, M. C. (2018). An individualized method for establishing and thinning multiple schedules of reinforcement following functional communication training. *Learning and Motivation, 62*, 91–102. https://doi.org/10.1016/j.lmot.2017.03.006

Carr, E. G. (1977). The motivation of self-injurious behavior: A review of some hypotheses. *Psychological Bulletin, 84*(4), 800–816. https://doi.org/10.1037/0033-2909.84.4.800

Carr, E. G., & Durand, V. M. (1985). Reducing behavior problems through functional communication training. *Journal of Applied Behavior Analysis, 18*(2), 111–126. https://doi.org/10.1901/jaba.1985.18-111

Carr, J. E., & LeBlanc, L. A. (2006). Noncontingent reinforcement as antecedent behavior support. In J. K. Luiselli (Ed.), *Antecedent assessment and intervention* (pp. 147–164). Baltimore: Paul H. Brookes.

Carr, J. E., Severtson, J. M., & Lepper, T. L. (2009). Noncontingent reinforcement is an empirically supported treatment for problem behavior exhibited by individuals with developmental disabilities. *Research in Developmental Disabilities, 30*(1), 44–57. https://doi.org/10.1016/j.ridd.2008.03.002

Chadwick, O., Kusel, Y., Cuddy, M., & Taylor, E. (2005). Psychiatric diagnoses and behaviour problems from childhood to early adolescence in young people with severe intellectual disabilities. *Psychological Medicine, 35*(5), 751–760. https://doi.org/10.1017/S0033291704003733

Chezan, L. C., Gable, R. A., McWhorter, G. Z., & White, S. D. (2017). Current perspectives on interventions for self-injurious behavior of children with autism spectrum disorder: A systematic review of the literature. *Journal of Behavioral Education, 26*(3), 293–329. https://doi.org/10.1007/s10864-017-9269-4

Cohen, I. L., Tsiouris, J. A., Flory, M. J., Kim, S. Y., Freedland, R., Heaney, G., … Brown, W. T. (2010). A large scale study of the psychometric characteristics of the IBR Modified Overt Aggression Scale: Findings and evidence for increased self-destructive behaviors in adult females with autism spectrum disorder. *Journal of Autism and Developmental Disorders, 40*(5), 599–609. https://doi.org/10.1007/s10803-009-0908-z

Cooper, S.-A., Smiley, E., Allan, L. M., Jackson, A., Finlayson, J., Mantry, D., & Morrison, J. (2009). Adults with intellectual disabilities: Prevalence, incidence and remission of self-injurious behaviour, and related factors. *Journal of Intellectual Disability Research, 53*(3), 200–216. https://doi.org/10.1111/j.1365-2788.2008.01060.x

Cowdery, G. E., Iwata, B. A., & Pace, G. M. (1990). Effects and side effects of DRO as treatment for self-injurious behavior. *Journal of Applied Behavior Analysis, 23*(4), 497–506. https://doi.org/10.1901/jaba.1990.23-497

Crosland, K. A., Zarcone, J. R., Lindauer, S. E., Valdovinos, M. G., Zarcone, T. J., Hellings, J. A., & Schroeder, S. R. (2003). Use of functional analysis methodology in the evaluation of medication effects. *Journal of Autism and Developmental Disorders, 33*(3), 271–279. https://doi.org/10.1023/A:1024402500425

Davies, L. E., & Oliver, C. (2016). Self-injury, aggression and destruction in children with severe intellectual disability: Incidence, persistence and novel, predictive behavioural risk markers. *Research in Developmental Disabilities, 49–50*, 291–301. https://doi.org/10.1016/j.ridd.2015.12.003

Day, H. M., Horner, R. H., & O'Neill, R. E. (1994). Multiple functions of problem behaviors: Assessment and intervention. *Journal of Applied Behavior Analysis, 27*(2), 279–289. https://doi.org/10.1901/jaba.1994.27-279

DeLeon, I. G., Anders, B. M., Rodriguez-Catter, V., & Neidert, P. L. (2000). The effects of noncontingent access to single-versus multiple-stimulus sets on self-injurious behavior. *Journal of Applied Behavior Analysis, 33*(4), 623–626. https://doi.org/10.1901/jaba.2000.33-623

Derby, K. M., Fisher, W. W., Piazza, C. C., Wilke, A. E., & Johnson, W. (1998). The effects of noncontingent and contingent attention for self-injury, manding, and collateral responses. *Behavior Modification, 22*(4), 474–484. https://doi.org/10.1177/01454455980224002

Dimian, A. F., Botteron, K. N., Dager, S. R., Elison, J. T., Estes, A. M., Pruett, J. R., … Wolff, J. J. (2017). Potential risk factors for the development of self-injurious behavior among infants at risk for autism spectrum disorder. *Journal of Autism and Developmental Disorders, 47*(5), 1403–1415. https://doi.org/10.1007/s10803-017-3057-9

Durand, V. M. (1999). Functional communication training using assistive devices: Recruiting natural communities of reinforcement. *Journal of Applied Behavior Analysis, 32*(3), 247–267. https://doi.org/10.1901/jaba.1999.32-247

Durand, V. M., & Moskowitz, L. (2015). Functional communication training: Thirty years of treating challenging behavior. *Topics in Early Childhood Special Education, 35*(2), 116–126. https://doi.org/10.1177/0271121415569509

Dymond, S., Dunsmoor, J. E., Vervliet, B., Roche, B., & Hermans, D. (2015). Fear generalization in humans: Systematic review and implications for anxiety disorder research. *Behavior Therapy, 46*(5), 561–582. https://doi.org/10.1016/j.beth.2014.10.001

Fallah, M. S., Shaikh, M. R., Neupane, B., Rusiecki, D., Bennett, T. A., & Beyene, J. (2019). Atypical antipsychotics for irritability in pediatric autism: A systematic review and network meta-analysis. *Journal of Child and Adolescent Psychopharmacology, 29*(3), 168–180. https://doi.org/10.1089/cap.2018.0115

Farmer, C. A., & Aman, M. G. (2013). Pharmacological intervention for disruptive behaviors in intellectual and developmental disabilities: The glass is half full. *International Review of Research in Developmental Disabilities, 44*, 281–325. https://doi.org/10.1016/B978-0-12-401662-0.00009-9

Findling, R. L., Aman, M. G., Eerdekens, M., Derivan, A., & Lyons, B. (2004). Long-term, open-label study of risperidone in children with severe disruptive behaviors and below-average IQ. *American Journal of Psychiatry, 161*(4), 677–684. https://doi.org/10.1176/appi.ajp.161.4.677

Findling, R. L., Mankoski, R., Timko, K., Lears, K., McCartney, T., McQuade, R. D., … Sheehan, J. J. (2014). A randomized controlled trial investigating the safety and efficacy of aripiprazole in the long-term maintenance treatment of pediatric patients with irritability associated with autistic disorder. *Journal of Clinical Psychiatry, 75*(1), 22–30. https://doi.org/10.4088/JCP.13m08500

Fisher, W. W., Greer, B. D., Craig, A. R., Retzlaff, B. J., Fuhrman, A. M., Lichtblau, K. R., & Saini, V. (2018). On the predictive validity of behavioral momentum theory for mitigating resurgence of problem behavior. *Journal of the Experimental Analysis of Behavior, 109*(1), 281–290. https://doi.org/10.1002/jeab.303

Fisher, W. W., Greer, B. D., Fuhrman, A. M., & Querim, A. C. (2015). Using multiple schedules during functional communication training to promote rapid transfer of treatment effects. *Journal of Applied Behavior Analysis, 48*(4), 713–733. https://doi.org/10.1002/jaba.254

Fisher, W. W., Greer, B. D., Mitteer, D. R., Fuhrman, A. M., Romani, P. W., & Zangrillo, A. N. (2018). Further evaluation of differential exposure to establishing operations during functional communication training. *Journal of Applied Behavior Analysis, 51*(2), 360–373. https://doi.org/10.1002/jaba.451

Fisher, W., Piazza, C., Cataldo, M., Harrell, R., Jefferson, G., & Conner, R. (1993). Functional communication training with and without extinction and punishment. *Journal of Applied Behavior Analysis, 26*(1), 23–36. https://doi.org/10.1901/jaba.1993.26-23

Fisher, W. W., Thompson, R. H., Hagopian, L. P., Bowman, L. G., & Krug, A. (2000). Facilitating tolerance of delayed reinforcement during functional communication training. *Behavior Modification, 24*(1), 3–29. https://doi.org/10.1177/0145445500241001

Fodstad, J. C., Kirsch, A., Faidley, M., & Bauer, N. (2018). Demonstration of parent training to address early self-injury in young children with intellectual and developmental delays. *Journal of Autism and Developmental Disorders, 48*(11), 3846–3857. https://doi.org/10.1007/s10803-018-3651-5

Fritz, J. N., Jackson, L. M., Stiefler, N. A., Wimberly, B. S., & Richardson, A. R. (2017). Noncontingent reinforcement without extinction plus differential reinforcement of alternative behavior during treatment of problem behavior. *Journal of Applied Behavior Analysis, 50*(3), 590–599. https://doi.org/10.1002/jaba.395

Fuhrman, A. M., Fisher, W. W., & Greer, B. D. (2016). A preliminary investigation on improving functional communication training by mitigating resurgence of destructive behavior. *Journal of Applied Behavior Analysis, 49*(4), 884–899. https://doi.org/10.1002/jaba.338

Ghaemmaghami, M., Hanley, G. P., Jessel, J., & Landa, R. (2018). Shaping complex functional communication responses. *Journal of Applied Behavior Analysis, 51*(3), 502–520. https://doi.org/10.1002/jaba.468

Goel, R., Hong, J. S., Findling, R. L., & Ji, N. Y. (2018). An update on pharmacotherapy of autism spectrum disorder in children and adolescents. *International Review of Psychiatry, 30*(1), 78–95. https://doi.org/10.1080/09540261.2018.1458706

Goh, H.-L., Iwata, B. A., & DeLeon, I. G. (2000). Competition between noncontingent and contingent reinforcement schedules during response acquisition. *Journal of Applied Behavior Analysis, 33*(2), 195–205. https://doi.org/10.1901/jaba.2000.33-195

Goh, H.-L., Iwata, B. A., Shore, B. A., DeLeon, I. G., Lerman, D. C., Ulrich, S. M., & Smith, R. G. (1995). An analysis of the reinforcing properties of hand mouthing. *Journal of Applied Behavior Analysis, 28*(3), 269–283. https://doi.org/10.1901/jaba.1995.28-269

González, M. L., Dixon, D. R., Rojahn, J., Esbensen, A. J., Matson, J. L., Terlonge, C., & Smith, K. R. (2009). The Behavior Problems Inventory: Reliability and factor validity in institutionalized adults with intellectual disabilities. *Journal of Applied Research in Intellectual Disabilities, 22*(3), 223–235. https://doi.org/10.1111/j.1468-3148.2008.00429.x

Goodman, W. K., Price, L. H., Rasmussen, S. A., Mazure, C., Fleischmann, R. L., Hill, C. L., … Charney, D. S. (1989). The Yale-Brown Obsessive Compulsive Scale: I. development, use, and reliability. *Archives of General Psychiatry, 46*(11), 1006–1011. https://doi.org/10.1001/archpsyc.1989.01810110048007

Gormez, A., Rana, F., & Varghese, S. (2014). Pharmacological interventions for self-injurious behaviour in adults with intellectual disabilities: Abridged republication of a Cochrane systematic review*. *Journal of Psychopharmacology, 28*(7), 624–632. https://doi.org/10.1177/0269881114531665

Greer, B. D., Fisher, W. W., Saini, V., Owen, T. M., & Jones, J. K. (2016). Functional communication training during reinforcement schedule thinning: An analysis of 25 applications. *Journal of Applied Behavior Analysis, 49*(1), 105–121. https://doi.org/10.1002/jaba.265

Gregori, E., Rispoli, M., Gerow, S., & Lory, C. (2018). Treatment of self-injurious behavior in adults with intellectual and developmental disabilities: A systematic review. *Journal of Developmental and Physical Disabilities, 30*(1), 111–139. https://doi.org/10.1007/s10882-017-9568-7

Hagopian, L. P., Boelter, E. W., & Jarmolowicz, D. P. (2011). Reinforcement schedule thinning following functional communication training: Review and recommendations. *Behavior Analysis in Practice, 4*(1), 4–16. https://doi.org/10.1007/BF03391770

Hagopian, L. P., Crockett, J. L., Van Stone, M., DeLeon, I. G., & Bowman, L. G. (2000). Effects of noncontingent reinforcement on problem behavior and stimulus engagement: The role of satiation, extinction, and alternative reinforcement. *Journal of Applied Behavior Analysis, 33*(4), 433–449. https://doi.org/10.1901/jaba.2000.33-433

Hagopian, L. P., Kuhn, S. A. C., Long, E. S., & Rush, K. S. (2005). Schedule thinning following communication training: Using competing stimuli to enhance tolerance to decrements in reinforcer density. *Journal of Applied Behavior Analysis, 38*(2), 177–193. https://doi.org/10.1901/jaba.2005.43-04

Hagopian, L. P., Rooker, G. W., & Zarcone, J. R. (2015). Delineating subtypes of self-injurious behavior maintained by automatic reinforcement. *Journal of Applied Behavior Analysis, 48* (3), 523–543. https://doi.org/10.1002/jaba.236

Hagopian, L. P., Rooker, G. W., & Yenokyan, G. (2018). Identifying predictive behavioral markers: A demonstration using automatically reinforced self-injurious behavior. *Journal of Applied Behavior Analysis, 51*(3), 443–465. https://doi.org/10.1002/jaba.477

Hanley, G. P., Iwata, B. A., & Thompson, R. H. (2001). Reinforcement schedule thinning following treatment with functional communication training. *Journal of Applied Behavior Analysis, 34*(1), 17–38. https://doi.org/10.1901/jaba.2001.34-17

Hassiotis, A., Robotham, D., Canagasabey, A., Marston, L., Thomas, B., & King, M. (2012). Brief report: Impact of applied behaviour analysis (ABA) on carer burden and community participation in challenging behaviour: Results from a randomised controlled trial. *Journal of Intellectual Disability Research, 56*(3), 285–290. https://doi.org/10.1111/j.1365-2788.2011.01467.x

Hausman, N., Kahng, S., Farrell, E., & Mongeon, C. (2009). Idiosyncratic functions: Severe problem behavior maintained by access to ritualistic behaviors. *Education and Treatment of Children, 32*(1), 77–87. https://doi.org/10.1353/etc.0.0051

Hellings, J. A., Weckbaugh, M., Nickel, E. J., Cain, S. E., Zarcone, J. R., Reese, R. M., … Cook, E. H. (2005). A double-blind, placebo-controlled study of valproate for aggression in youth with pervasive developmental disorders. *Journal of Child and Adolescent Psychopharmacology, 15*(4), 682–692. https://doi.org/10.1089/cap.2005.15.682

Hellings, J. A., Zarcone, J. R., Reese, R. M., Valdovinos, M. G., Marquis, J. G., Fleming, K. K., & Schroeder, S. R. (2006). A crossover study of risperidone in children, adolescents and adults with mental retardation. *Journal of Autism and Developmental Disorders, 36*(3), 401–411. https://doi.org/10.1007/s10803-006-0078-1

Henry, C. A., Shervin, D., Neumeyer, A., Steingard, R., Spybrook, J., Choueiri, R., & Bauman, M. (2009). Retrial of selective serotonin reuptake inhibitors in children with pervasive developmental disorders: A retrospective chart review. *Journal of Child and Adolescent Psychopharmacology, 19*(2), 111–117. https://doi.org/10.1089/cap.2008.037

Hoch, H., McComas, J. J., Thompson, A. L., & Paone, D. (2002). Concurrent reinforcement schedules: Behavior change and maintenance without extinction. *Journal of Applied Behavior Analysis, 35*(2), 155–169. https://doi.org/10.1901/jaba.2002.35-155

Hoffman, K., & Falcomata, T. S. (2014). An evaluation of resurgence of appropriate communication in individuals with autism who exhibit severe problem behavior. *Journal of Applied Behavior Analysis, 47*(3), 651–656. https://doi.org/10.1002/jaba.144

Hollander, E., Chaplin, W., Soorya, L., Wasserman, S., Novotny, S., Rusoff, J., … Anagnostou, E. (2010). Divalproex sodium vs placebo for the treatment of irritability in children and adolescents with autism spectrum disorders. *Neuropsychopharmacology, 35*(4), 990–998. https://doi.org/10.1038/npp.2009.202

Horner, R. H., & Day, H. M. (1991). The effects of response efficiency on functionally equivalent competing behaviors. *Journal of Applied Behavior Analysis, 24*(4), 719–732. https://doi.org/10.1901/jaba.1991.24-719

Horner, R. H., Day, H. M., & Day, J. R. (1997). Using neutralizing routines to reduce problem behaviors. *Journal of Applied Behavior Analysis, 30*(4), 601–614. https://doi.org/10.1901/jaba.1997.30-601

Horner, R. H., Day, H. M., Sprague, J. R., O'Brien, M., & Heathfield, L. T. (1991). Interspersed requests: A nonaversive procedure for reducing aggression and self-injury during instruction. *Journal of Applied Behavior Analysis, 24*(2), 265–278. https://doi.org/10.1901/jaba.1991.24-265

Howes, O. D., Rogdaki, M., Findon, J. L., Wichers, R. H., Charman, T., King, B. H., … Murphy, D. G. (2018). Autism spectrum disorder: Consensus guidelines on assessment, treatment and research from the British Association for Psychopharmacology. *Journal of Psychopharmacology, 32*(1), 3–29. https://doi.org/10.1177/0269881117741766

Ichikawa, H., Hiratani, M., Yasuhara, A., Tsujii, N., Oshimo, T., Ono, H., & Tadori, Y. (2018). An open-label extension long-term study of the safety and efficacy of aripiprazole for irritability in children and adolescents with autistic disorder in Japan. *Psychiatry and Clinical Neurosciences, 72*(2), 84–94. https://doi.org/10.1111/pcn.12607

Ichikawa, H., Mikami, K., Okada, T., Yamashita, Y., Ishizaki, Y., Tomoda, A., … Tadori, Y. (2017). Aripiprazole in the treatment of irritability in children and adolescents with autism spectrum disorder in Japan: A randomized, double-blind, placebo-controlled study. *Child Psychiatry and Human Development, 48*(5), 796–806. https://doi.org/10.1007/s10578-016-0704-x

Ingvarsson, E. T., Kahng, S. W., & Hausman, N. L. (2008). Some effects of noncontingent positive reinforcement on multiply controlled problem behavior and compliance in a demand context. *Journal of Applied Behavior Analysis, 41*(3), 435–440. https://doi.org/10.1901/jaba.2008.41-435

Iwata, B. A., Dorsey, M. F., Slifer, K. J., Bauman, K. E., & Richman, G. S. (1982). Toward a functional analysis of self-injury. *Analysis and Intervention in Developmental Disabilities, 2*(1), 3–20. https://doi.org/10.1016/0270-4684(82)90003-9

Iwata, B. A., Pace, G. M., Dorsey, M. F., Zarcone, J. R., Vollmer, T. R., Smith, R. G., … Willis, K. D. (1994). The functions of self-injurious behavior: An experimental-epidemiological

analysis. *Journal of Applied Behavior Analysis, 27*(2), 215–240. https://doi.org/10.1901/jaba.1994.27-215
Iwata, B. A., Roscoe, E. M., Zarcone, J. R., & Richman, D. M. (2002). Environmental determinants of self-injurious behavior. In S. R. Schroeder, M. L. Oster-Granite, & T. Thompson (Eds.), *Self-injurious behavior: Gene-brain-behavior relationships* (pp. 93–103). Washington, DC: American Psychological Association.
Janowsky, D. S., Shetty, M., Barnhill, J., Elamir, B., & Davis, J. M. (2005). Serotonergic antidepressant effects on aggressive, self-injurious and destructive/disruptive behaviours in intellectually disabled adults: A retrospective, open-label, naturalistic trial. *International Journal of Neuropsychopharmacology, 8*(1), 37–48. https://doi.org/10.1017/S146114570400481X
Jennett, H. K., & Hagopian, L. P. (2008). Identifying empirically supported treatments for phobic avoidance in individuals with intellectual disabilities. *Behavior Therapy, 39*(2), 151–161. https://doi.org/10.1016/j.beth.2007.06.003
Kahng, S., Iwata, B. A., DeLeon, I. G., & Wallace, M. D. (2000). A comparison of procedures for programming noncontingent reinforcement schedules. *Journal of Applied Behavior Analysis, 33*(2), 223–231. https://doi.org/10.1901/jaba.2000.33-223
Kelley, M. E., Nadler, C. B., Rey, C., Cowie, S., & Podlesnik, C. A. (2017). Noncontingent reinforcement competes with response performance. *Journal of the Experimental Analysis of Behavior, 107*(3), 343–353. https://doi.org/10.1002/jeab.255
Kimball, R. T., Kelley, M. E., Podlesnik, C. A., Forton, A., & Hinkle, B. (2018). Resurgence with and without an alternative response. *Journal of Applied Behavior Analysis, 51*(4), 854–865. https://doi.org/10.1002/jaba.466
King, B. H., Hollander, E., Sikich, L., McCracken, J. T., Scahill, L., Bregman, J. D., … Ritz, L. (2009). Lack of efficacy of citalopram in children with autism spectrum disorders and high levels of repetitive behavior: Citalopram ineffective in children with autism. *Archives of General Psychiatry, 66*(6), 583–590. https://doi.org/10.1001/archgenpsychiatry.2009.30
König, I. R., Fuchs, O., Hansen, G., von Mutius, E., & Kopp, M. V. (2017). What is precision medicine? *The European Respiratory Journal, 50*(4), 1700391. https://doi.org/10.1183/13993003.00391-2017
Kunnavatana, S. S., Wolfe, K., & Aguilar, A. N. (2018). Assessing mand topography preference when developing a functional communication training intervention. *Behavior Modification, 42*(3), 364–381. https://doi.org/10.1177/0145445517751437
Kurtz, P. F., Boelter, E. W., Jarmolowicz, D. P., Chin, M. D., & Hagopian, L. P. (2011). An analysis of functional communication training as an empirically supported treatment for problem behavior displayed by individuals with intellectual disabilities. *Research in Developmental Disabilities, 32*(6), 2935–2942. https://doi.org/10.1016/j.ridd.2011.05.009
Lalli, J. S., Casey, S., & Kates, K. (1995). Reducing escape behavior and increasing task completion with functional communication training, extinction and response chaining. *Journal of Applied Behavior Analysis, 28*(3), 261–268. https://doi.org/10.1901/jaba.1995.28-261
Lalli, J. S., Vollmer, T. R., Progar, P. R., Wright, C., Borrero, J., Daniel, D., … May, W. (1999). Competition between positive and negative reinforcement in the treatment of escape behavior. *Journal of Applied Behavior Analysis, 32*(3), 285–296. https://doi.org/10.1901/jaba.1999.32-285
Lambert, J. M., Bloom, S. E., Samaha, A. L., & Dayton, E. (2017). Serial functional communication training: Extending serial DRA to mands and problem behavior. *Behavioral Interventions, 32*(4), 311–325. https://doi.org/10.1002/bin.1493
Lambert, J. M., Bloom, S. E., Samaha, A. L., Dayton, E., & Rodewald, A. M. (2015). Serial alternative response training as intervention for target response resurgence. *Journal of Applied Behavior Analysis, 48*(4), 765–780. https://doi.org/10.1002/jaba.253
Lamy, M., & Erickson, C. A. (2018). Pharmacological management of behavioral disturbances in children and adolescents with autism spectrum disorders. *Current Problems in Pediatric and Adolescent Health Care, 48*(10), 250–264. https://doi.org/10.1016/j.cppeds.2018.08.015

Lang, R., Sigafoos, J., van der Meer, L., O'Reilly, M. F., Lancioni, G. E., & Didden, R. (2013). Early signs and early behavioral intervention of challenging behavior. *International Review of Research in Developmental Disabilities, 44*, 1–35. https://doi.org/10.1016/B978-0-12-401662-0.00001-4

Layng, T. V. J., Andronis, P. T., & Goldiamond, I. (1999). Animal models of psychopathology: The establishment, maintenance, attenuation, and persistence of head-banging by pigeons. *Journal of Behavior Therapy and Experimental Psychiatry, 30*(1), 45–61. https://doi.org/10.1016/S0005-7916(99)00003-8

LeBlanc, J. C., Binder, C. E., Armenteros, J. L., Aman, M. G., Wang, J. S., Hew, H., & Kusumakar, V. (2005). Risperidone reduces aggression in boys with a disruptive behaviour disorder and below average intelligence quotient: Analysis of two placebo-controlled randomized trials. *International Clinical Psychopharmacology, 20*(5), 275–283. https://doi.org/10.1097/01.yic.0000166403.03732.72

Lerman, D. C., Iwata, B. A., & Wallace, M. D. (1999). Side effects of extinction: Prevalence of bursting and aggression during the treatment of self-injurious behavior. *Journal of Applied Behavior Analysis, 32*(1), 1–8. https://doi.org/10.1901/jaba.1999.32-1

Liggett, A. P., Nastri, R., & Podlesnik, C. A. (2018). Assessing the combined effects of resurgence and reinstatement in children diagnosed with autism spectrum disorder. *Journal of the Experimental Analysis of Behavior, 109*(2), 408–421. https://doi.org/10.1002/jeab.315

Lindberg, J. S., Iwata, B. A., Roscoe, E. M., Worsdell, A. S., & Hanley, G. P. (2003). Treatment efficacy of noncontingent reinforcement during brief and extended application. *Journal of Applied Behavior Analysis, 36*(1), 1–19. https://doi.org/10.1901/jaba.2003.36-1

Lindsay, W. R., Richardson, I., & Michie, A. M. (1989). Short-term generalised effects of relaxation training on adults with moderate and severe mental handicaps. *Mental Handicap Research, 2*(2), 197–206. https://doi.org/10.1111/j.1468-3148.1989.tb00027.x

Love, J. R., Carr, J. E., & LeBlanc, L. A. (2009). Functional assessment of problem behavior in children with autism spectrum disorders: A summary of 32 outpatient cases. *Journal of Autism and Developmental Disorders, 39*(2), 363–372. https://doi.org/10.1007/s10803-008-0633-z

Luczynski, K. C., & Hanley, G. P. (2013). Prevention of problem behavior by teaching functional communication and self-control skills to preschoolers. *Journal of Applied Behavior Analysis, 46*(2), 355–368. https://doi.org/10.1002/jaba.44

Lundqvist, L.-O. (2011). Psychometric properties and factor structure of the Behavior Problems Inventory (BPI-01) in a Swedish community population of adults with intellectual disability. *Research in Developmental Disabilities, 32*(6), 2295–2303. https://doi.org/10.1016/j.ridd.2011.07.037

Mace, F. C., & Mauk, J. E. (1995). Bio-behavioral diagnosis and treatment of self-injury. *Mental Retardation and Developmental Disabilities Research Reviews, 1*(2), 104–110. https://doi.org/10.1002/mrdd.1410010206

Makrygianni, M. K., Gena, A., Katoudi, S., & Galanis, P. (2018). The effectiveness of applied behavior analytic interventions for children with autism spectrum disorder: A meta-analytic study. *Research in Autism Spectrum Disorders, 51*, 18–31. https://doi.org/10.1016/j.rasd.2018.03.006

Marcus, R. N., Owen, R., Kamen, L., Manos, G., McQuade, R. D., Carson, W. H., & Aman, M. G. (2009). A placebo-controlled, fixed-dose study of aripiprazole in children and adolescents with irritability associated with autistic disorder. *Journal of the American Academy of Child and Adolescent Psychiatry, 48*(11), 1110–1119. https://doi.org/10.1097/CHI.0b013e3181b76658

Marcus, R. N., Owen, R., Manos, G., Mankoski, R., Kamen, L., McQuade, R. D., … Aman, M. G. (2011a). Aripiprazole in the treatment of irritability in pediatric patients (aged 6-17 years) with autistic disorder: Results from a 52-week, open-label study. *Journal of Child and Adolescent Psychopharmacology, 21*(3), 229–236. https://doi.org/10.1089/cap.2009.0121

Marcus, R. N., Owen, R., Manos, G., Mankoski, R., Kamen, L., McQuade, R. D., … Findling, R. L. (2011b). Safety and tolerability of aripiprazole for irritability in pediatric patients with autistic disorder: A 52-week, open-label, multicenter study. *Journal of Clinical Psychiatry, 72*(9), 1270–1276. https://doi.org/10.4088/JCP.09m05933

Marcus, B. A., & Vollmer, T. R. (1996). Combining noncontingent reinforcement and differential reinforcement schedules as treatment for aberrant behavior. *Journal of Applied Behavior Analysis, 29*(1), 43–51. https://doi.org/10.1901/jaba.1996.29-43

Marshburn, E. C., & Aman, M. G. (1992). Factor validity and norms for the Aberrant Behavior Checklist in a community sample of children with mental retardation. *Journal of Autism and Developmental Disorders, 22*(3), 357–373. https://doi.org/10.1007/BF01048240

Mascitelli, A. N., Rojahn, J., Nicolaides, V. C., Moore, L., Hastings, R. P., & Christian-Jones, C. (2015). The Behaviour Problems Inventory-short form: Reliability and factorial validity in adults with intellectual disabilities. *Journal of Applied Research in Intellectual Disabilities, 28*(6), 561–571. https://doi.org/10.1111/jar.12152

McCord, B. E., Iwata, B. A., Galensky, T. L., Ellingson, S. A., & Thomson, R. J. (2001). Functional analysis and treatment of problem behavior evoked by noise. *Journal of Applied Behavior Analysis, 34*(4), 447–462. https://doi.org/10.1901/jaba.2001.34-447

McCracken, J. T., McGough, J., Shah, B., Cronin, P., Hong, D., Aman, M. G., … McMahon, D. (2002). Risperidone in children with autism and serious behavioral problems. *New England Journal of Medicine, 347*(5), 314–321. https://doi.org/10.1056/NEJMoa013171

McDougle, C. J., Holmes, J. P., Carlson, C., Pelton, G. H., Cohen, D. J., & Price, L. H. (1998). A double-blind, placebo-controlled study of risperidone in adults with autistic disorder and other pervasive developmental disorders. *Archives of General Psychiatry, 55*(7), 633–641. https://doi.org/10.1001/archpsyc.55.7.633

McGill, P. (1999). Establishing operations: Implications for the assessment, treatment and prevention of problem behavior. *Journal of Applied Behavior Analysis, 32*(3), 393–418. https://doi.org/10.1901/jaba.1999.32-393

McNamara, R., Randell, E., Gillespie, D., Wood, F., Felce, D., Romeo, R., … Kerr, M. (2017). A pilot randomised controlled trial of community-led antipsychotic drug reduction for adults with learning disabilities. *Health Technology Assessment, 21*(47), 1–122. https://doi.org/10.3310/hta21470

McQuire, C., Hassiotis, A., Harrison, B., & Pilling, S. (2015). Pharmacological interventions for challenging behaviour in children with intellectual disabilities: A systematic review and meta-analysis. *BMC Psychiatry, 15*(1), 303. https://doi.org/10.1186/s12888-015-0688-2

McQuire, C., Hassiotis, A., Harrison, B., & Pilling, S. (2016). Erratum to: Pharmacological interventions for challenging behaviour in children with intellectual disabilities: A systematic review and meta-analysis [BMC Psychiatry, 15, (2015), 303]. *BMC Psychiatry, 16*(1). https://doi.org/10.1186/s12888-015-0704-6

Mehta, H., & Glover, G. (2019). *Psychotropic drugs and people with learning disabilities or autism*. London: Public Health England. Retrieved from https://www.gov.uk/government/publications/psychotropic-drugs-and-people-with-learning-disabilities-or-autism

Michael, J. (2000). Implications and refinements of the establishing operation concept. *Journal of Applied Behavior Analysis, 33*(4), 401–410. https://doi.org/10.1901/jaba.2000.33-401

Miltenberger, R. G. (2006). Antecedent interventions for challenging behaviors maintained by escape from instructional activities. In J. K. Luiselli (Ed.), *Antecedent assessment and intervention* (pp. 101–124). Baltimore, MD: Paul H. Brookes.

Minshawi, N. F., Hurwitz, S., Morriss, D., & McDougle, C. J. (2015). Multidisciplinary assessment and treatment of self-injurious behavior in autism spectrum disorder and intellectual disability: Integration of psychological and biological theory and approach. *Journal of Autism and Developmental Disorders, 45*(6), 1541–1568. https://doi.org/10.1007/s10803-014-2307-3

Mirenda, P. (1997). Supporting individuals with challenging behavior through functional communication training and AAC: Research review. *AAC: Augmentative and Alternative Communication, 13*(4), 207–225. https://doi.org/10.1080/07434619712331278048

Neely, L., Garcia, E., Bankston, B., & Green, A. (2018). Generalization and maintenance of functional communication training for individuals with developmental disabilities: A systematic and quality review. *Research in Developmental Disabilities, 79*, 116–129. https://doi.org/10.1016/j.ridd.2018.02.002

Nevill, R. E., Lecavalier, L., & Stratis, E. A. (2018). Meta-analysis of parent-mediated interventions for young children with autism spectrum disorder. *Autism, 22*(2), 84–98. https://doi.org/10.1177/1362361316677838
O'Reilly, M., Rispoli, M., Davis, T., Machalicek, W., Lang, R., Sigafoos, J., … Didden, R. (2010). Functional analysis of challenging behavior in children with autism spectrum disorders: A summary of 10 cases. *Research in Autism Spectrum Disorders, 4*(1), 1–10. https://doi.org/10.1016/j.rasd.2009.07.001
O'Reilly, M., Sigafoos, J., Lancioni, G., Edrisinha, C., & Andrews, A. (2005). An examination of the effects of a classroom activity schedule on levels of self-injury and engagement for a child with severe autism. *Journal of Autism and Developmental Disorders, 35*(3), 305–311. https://doi.org/10.1007/s10803-005-3294-1
Oliver, C., & Head, D. (1990). Self-injurious behaviour in people with learning disabilities: Determinants and interventions. *International Review of Psychiatry, 2*(1), 101–116. https://doi.org/10.3109/09540269009028276
Olson, L., & Houlihan, D. (2000). A review of behavioral treatments used for Lesch-Nyhan syndrome. *Behavior Modification, 24*(2), 202–222. https://doi.org/10.1177/0145445500242003
Owen, R., Sikich, L., Marcus, R. N., Corey-Lisle, P., Manos, G., McQuade, R. D., … Findling, R. L. (2009). Aripiprazole in the treatment of irritability in children and adolescents with autistic disorder. *Pediatrics, 124*(6), 1533–1540. https://doi.org/10.1542/peds.2008-3782
Pace, G. M., Iwata, B. A., Cowdery, G. E., Andree, P. J., & McIntyre, T. (1993). Stimulus (instructional) fading during extinction of self-injurious escape behavior. *Journal of Applied Behavior Analysis, 26*(2), 205–212. https://doi.org/10.1901/jaba.1993.26-205
Patra, S., Nebhinani, N., Viswanathan, A., & Kirubakaran, R. (2019). Atomoxetine for attention deficit hyperactivity disorder in children and adolescents with autism: A systematic review and meta-analysis. *Autism Research, 12*(4), 542–552. https://doi.org/10.1002/aur.2059
Pearson, D. A., Santos, C. W., Roache, J. D., Casat, C. D., Loveland, K. A., Lachar, D., … Cleveland, L. A. (2003). Treatment effects of methylphenidate on behavioral adjustment in children with mental retardation and ADHD. *Journal of the American Academy of Child and Adolescent Psychiatry, 42*(2), 209–216. https://doi.org/10.1097/00004583-200302000-00015
Petscher, E. S., Rey, C., & Bailey, J. S. (2009). A review of empirical support for differential reinforcement of alternative behavior. *Research in Developmental Disabilities, 30*(3), 409–425. https://doi.org/10.1016/j.ridd.2008.08.008
Phillips, C. L., Iannaccone, J. A., Rooker, G. W., & Hagopian, L. P. (2017). Noncontingent reinforcement for the treatment of severe problem behavior: An analysis of 27 consecutive applications. *Journal of Applied Behavior Analysis, 50*(2), 357–376. https://doi.org/10.1002/jaba.376
Pipkin, C. S. P., Vollmer, T. R., & Sloman, K. N. (2010). Effects of treatment integrity failures during differential reinforcement of alternative behavior: A translational model. *Journal of Applied Behavior Analysis, 43*(1), 45–70. https://doi.org/10.1901/jaba.2010.43-47
Podlesnik, C. A., Kelley, M. E., Jimenez-Gomez, C., & Bouton, M. E. (2017). Renewed behavior produced by context change and its implications for treatment maintenance: A review. *Journal of Applied Behavior Analysis, 50*(3), 675–697. https://doi.org/10.1002/jaba.400
Politte, L. C., & McDougle, C. J. (2014). Atypical antipsychotics in the treatment of children and adolescents with pervasive developmental disorders. *Psychopharmacology, 231*(6), 1023–1036. https://doi.org/10.1007/s00213-013-3068-y
Posey, D. J., Erickson, C. A., Stigler, K. A., & McDougle, C. J. (2006). The use of selective serotonin reuptake inhibitors in autism and related disorders. *Journal of Child and Adolescent Psychopharmacology, 16*(1–2), 181–186. https://doi.org/10.1089/cap.2006.16.181
Posey, D. J., Stigler, K. A., Erickson, C. A., & McDougle, C. J. (2008). Antipsychotics in the treatment of autism. *Journal of Clinical Investigation, 118*(1), 6–14. https://doi.org/10.1172/JCI32483
Ramerman, L., de Kuijper, G., Scheers, T., Vink, M., Vrijmoeth, P., & Hoekstra, P. J. (2019). Is risperidone effective in reducing challenging behaviours in individuals with intellectual disabilities after 1 year or longer use? A placebo-controlled, randomised, double-blind discontinuation

study. *Journal of Intellectual Disability Research, 63*(5), 418–428. https://doi.org/10.1111/jir.12584

Reese, R. M., Richman, D. M., Belmont, J. M., & Morse, P. (2005). Functional characteristics of disruptive behavior in developmentally disabled children with and without autism. *Journal of Autism and Developmental Disorders, 35*(4), 419–428. https://doi.org/10.1007/s10803-005-5032-0

Reichow, B., Volkmar, F. R., & Bloch, M. H. (2013). Systematic review and meta-analysis of pharmacological treatment of the symptoms of attention-deficit/hyperactivity disorder in children with pervasive developmental disorders. *Journal of Autism and Developmental Disorders, 43*(10), 2435–2441. https://doi.org/10.1007/s10803-013-1793-z

Research Units on Paediatric Psychopharmacology Autism Network. (2005). Risperidone treatment of autistic disorder: Longer-term benefits and blinded discontinuation after 6 months. *American Journal of Psychiatry, 162*(7), 1361–1369. https://doi.org/10.1176/appi.ajp.162.7.1361

Rezaei, V., Mohammadi, M. R., Ghanizadeh, A., Sahraian, A., Tabrizi, M., Rezazadeh, S. A., & Akhondzadeh, S. (2010). Double-blind, placebo-controlled trial of risperidone plus topiramate in children with autistic disorder. *Progress in Neuro-Psychopharmacology and Biological Psychiatry, 34*(7), 1269–1272. https://doi.org/10.1016/j.pnpbp.2010.07.005

Richman, D. M., Barnard-Brak, L., Grubb, L., Bosch, A., & Abby, L. (2015). Meta-analysis of noncontingent reinforcement effects on problem behavior. *Journal of Applied Behavior Analysis, 48*(1), 131–152. https://doi.org/10.1002/jaba.189

Richman, D. M., Wacker, D. P., & Winborn, L. (2001). Response efficiency during functional communication training: Effects of effort on response allocation. *Journal of Applied Behavior Analysis, 34*(1), 73–76. https://doi.org/10.1901/jaba.2001.34-73

Rispoli, M., Camargo, S., Machalicek, W., Lang, R., & Sigafoos, J. (2014). Functional communication training in the treatment of problem behavior maintained by access to rituals. *Journal of Applied Behavior Analysis, 47*(3), 580–593. https://doi.org/10.1002/jaba.130

Ritter, W. A., Barnard-Brak, L., Richman, D. M., & Grubb, L. M. (2018). The influence of function, topography, and setting on noncontingent reinforcement effect sizes for reduction in problem behavior: A meta-analysis of single-case experimental design data. *Journal of Behavioral Education, 27*(1), 1–22. https://doi.org/10.1007/s10864-017-9277-4

Robb, A. S., Andersson, C., Bellocchio, E. E., Manos, G., Rojas-Fernandez, C., Mathew, S., … Mankoski, R. (2011). Safety and tolerability of aripiprazole in the treatment of irritability associated with autistic disorder in pediatric subjects (6-17 years old): Results from a pooled analysis of 2 studies. *Primary Care Companion to the Journal of Clinical Psychiatry, 13*(1), e1–e9. https://doi.org/10.4088/PCC.10m01008gry

Roberts, M. L., Mace, F. C., & Daggett, J. A. (1995). Preliminary comparison of two negative reinforcement schedules to reduce self-injury. *Journal of Applied Behavior Analysis, 28*(4), 579–580. https://doi.org/10.1901/jaba.1995.28-579

Rojahn, J. (1984). Self-injurious behavior in institutionalized, severely/profoundly retarded adults-prevalence data and staff agreement. *Journal of Behavioral Assessment, 6*(1), 13–27. https://doi.org/10.1007/BF01321457

Rojahn, J. (1986). Self-injurious and stereotypic behavior of noninstitutionalized mentally retarded people: Prevalence and classification. *American Journal of Mental Deficiency, 91*(3), 268–276.

Rojahn, J., & Helsel, W. J. (1991). The Aberrant Behavior Checklist with children and adolescents with dual diagnosis. *Journal of Autism and Developmental Disorders, 21*(1), 17–28. https://doi.org/10.1007/BF02206994

Rojahn, J., Matlock, S. T., & Tassé, M. J. (2000). The Stereotyped Behavior Scale: Psychometric properties and norms. *Research in Developmental Disabilities, 21*(6), 437–454. https://doi.org/10.1016/S0891-4222(00)00057-3

Rojahn, J., Matson, J. L., Lott, D., Esbensen, A. J., & Smalls, Y. (2001). The Behavior Problems Inventory: An instrument for the assessment of self-injury, stereotyped behavior, and aggression/destruction in individuals with developmental disabilities. *Journal of Autism and Developmental Disorders, 31*(6), 577–588. https://doi.org/10.1023/A:1013299028321

Rojahn, J., Rowe, E. W., Macken, J., Gray, A., Delitta, D., Booth, A., & Kimbrell, K. (2010). Psychometric evaluation of the Behavior Problems Inventory-01 and the Nisonger Child Behavior Rating Form with children and adolescents. *Journal of Mental Health Research in Intellectual Disabilities, 3*(1), 28–50. https://doi.org/10.1080/19315860903558168

Rojahn, J., Rowe, E. W., Sharber, A. C., Hastings, R., Matson, J. L., Didden, R., … Dumont, E. L. M. (2012a). The Behavior Problems Inventory-short form for individuals with intellectual disabilities: Part I: Development and provisional clinical reference data. *Journal of Intellectual Disability Research, 56*(5), 527–545. https://doi.org/10.1111/j.1365-2788.2011.01507.x

Rojahn, J., Rowe, E. W., Sharber, A. C., Hastings, R., Matson, J. L., Didden, R., … Dumont, E. L. M. (2012b). The Behavior Problems Inventory-short form for individuals with intellectual disabilities: Part II: Reliability and validity. *Journal of Intellectual Disability Research, 56*(5), 546–565. https://doi.org/10.1111/j.1365-2788.2011.01506.x

Rojahn, J., Schroeder, S. R., & Hoch, T. A. (2008). *Self-injurious behavior in intellectual disabilities*. Amsterdam: Elsevier.

Rojahn, J., Tassé, M. J., & Sturmey, P. (1997). The Stereotyped Behavior scale for adolescents and adults with mental retardation. *American Journal on Mental Retardation, 102*(2), 137–146. https://doi.org/10.1352/0895-8017(1997)102<0137:TSBSFA>2.0.CO;2

Rooker, G. W., Bonner, A. C., Dillon, C. M., & Zarcone, J. R. (2018). Behavioral treatment of automatically reinforced SIB: 1982 – 2015. *Journal of Applied Behavior Analysis, 51*(4), 974–997. https://doi.org/10.1002/jaba.492

Rosen, T. E., Connell, J. E., & Kerns, C. M. (2016). A review of behavioral interventions for anxiety-related behaviors in lower-functioning individuals with autism. *Behavioral Interventions, 31*(2), 120–143. https://doi.org/10.1002/bin.1442

Royal College of Psychiatrists Faculty of Psychiatry of Intellectual Disability (n.d.). Stopping overuse of medication in people with learning disability (STOMP). London: Royal College of Psychiatrists. Retrieved July 1, 2019, from https://www.rcpsych.ac.uk/docs/default-source/members/faculties/intellectual-disability/id-stomp-faculty-psychiatry-intellectual-disability-(002).pdf?sfvrsn=3c4c644b_2

Saini, V., Fisher, W. W., & Pisman, M. D. (2017). Persistence during and resurgence following noncontingent reinforcement implemented with and without extinction. *Journal of Applied Behavior Analysis, 50*(2), 377–392. https://doi.org/10.1002/jaba.380

Saini, V., Miller, S. A., & Fisher, W. W. (2016). Multiple schedules in practical application: Research trends and implications for future investigation. *Journal of Applied Behavior Analysis, 49*(2), 421–444. https://doi.org/10.1002/jaba.300

Saini, V., Sullivan, W. E., Baxter, E. L., DeRosa, N. M., & Roane, H. S. (2018). Renewal during functional communication training. *Journal of Applied Behavior Analysis, 51*(3), 603–619. https://doi.org/10.1002/jaba.471

Sandman, C. A., & Kemp, A. S. (2011). Opioid antagonists may reverse endogenous opiate “dependence” in the treatment of self-injurious behavior. *Pharmaceuticals, 4*(2), 366–381. https://doi.org/10.3390/ph4020366

Sandman, C. A., Touchette, P., Lenjavi, M., Marion, S., & Chicz-DeMet, A. (2003). β-Endorphin and ACTH are dissociated after self-injury in adults with developmental disabilities. *American Journal on Mental Retardation, 108*(6), 414–424 + 438. https://doi.org/10.1352/0895-8017(2003)108<414:EAAADA>2.0.CO;2

Sandman, C. A., Touchette, P. E., Marion, S. D., & Chicz-DeMet, A. (2008). The role of proopiomelanocortin (POMC) in sequentially dependent self-injurious behavior. *Developmental Psychobiology, 50*(7), 680–689. https://doi.org/10.1002/dev.20323

Sandman, C. A., Touchette, P., Marion, S., Lenjavi, M., & Chicz-Demet, A. (2002). Disregulation of proopiomelanocortin and contagious maladaptive behavior. *Regulatory Peptides, 108*(2–3), 179–185. https://doi.org/10.1016/S0167-0115(02)00097-6

Sawyer, A., Lake, J. K., Lunsky, Y., Liu, S.-K., & Desarkar, P. (2014). Psychopharmacological treatment of challenging behaviours in adults with autism and intellectual disabilities: A systematic review. *Research in Autism Spectrum Disorders, 8*(7), 803–813. https://doi.org/10.1016/j.rasd.2014.03.021

Schmidt, J. D., Luiselli, J. K., Rue, H., & Whalley, K. (2013). Graduated exposure and positive reinforcement to overcome setting and activity avoidance in an adolescent with autism. *Behavior Modification, 37*(1), 128–142. https://doi.org/10.1177/0145445512456547

Shabani, D. B., & Fisher, W. W. (2006). Stimulus fading and differential reinforcement for the treatment of needle phobia in a youth with autism. *Journal of Applied Behavior Analysis, 39*(4), 449–452. https://doi.org/10.1901/jaba.2006.30-05

Shea, S., Turgay, A., Carroll, A., Schulz, M., Orlik, H., Smith, I., & Dunbar, F. (2004). Risperidone in the treatment of disruptive behavioral symptoms in children with autistic and other pervasive developmental disorders. *Pediatrics, 114*(5), e634–e641. https://doi.org/10.1542/peds.2003-0264-F

Sheehan, R., & Hassiotis, A. (2017). Reduction or discontinuation of antipsychotics for challenging behaviour in adults with intellectual disability: A systematic review. *The Lancet Psychiatry, 4*(3), 238–256. https://doi.org/10.1016/S2215-0366(16)30191-2

Shirley, M. J., Iwata, B. A., Kahng, S., Mazaleski, J. L., & Lerman, D. C. (1997). Does functional communication training compete with ongoing contingencies of reinforcement? An analysis during response acquisition and maintenance. *Journal of Applied Behavior Analysis, 30*(1), 93–104. https://doi.org/10.1901/jaba.1997.30-93

Shore, B. A., Iwata, B. A., DeLeon, I. G., Kahng, S. W., & Smith, R. G. (1997). An analysis of reinforcer substitutability using object manipulation and self-injury as competing responses. *Journal of Applied Behavior Analysis, 30*(1), 21–41. https://doi.org/10.1901/jaba.1997.30-21

Siegel, M., & Beaulieu, A. A. (2012). Psychotropic medications in children with autism spectrum disorders: A systematic review and synthesis for evidence-based practice. *Journal of Autism and Developmental Disorders, 42*(8), 1592–1605. https://doi.org/10.1007/s10803-011-1399-2

Slocum, S. K., Grauerholz-Fisher, E., Peters, K. P., & Vollmer, T. R. (2018). A multicomponent approach to thinning reinforcer delivery during noncontingent reinforcement schedules. *Journal of Applied Behavior Analysis, 51*(1), 61–69. https://doi.org/10.1002/jaba.427

Snyder, R., Turgay, A., Aman, M., Binder, C., Fisman, S., & Carroll, A. (2002). Effects of risperidone on conduct and disruptive behavior disorders in children with subaverage IQs. *Journal of the American Academy of Child and Adolescent Psychiatry, 41*(9), 1026–1036. https://doi.org/10.1097/00004583-200209000-00002

Steege, M. W., Wacker, D. P., Berg, W. K., Cigrand, K. K., & Cooper, L. J. (1989). The use of behavioral assessment to prescribe and evaluate treatments for severely handicapped children. *Journal of Applied Behavior Analysis, 22*(1), 23–33. https://doi.org/10.1901/jaba.1989.22-23

Stokes, T. F., & Baer, D. M. (1977). An implicit technology of generalization. *Journal of Applied Behavior Analysis, 10*(2), 349–367. https://doi.org/10.1901/jaba.1977.10-349

Symons, F. J., Hoch, J., Dahl, N. A., & McComas, J. J. (2003). Sequential and matching analyses of self-injurious behavior: A case of overmatching in the natural environment. *Journal of Applied Behavior Analysis, 36*(2), 267–270. https://doi.org/10.1901/jaba.2003.36-267

Tarrant, N., Roy, M., Deb, S., Odedra, S., Retzer, A., & Roy, A. (2018). The effectiveness of methylphenidate in the management of attention deficit hyperactivity disorder (ADHD) in people with intellectual disabilities: A systematic review. *Research in Developmental Disabilities, 83*, 217–232. https://doi.org/10.1016/j.ridd.2018.08.017

Tassé, M. J., Aman, M. G., Hammer, D., & Rojahn, J. (1996). The Nisonger Child Behavior Rating Form: Age and gender effects and norms. *Research in Developmental Disabilities, 17*(1), 59–75. https://doi.org/10.1016/0891-4222(95)00037-2

Thompson, T., & Symons, F. J. (1999). Neurobehavioral mechanisms of drug action. In N. A. Wieseler & R. H. Hanson (Eds.), *Challenging behavior of persons with mental health disorders and severe developmental disabilities* (pp. 125–150). Washington, DC: American Association on Mental Retardation.

Tiger, J. H., Hanley, G. P., & Bruzek, J. (2008). Functional communication training: A review and practical guide. *Behavior Analysis in Practice, 1*(1), 16–23. https://doi.org/10.1007/BF03391716

Tomlin, M., & Reed, P. (2012). Effects of fixed-time reinforcement delivered by teachers for reducing problem behavior in special education classrooms. *Journal of Behavioral Education, 21*(2), 150–162. https://doi.org/10.1007/s10864-012-9147-z

Torres-Viso, M., Strohmeier, C. W., & Zarcone, J. R. (2018). Functional analysis and treatment of problem behavior related to mands for rearrangement. *Journal of Applied Behavior Analysis, 51*(1), 158–165. https://doi.org/10.1002/jaba.437

Turgay, A., Binder, C., Snyder, R., & Fisman, S. (2002). Long-term safety and efficacy of risperidone for the treatment of disruptive behavior disorders in children with subaverage IQs. *Pediatrics, 110*(3), e34. https://doi.org/10.1542/peds.110.3.e34

Van Camp, C. M., Lerman, D. C., Kelley, M. E., Contrucci, S. A., & Vorndran, C. M. (2000). Variable-time reinforcement schedules in the treatment of socially maintained problem behavior. *Journal of Applied Behavior Analysis, 33*(4), 545–557. https://doi.org/10.1901/jaba.2000.33-545

Van Camp, C. M., Vollmer, T. R., & Daniel, D. (2001). A systematic evaluation of stimulus preference, response effort, and stimulus control in the treatment of automatically reinforced self-injury. *Behavior Therapy, 32*(3), 603–613. https://doi.org/10.1016/S0005-7894(01)80037-X

van Ingen, D. J., Moore, L. L., Zaja, R. H., & Rojahn, J. (2010). The Behavior Problems Inventory (BPI-01) in community-based adults with intellectual disabilities: Reliability and concurrent validity vis-à-vis the Inventory for Client and Agency Planning (ICAP). *Research in Developmental Disabilities, 31*(1), 97–107. https://doi.org/10.1016/j.ridd.2009.08.004

Vollmer, T. R., Iwata, B. A., Zarcone, J. R., Smith, R. G., & Mazaleski, J. L. (1993). The role of attention in the treatment of attention-maintained self-injurious behavior: Noncontingent reinforcement and differential reinforcement of other behavior. *Journal of Applied Behavior Analysis, 26*(1), 9–21. https://doi.org/10.1901/jaba.1993.26-9

Vollmer, T. R., Marcus, B. A., & LeBlanc, L. (1994). Treatment of self-injury and hand mouthing following inconclusive functional analyses. *Journal of Applied Behavior Analysis, 27*(2), 331–344. https://doi.org/10.1901/jaba.1994.27-331

Vollmer, T. R., Marcus, B. A., & Ringdahl, J. E. (1995). Noncontingent escape as treatment for self-injurious behavior maintained by negative reinforcement. *Journal of Applied Behavior Analysis, 28*(1), 15–26. https://doi.org/10.1901/jaba.1995.28-15

Vollmer, T. R., Progar, P. R., Lalli, J. S., Van Camp, C. M., Sierp, B. J., Wright, C. S., … Eisenschink, K. J. (1998). Fixed-time schedules attenuate extinction-induced phenomena in the treatment of severe aberrant behavior. *Journal of Applied Behavior Analysis, 31*(4), 529–542. https://doi.org/10.1901/jaba.1998.31-529

Wacker, D. P., Steege, M. W., Northup, J., Sasso, G., Berg, W., Reimers, T., … Donn, L. (1990). A component analysis of functional communication training across three topographies of severe behavior problems. *Journal of Applied Behavior Analysis, 23*(4), 417–429. https://doi.org/10.1901/jaba.1990.23-417

Walker, V. L., & Snell, M. E. (2013). Effects of augmentative and alternative communication on challenging behavior: A meta-analysis. *AAC: Augmentative and Alternative Communication, 29*(2), 117–131. https://doi.org/10.3109/07434618.2013.785020

Wallace, M. D., Iwata, B. A., Hanley, G. P., Thompson, R. H., & Roscoe, E. M. (2012). Noncontingent reinforcement: A further examination of schedule effects during treatment. *Journal of Applied Behavior Analysis, 45*(4), 709–719. https://doi.org/10.1901/jaba.2012.45-709

Ward, F., Tharian, P., Roy, M., Deb, S., & Unwin, G. L. (2013). Efficacy of beta blockers in the management of problem behaviours in people with intellectual disabilities: A systematic review. *Research in Developmental Disabilities, 34*(12), 4293–4303. https://doi.org/10.1016/j.ridd.2013.08.015

Winborn, L., Wacker, D. P., Richman, D. M., Asmus, J., & Geier, D. (2002). Assessment of mand selection for functional communication training packages. *Journal of Applied Behavior Analysis, 35*(3), 295–298. https://doi.org/10.1901/jaba.2002.35-295

Wolf, M., Risley, T., & Mees, H. (1963). Application of operant conditioning procedures to the behaviour problems of an autistic child. *Behaviour Research and Therapy, 1*(2–4), 305–312. https://doi.org/10.1016/0005-7967(63)90045-7

Worsdell, A. S., Iwata, B. A., Hanley, G. P., Thompson, R. H., & Kahng, S. W. (2000). Effects of continuous and intermittent reinforcement for problem behavior during functional communication training. *Journal of Applied Behavior Analysis, 33*(2), 167–179. https://doi.org/10.1901/jaba.2000.33-167

Zarcone, J. R., Hellings, J. A., Crandall, K., Matthew Reese, R., Marquis, J., Fleming, K., ... Schroeder, S. R. (2001). Effects of risperidone on aberrant behavior of persons with developmental disabilities: I. A double-blind crossover study using multiple measures. *American Journal on Mental Retardation, 106*(6), 525–538. https://doi.org/10.1352/0895-8017(2001)106<0525:EOROAB>2.0.CO;2

Zarcone, J. R., Iwata, B. A., Mazaleski, J. L., & Smith, R. G. (1994). Momentum and extinction effects on self-injurious escape behavior and noncompliance. *Journal of Applied Behavior Analysis, 27*(4), 649–658. https://doi.org/10.1901/jaba.1994.27-649

Zarcone, J. R., Iwata, B. A., Smith, R. G., Mazaleski, J. L., & Lerman, D. C. (1994). Reemergence and extinction of self-injurious escape behavior during stimulus (instructional) fading. *Journal of Applied Behavior Analysis, 27*(2), 307–316. https://doi.org/10.1901/jaba.1994.27-307

Zarcone, J. R., Lindauer, S. E., Morse, P. S., Crosland, K. A., Valdovinos, M. G., McKerchar, T. L., ... Schroeder, S. R. (2004). Effects of risperidone on destructive behavior of persons with developmental disabilities: III. Functional analysis. *American Journal on Mental Retardation, 109*(4), 310–321. https://doi.org/10.1352/0895-8017(2004)109<310:EORODB>2.0.CO;2

Chapter 7
Assessment and Intervention with Self-Restraint

7.1 Introduction

One of the most striking features of Nyhan's (1976) early descriptions of the behavior of children with Lesch-Nyhan syndrome (LNS) concerned the terror they experienced when protective equipment or restraints were removed and they were free to engage in self-injurious behavior (SIB). In a later report on 19 children and teenagers with LNS (Christie et al., 1982), Nyhan again emphasized the agitation they experienced when their restraints were removed. Christie et al. (1982) also observed however that as children with LNS became older, many learned to control their own SIB, for example, by sitting on their hands or placing their hands behind their backs. Christie et al. (1982) described one 18-year-old who, when his restraints were removed at his own request, would exhort his right hand to "be good." Nyhan (Shear, Nyhan, Kirman, & Stern, 1971) reported a similar phenomenon in the SIB of a boy with Cornelia de Lange syndrome (CdLS), who at around 5 years of age began to bite his thumbs, sometimes with sufficient force to break the skin. His mother attempted to discourage this behavior by placing small plastic tubes (hair rollers) over his thumbs. Shear et al. (1971) noted that although the boy could remove the tubes if he wished, he became used to keeping them on and would become unhappy if he was without them.

Roughly contemporaneously with these descriptions of the behavior of children with LNS and CdLS, reports of early attempts to use behavioral techniques to reduce SIB in people with intellectual disabilities (IDs) mentioned the emergence of similar behaviors in response to behavioral treatment. Myers Jr. and Deibert (1971) used a differential reinforcement of other behavior (DRO) approach with food as the reinforcer to reduce the head-hitting of an 11-year-old boy with an ID and severe visual handicap. Prior to the behavioral intervention, attempts had been made to use a padded football helmet with a face guard as protective equipment, but the boy removed it. During the behavioral intervention however, the boy would tolerate

F. Furniss, A. B. Biswas, *Self-Injurious Behavior in Individuals with Neurodevelopmental Conditions*, Autism and Child Psychopathology Series,
https://doi.org/10.1007/978-3-030-36016-0_7

wearing the helmet and would put his arms through the face guard as if to prevent himself from hitting his head. If the helmet was removed, he again engaged in SIB. The DRO intervention was eventually used to teach him to refrain from SIB when the helmet was removed. Attempts by people with IDs to prevent themselves from engaging in SIB were not however reported only as a direct consequence of behavioral interventions. Ball, Sibbach, Jones, Steele, and Frazier (1975) noted that prior to their intervention with a girl who pinched, bit, and hit herself, she sometimes attempted to restrain herself from engaging in SIB by sitting on her hands or tucking them into her trousers.

Lovaas and Simmons (1969) also observed similar behaviors in children with IDs and noted that although they might be thought of as self-restraint (SR), in some cases these behaviors may have been encouraged by parents, as if they were the target behavior of a differential reinforcement of incompatible behavior (DRI) intervention. One 5-year-old boy with a severe ID who hit his temple and forehead with his fists and knuckles had, for example, been taught by his mother to hold a cup in each hand to prevent this behavior. Over the course of the next 2 years however, his behavior worsened to the point where he was continuously restrained and became very frightened and agitated if restraints were removed.

These self-restraining behaviors vary considerably both in topography and in the extent to which they pose a physical impediment to a person engaging in SIB. Some behaviors, such as wrapping items of clothing repeatedly round the hands, or keeping the arms inside the body of a tightly buttoned shirt or other top, substantially increase the amount of effort required to engage in a behavior such as hand-to-head hitting. Others however, such as holding a small object in the hand, may have no such direct physical effect on the effort required to engage in SIB, but nevertheless appear to exert substantial control over the behavior. Although self-restraining behaviors can reduce physical harm from SIB, in some cases they can also have negative consequences. In the short term, some may make it difficult or impossible for the person to engage in many constructive activities. Since people may engage in SR for a very high proportion of their time (Rojahn, Mulick, McCoy, & Schroeder, 1978), this loss of opportunities could have a substantial long-term effect on quality of life. Topographies of SR are often idiosyncratic and can be unusual, such as the use of the helmet described by Myers Jr. and Deibert (1971), with the potential to draw negative social consequences. In the longer term, some forms of self-restraint may themselves result in physical harm. Foxx and Dufrense (1984), for example, describe a situation in which a man with a severe ID was self-restraining using rigid arm splints to the point where his arm muscles were beginning to atrophy. Finally, although a causal chain does not seem to have been established in any one case, it appears that for some people use of relatively limited forms of SR may be a step toward dependence on much more intrusive restraint to prevent SIB (Lovaas & Simmons, 1969). Despite these concerns, there is relatively little research into SR, which remains poorly understood. This chapter reviews the limited evidence available on the phenomenology and prevalence of SR, together with theory and research on its functional dynamics. Finally, we will discuss options for assessment and treatment.

7.2 Phenomenology and Prevalence of Self-Restraint

In an early review of research on SR, Isley, Kartsonis, McCurley, Eager Weisz, and Roberts (1991) proposed that the many different topographies observed can usefully be considered as falling into three major categories. The first of these involves restricting the movement of body parts by wrapping or entangling them in inanimate objects, most frequently clothing (of the person engaging in SR or of another person). The second category comprises behaviors in which one part of the body is used to restrain another, e.g., by clasping hands together, sitting on hands, or trapping an arm between one's back and a chair. The third category of SR consists of self-applying, or requesting application of, protective equipment or restraints, or holding particular objects. Oliver, Murphy, Hall, Arron, and Leggett (2003) suggested that clinging to other people, requesting physical restraint, requesting hands to be held and so one might be considered a further category of SR.

In contrast to the substantial number of studies on the prevalence of SIB, few have provided prevalence estimates for SR. Isley et al. (1991) reported that approximately 4% of residents of an 858-place institutional residential service for people with IDs engaged in SR. Fovel, Lash, Barron Jr., and Roberts (1989) surveyed the residents of another large residential service on two occasions, at an interval of 3 years. Of the 669 people who were resident in the service at both time points, 20 were identified as engaging in SR at both time points, with a further 14 engaging in SR at only one time point, giving a possible overall prevalence range between 2.99 and 5.08%. Fovel et al. (1989) noted that of the people who engaged in SR at both time points, 90% engaged in SIB, and of the people who engaged in SR at only one time, 71% engaged in SIB, whereas the overall prevalence of SIB among residents was only 28%. Rojahn (1986) surveyed 25,872 people with IDs using community-based services in Germany and identified 431 who engaged in SIB. A total of 12% of people who engaged in SIB, and 5% of a control group drawn from those reported not to show SIB, engaged in SR. In Rojahn's (1986) study, SR was defined as comprising only self-restraint of the arms in one's own clothing, and the only specific topography of SIB significantly associated with SR was self-pinching.

Few studies have examined the prevalences and associations with SIB of specific topographies of SR. Powell, Bodfish, Parker, Crawford, and Lewis (1996) examined SR in 99 adults with severe IDs who were reported to engage in SIB comprising head-hitting, hitting the self against a surface or object, hitting the self with an object, or self-pulling, self-rubbing or self-scratching, or inserting fingers or objects (e.g., eye-poking), which was repetitive and had potential to cause injury. Overall, 46% of these individuals were reported to engage in SR. Within the group of 46 persons who engaged in SR, 52% engaged in only one form of SR, 20% engaged in two forms, 13% engaged in three forms, 9% engaged in four forms, and 6.5% engaged in five forms. The most common individual topographies of SR were holding/squeezing objects, holding onto other people or their clothing, positioning the body so as to restrain a body part, and wrapping oneself in clothing, all of which were engaged in by over 20% of the people who engaged in SR. With the first two of these topographies excluded from consideration, the proportion of the group engaging in SR was reduced to 22%. Powell et al. (1996) also showed that of the 46 individuals who engaged in SIB and SR, 57% also showed compulsions, whereas for the 53 people who engaged in SIB without SR, only 33% showed compulsions, revealing a significant association between presence of SR within SIB and presence of compulsions. Powell et al. (1996) also examined the reactions of ten people showing SIB and SR, and a control group of ten who engaged in SIB without SR but had a highly preferred object, to brief physical interruption of their SR or removal of the object. In response to the interruption, people who engaged in SR were significantly more likely than those who did not to persist in the behavior (SR or holding the object), return immediately to the behavior when the interruption was over, engage in SIB and/or negative vocalizations, and show anxiety. In a second study of specific topographies of SR, Oliver et al. (2003) used the Self-Restraint Questionnaire (SRQ), a 23-item instrument developed specifically for the study. The SRQ has four subscales based on the categories of SR proposed by Isley et al. (1991), i.e., use of clothing or materials (nine items), use of body (nine items), use of objects (three items), and use of other people (two items). In addition to specifying topographies of SR in greater detail than measures used in previous studies, the SRQ also includes a rating of the frequency of occurrence of each item on a five-point scale ranging from "never" to "all of the time." The participants in Oliver et al.'s (2003) study were 88 individuals with IDs who had been identified in a previous study as engaging in SIB which resulted in actual tissue damage or had the potential to do so were it not for the use of specific interventions or protective equipment. For the purpose of some analyses, participants were divided into 41 individuals who used protective devices or equipment of various kinds and 47 who did not. Overall, 67 individuals (76.1%) engaged in at least one form of SR at least some of the time, comprising 58.5% of those using protective devices and 91.5% of those who did not. Engagement in SR was significantly associated with non-use of protective equipment. Individual topographies of SR engaged in by at least 20% of participants who did not use protective devices were entwining hands in clothes, pulling sleeves over hands, putting hands into trousers, putting hands into pockets, carrying an object everywhere, sitting on hands, putting hands between legs, folding arms, locking fingers together, asking for the hands to be held, and asking for arms to be held. Individuals not using protective devices engaged in a significantly higher number of forms of SR than those who used protective devices, and subscale scores on the SRQ were higher for the no protective devices group for use of clothing, use of body, and use of other people, but not use of objects.

Oliver and his colleagues have also begun to investigate prevalences of SR among people with specific neurodevelopmental conditions (NDCs). Hyman, Oliver, and Hall (2002) used the Self Restraint Checklist (SRC) previously employed by Powell et al. (1996) to assess the prevalence of SR in a sample of 88 children and adults with Cornelia de Lange syndrome (CdLS), of whom 56 (63.6%) were reported to have engaged in SIB within the last month. Of the 88 participants, 47 (53.4%) were reported to show at least 1 form of SR from the 7 topographies included on the SRC. The most common forms of SR reported were holding on to other people or their clothing and holding or squeezing objects, but wrapping body parts in clothing (or holding on to one's own clothing) and choosing to wear a particular item of clothing were also present for over one quarter of the people who engaged in SR. The proportion of people who engaged in SR who showed only one topography of SR was 47.8%, with only two people showing more than three forms. Analyses of subgroups of participants aged 12 and under and 13 and over showed that presence of SR was associated with the older age range and that individuals 13 years of age and over showed more topographies of SR than younger people. Although 11 people of the total group were reported to engage in SR without SIB, presence of SR was significantly associated with presence of SIB. Hyman et al. (2002) also assessed compulsive behaviors in their participants and found that individuals who engaged in both SR and SIB showed a greater number of compulsive behaviors than those who engaged in either SR or SIB alone or those who engaged in neither behavior.

More recently, Richards, Davies, and Oliver (2017) investigated the relationship between SR and SIB in a large sample of 208 children and 216 adults with autism spectrum conditions (ASCs) who were receiving services from a major service provider in the UK. The prevalence of SIB was 46% among the children and 49% among the adults, while the corresponding prevalences of SR were 41 and 43%. Substantial numbers of people in both groups (30 children and 31 adults) were reported to engage in SR in the absence of SIB; nevertheless, the presence of SR was significantly associated with the presence of SIB for both age groups. The presence of one particular topography of SR (holding onto other people or their clothing) was significantly associated with membership of the younger age group. Logistic regression analyses showed that for the children, measures of overactivity/impulsivity and repetitive/restricted behaviors, in addition to the presence of SIB, were independently associated with the presence of SR. For the adults however the presence of SIB was the only factor associated with presence of SR with other variables controlled.

The findings of Richards et al. (2017) offer a possible insight into the development of SR, of which almost nothing is known. The finding that holding onto other people or their clothing was associated with (younger) age, taken together with the reported independent association of overactivity/impulsivity with SR among the children but not the adults, suggests a hypothesis that children experiencing difficulties in controlling their SIB might seek forms of assistance in preventing the behavior from carers, which then evolve into SR (Richards et al., 2017). This possibility seems compatible with case reports of parents having encouraged early forms of SR in children who engaged in SIB (Lovaas & Simmons, 1969; Shear et al., 1971).

7.3 Functional Dynamics of Self-Restraint

As mentioned above, several early accounts of the development of SR suggested that the behaviors concerned might initially have been encouraged by parents (Lovaas & Simmons, 1969; Shear et al., 1971). The developmental course of SR has however received very little research attention, and theoretical accounts and hypotheses regarding the functional dynamics of SR have focused mainly on possible relationships between SR and SIB (Fisher & Iwata, 1996; Isley et al., 1991; Smith, Iwata, Vollmer, & Pace, 1992). One hypothesis is that SR may be reinforced by termination or avoidance of SIB (or aversive consequences of SIB). Fisher and Iwata (1996) suggested that in many cases SIB may be controlled by both positive and aversive consequences and that SR may emerge when the effects of reinforcement of SIB are outweighed by its aversive consequences. Hagopian (Hagopian, Rooker, & Yenokyan, 2018; Hagopian, Rooker, & Zarcone, 2015; Hagopian, Rooker, Zarcone, Bonner, & Arevalo, 2017) has further proposed that SIB which automatically (i.e., by mechanical and biological mechanisms rather than via social effects) produces both reinforcing and aversive consequences may often be accompanied by SR. A second hypothesis is that access to self-restraint may reinforce SIB (Rooker & Roscoe, 2005; Smith, Lerman, & Iwata, 1996). The foundation for this proposal was provided by a study involving three people with very severe IDs with extensive experience of being placed in restraints by people supporting them to limit physical harm resulting from their SIB (Favell, McGimsey, & Jones, 1978). Favell et al. (1978) showed that treatment packages which included making access to restraint contingent on progressively increased periods of time in which the people concerned refrained from SIB reduced levels of SIB for all three. Favell et al. (1978) noted that the treatment packages employed included other components including social interaction and toy play during periods out of restraints and additionally observed that the process of applying restraints to the people concerned also necessarily involved social interaction. They speculated however that restraint may have acted as a positive reinforcer, possibly because of a history of association either with social interaction or with escape from or avoidance of task demands. Favell et al. (1978) provided some evidence to support this possibility by demonstrating that contingent restraint could be used to reinforce performance on a simple task, suggesting the possibility that access to SR, especially if this requires access to specific items, might reinforce SIB. The third hypothesis is that SR and SIB may be functionally equivalent members of the same response class, maintained by positive or negative social reinforcement or automatic reinforcement (Derby, Fisher, & Piazza, 1996). Fourthly, SR may be a member of a distinct operant class from SIB, maintained by different consequences (Rapp & Miltenberger, 2000). Finally it has been proposed that SR may be negatively reinforced by termination of an aversive emotional state (anxiety) predictive of "compulsive" SIB (Hyman et al., 2002; King, 1993).

Several of these hypotheses have received some support from a number of experimental case studies. Fisher, Grace, and Murphy (1996) showed that physically blocking the SIB of a 19-year-old with a severe ID reduced levels of SR, consistent with the proposal that SR was reinforced by avoidance of SIB, and that eliminating the presumed aversive effects of SIB made its avoidance less reinforcing. Scheithauer, O'Connor, and Toby (2015) similarly found that the SR of a 12-year-old girl with Down syndrome was reduced when the force with which she was able to engage in SIB was reduced by semi-flexible arm splints, which again were presumed to reduce the aversive effects of SIB. This hypothesis has also received some support from a naturalistic observational study by Forman, Hall, and Oliver (2002), who observed SIB (face-hitting and mouth-poking), SR, and social environmental events in a 26-year-old man with profound intellectual disabilities. Forman et al. (2002) analyzed relationships between SR, SIB, carer attention, carer "denials" (preventing the participant from accessing an activity or object), and task demand. The probabilities of carer attention, demands, and denials were consistently low immediately before, during, and immediately after episodes of SR and both forms of SIB, suggesting that these behaviors were not related to caregiver behaviors. One topography of SIB (face-hitting) similarly occurred at low levels before, during and after SR, but a second topography (mouth-poking) increased significantly in probability immediately before the onset of SR and occurred with close to zero probability during SR (despite SR and mouth-poking being physically compatible). Forman et al. (2002) interpreted these data as supporting the hypothesis that their participant's SR might be reinforced by escape from SIB and concluded that neither the SR nor the SIB of their participant was socially reinforced.

With regard to the second hypothesis, that access to SR may reinforce SIB, Smith et al. (1996) demonstrated that the SIB of a 32-year-old woman increased when access to SR was contingent on SIB, consistent with the suggestion that SR reinforced SIB. Vollmer and Vorndran (1998) replicated this finding with a 29-year-old woman with a severe ID and further showed that her SIB reduced when access to her preferred means of SR was contingent on a communicative response and not on SIB. With regard to the third hypothesis, Derby et al. (1996) evaluated the possibility that SR and SIB might be functionally equivalent by comparing levels of the two behaviors engaged in by a 12-year-old with a profound ID when attention was contingent on either SIB or SR or presented noncontingently. Contingent attention was shown to increase levels of either behavior. With regard to the final hypothesis that SR and SIB might be functionally independent, Rapp and Miltenberger (2000) produced evidence to suggest that the SIB and SR of an 11-year-old with a severe ID were maintained by distinct consequences. Although experimental support for the suggestion that SR is maintained by escape from or avoidance of a negative emotional state associated with "compulsive" SIB is lacking, the findings of Powell et al. (1996) and Hyman et al. (2002) of an association between coexisting SR and SIB and compulsive behaviors may offer some support for this hypothesis.

The single-case experimental studies described above have produced evidence consistent both with the possibility that SR may be a socially reinforced behavior, in some cases functionally equivalent to SIB, and with the possibility that SR may reinforce SIB or be reinforced by escape from SIB. It seems possible therefore that contingencies between SR and social consequences and between SR and SIB may both be important in maintaining SR. Smith et al. (1992) attempted to distinguish between these different sources of control using the experimental functional analysis (EFA; see Chap. 5 for further details) method of Iwata, Dorsey, Slifer, Bauman, and Richman (1982). Smith et al. (1992) worked with five people with profound IDs with long histories of engaging in SIB and SR. The investigators observed the behaviors of their participants during the four standard EFA conditions of Iwata et al. (1982). However, for the three people for whom it was possible, each EFA condition comprised two sub-conditions; in one of these, the materials necessary for the person to engage in SR were available, and in the second sub-condition, they were absent. In each condition, reinforcement contingencies were programmed according to the EFA condition for SIB, but no systematic contingencies were in effect for SR. Smith et al. (1992) reasoned that if SR were maintained by escape from or avoidance of SIB, the availability of SR should reduce the level of SIB seen in the EFA condition in which SIB most commonly occurs. Further, the hypothesis of SR being maintained by escape from SIB would suggest that SR should increase, and SIB decrease, in the condition with the highest rate of SIB when SR becomes available, and conditions which do not result in high rates of SIB should also not produce high rates of SR. By contrast, if SIB and SR were functionally equivalent, in early EFA sessions, the EFA condition which results in the highest rate of SIB without restraint should, when restraint is available, result in somewhat lower levels of SIB but high levels of SR, as the two responses are functionally interchangeable. As assessment progresses over sessions however, the lack of programmed reinforcement for SR should result in decreased levels of SR and a recovery of levels of SIB in that condition. Smith et al. (1992) were unable to implement sessions without restraint available for two of their participants, who self-restrained using their usual clothing. For one participant, the EFA indicated that his SIB was maintained by escape from task demands, but the function of his SR was not clear. For a second participant, levels of SIB were high across all conditions without SR and low across all conditions with SR. For the third person, the EFA indicated that SIB was maintained by escape from task demands. This participant self-restrained using his everyday clothing. His level of SR decreased across EFA sessions, but with the decrease in the task demand condition lagging behind decreases in other conditions. Smith et al. (1992) argued that these results suggested that this person's SIB and SR had the common function of resulting in escape from task demands, with the decline in SR over sessions resulting from the fact that SR had lost this function under assessment conditions. For the final two participants, levels of SIB were high and variable across all conditions, making it impossible to draw firm conclusions regarding the functions of both the SIB and the SR engaged in by these participants. Smith et al. (1992) concluded that the functions of SR, as for SIB, were likely to vary between individuals and that successful intervention with SR would require assessment of the function of the behavior for each individual.

7.4 Assessment of Self-Restraint

7.4.1 Identifying Self-Restraint

Despite the high prevalence and potentially serious long-term consequences of SR, methods for its assessment, and reports of successful intervention, are relatively few. The 7-item SRC (Powell et al., 1996) or the 23-item SRQ (Oliver et al., 2003) can be used to identify individuals who engage in SR. The SRC, which is completed simply by endorsing (or not) each item, has an interrater reliability of 91% for overall presence of SR, with interrater reliability for individual items ranging from 75 to 100%, with a mean of 90.3% (Powell et al., 1996). Items on the SRQ are scored on a five-point scale, and Oliver et al. (2003) assessed interrater reliability using intraclass correlation coefficients (ICCs) which ranged from close to zero to 0.89 across items, with a mean of 0.49. The ICCs for the four subscale scores were 0.87, 0.17, 0.72, and 0.61 for use of clothing or materials, use of body, use of objects, and use of other people (Oliver et al., 2003). Lower agreement regarding use of body is perhaps to be expected given that items can be scored as occurring "some of the time," and the topographies rated include some which may or may not represent SR (e.g., "folds arms"). Oliver et al. (2003) also carried out a small study of the validity of the SRQ by directly observing 14 individuals for three 30-min session distributed across the day and determining agreement between items endorsed (scoring above 0) on the SRQ and topographies seen during the observations. Percentage agreement across items ranged from 64.2 to 100% (mean 89.6%). Although there were obviously differences between the participant groups, Oliver et al.'s (2003) study using the SRQ reported a higher percentage of people engaging in SR than the studies of Powell et al. (1996), Hyman et al. (2002), and Richards et al. (2017). This may be due to the greater number of topographies included in the SRQ and the fact that items can be endorsed even if they occur only some of the time.

7.4.2 Functional Assessment of Self-Restraint

Functional assessment of SR can be difficult because many people who engage in SR do for very high proportions of their waking day. A person who restrains their hands by tangling them in clothing may, for example, release them only to eat or engage in basic self-care, and some individuals who self-restrain by holding objects may continue to do so even during such activities. Smith et al. (1992) did not conduct EFAs on the SR of their participants, but did observe the levels of their SR as contingencies applying to SIB were changed. Two of their participants engaged in SR almost continuously across all sessions in which SR was possible, while one showed highly variable levels of SR across conditions, with no sign that levels were reducing over sessions. As noted above, one participant however initially showed high levels of SR in all conditions, with levels decreasing across conditions, but with the decrease in "task demand" sessions lagging behind that in other conditions. Smith et al. (1992) interpreted this pattern of results as suggesting that the participant's SR was probably maintained by escape from, or avoidance of, task demands. The SR of the final participant was initially highly variable across conditions, but decreased in all conditions as sessions progressed. Since no reinforcement contingency was being applied, Smith et al. interpreted this pattern of results as indicative of the behavior being maintained by some form of socially mediated reinforcement. The study of Smith et al. (1992) demonstrates that observation of SR during EFAs in which the consequences of SIB are manipulated can also provide information relevant to understanding the functions of the SR. In general, however, possible functions of SR must be inferred from the function(s) of the SIB which it accompanies, the observed relationship between the person's SIB and SR, and the person's responses to attempts to distract them from, or persuade them to briefly refrain from, engaging in SR.

7.5 Intervention with Self-Restraint

Despite the difficulties involved in undertaking functional assessment of SR, a small number of studies have reported on interventions to reduce the behavior. On the hypothesis that SR is maintained by escape from SIB, reducing levels of SIB should of course also reduce levels of SR. In an early application of this logic, Silverman, Watanabe, Marshall, and Baer (1984) showed that when use of a padded helmet reduced the head-hitting, and padded slippers reduced the self-kicking, of a 13-year-old boy with a severe ID, relevant forms of SR (arm restraint for head-hitting and leg restraint for self-kicking) were correspondingly selectively reduced. Silverman et al. (1984) argued that this outcome was consistent with the boy's SR being reinforced by avoidance of SIB, but also with other possible relationships between behaviors. The intervention used also included differential reinforcement of alternative behavior, including prompts to engage in activities and contingent music for winding a toy radio and engaging in other activities. Silverman et al. (1984) noted however that as sessions progressed, the boy developed ways of engaging in these activities while still maintaining some level of SR. As noted above, Fisher et al. (1996) showed that physically blocking the SIB of a 19-year-old with a severe ID, thereby presumably preventing its aversive effects, reduced levels of SR, again supporting the possibility that for some individuals successful interventions to reduce SIB should also indirectly weaken the maintenance of SR.

Derby et al. (1996) demonstrated that contingent attention increased levels of both attempted SIB (hand and knee to head blows) and SR (holding on to the hand of another person with her hands directly in front of her knees) engaged in by a 12-year-old girl with a profound ID. Derby et al. (1996) then also showed that providing social interaction noncontingently reduced both behaviors to low levels and suggested that providing social interaction noncontingently would therefore be an appropriate intervention for the girl's SR and SIB. They did not however report data from any extended application of such intervention.

The majority of studies which have reported on interventions to reduce SR have focused on SR which involves use of an object and have used stimulus fading approaches in attempts to reduce the level of restraint involved and/or increase the social acceptability of the restraints used. In an early study, Foxx and Dufrense (1984) described an extended intervention to reduce the SIB of "Harry," a young man with a severe ID who was reported to have engaged in SIB from early in infancy. According to Foxx and Dufrense (1984), Harry's mother reported having placed cardboard tubes over his arms when he was only 2 weeks old to prevent him from striking his face with his fists. At the time of the intervention, Harry was 22 years old and engaged in SIB comprising striking his nose, head, and thighs with his fists and biting his arms. He had long experience of external restraints being used to control his SIB and at the beginning of the intervention was wearing arm splints continuously apart from one 0.5 h period each day. During the course of an intervention intended to enable him to refrain from SIB without having the splints on, Harry began to attempt to self-restrain using either his own clothing or the clothing of other people who were with him. This SR, rather in keeping with philosophies of institutional care at the time, was initially simply prevented by modifying his clothing. Harry however started to self-restrain by holding an object in each hand. On one occasion when he was holding a drinking glass in each hand, the opportunity was taken to begin a process of fading in which he was provided with progressively smaller plastic glasses, and then cut-down plastic glasses, until after 20 days Harry was self-restraining using two plastic glass rims. It was then suggested to him that he could self-restrain by wearing a wristwatch and interlocking his fingers, but Harry expressed a preference for using a pair of eyeglasses as a means of restraint. As his eyesight was good, a pair of spectacles with plain glass lenses were provided for him. Foxx and Dufrense reported that 4.5 years later, he engaged in SIB infrequently and with low intensity and had a much improved quality of life. Despite its age, Foxx and Dufrense's (1984) report demonstrates an early insight into the clinical relevance of transfer of control between stimuli by associative, categorical, and semantic processes and illustrates the benefit of developing an intervention which builds on the person's own methods of coping with SIB.

Pace, Iwata, Edwards, and McCosh (1986) worked with an 18-year-old man whose SIB involved hand, arm, and shoulder biting and hand and leg scratching. Before intervention, the young man was self-restraining by holding rigid plastic tubes in place on his arms 24 h a day. Initial attempts to decrease his use of SR by prompting him to remove the tubes and providing praise and physical contact during restraint-free periods were successful in reducing his use of the restraints, but also resulted in increased levels of SIB. Pace et al. (1986) then continued the intervention while simultaneously reducing the length of the tubes from 47 to 5 cm in eight steps over a period of 22 days. When the tubes were 5 cm long, the young man was no longer prompted to remove them, but they were then first covered in fabric and then replaced by tennis wrist bands. Throughout this process SIB reduced to the levels which had been observed while the young man was fully self-restraining, and he was reported to be restraint-free and engaging in low levels of SIB at follow-up 2 years later.

Such restraint fading approaches may appear applicable only in situations when a person is using external mechanical restraints or objects. Pace et al. (1986), working with a second young person whose SIB comprised vigorous self-scratching and who self-restrained using his own body and clothing, succeeded in replacing his SR by introducing air splints in which the degree of arm flexion possible could be varied by altering the air pressure. Pace et al. (1986) successfully reduced the air pressure to the point where the boy could easily play with toys, while maintaining low levels of SR and SIB, despite the fact that both behaviors were physically possible. When the splints were fully deflated however, the boy again started to engage in SR and ceased involvement in toy play. Although Pace et al. (1986) were therefore successful in transferring the control of SIB from SR using the boy's clothes and body to a form of restraint which could be more easily faded, the splints had to be maintained (at very low pressure) to successfully substitute for the previous forms of SR. Lerman, Iwata, Smith, and Vollmer (1994) used a similar approach in working with a 20-year-old man with a severe ID whose SIB included neck, arm, and shoulder scratching and head, ear, and chin hitting. His SR included wrapping his arms in his own shirt and holding objects between his head and shoulders. Lerman et al. (1994) used a fading process to substitute wearing a headband and wristbands for the young man's previous forms of SR. At this stage in the intervention however, the young man was still self-restraining by placing his hands or fingers under the headband; however, his engagement in this form of SR was reduced while maintaining SIB at low levels by using differential reinforcement to encourage him to engage in activities including manual signing. He continued however to self-restrain by placing one hand under the headband. Banda, McAfee, and Hart (2012) similarly used restraint fading, in conjunction with dense noncontingent social reinforcement during periods without SIB, and minimizing social responses to SIB, to reduce SR while maintaining low levels of SIB (head-hitting) by a teenager with Tourette syndrome. The young man had been self-restraining by using one or more blankets. During intervention he was provided with a single blanket which was progressively reduced in size. Following intervention, the young man sometimes held a blanket in class, but asking him to put it down did not result in SIB, and his mother reported that she needed only to give him a small blanket or hand towel to use as a preventative strategy in stressful situations.

The emphasis on stimulus fading interventions, or on the possibility that SR is reinforced by termination or avoidance of the aversive consequences of SIB, has led to relative neglect of the hypotheses that SR might be reinforced by other consequences. Derby et al. (1996) proposed that for some people SR might be reinforced by socially mediated consequences, or by automatic reinforcement unrelated to the cessation of SIB, and that in such cases of SR reinforcement-based interventions such as fixed-time or variable-time schedules of reinforcement could be used to reduce the behavior. Powers, Roane, and Kelley (2007) reported that SR emerged as a novel behavior when the SIB of a 16-year-old girl with a moderate ID was reduced by arm splints in the absence of any programmed contingencies for either SR or SIB. Use of the arm splints greatly reduced the frequency with which she hit her head, despite the fact that although they physically prevented the girl from hitting her eyes, she could still hit other head areas. When the splints were in place, however, the girl started to remove the straps which held them in place, wrapping them around her fingers. This behavior (together with SIB) was reduced to zero levels when use of the arm splints was accompanied by giving her continuous access to five toys which had been identified as highly preferred in a stimulus preference assessment.

7.6 Self-Restraint: Summary and Conclusions

Despite the fact that SR appears to be a common problem among people NDCs who engage in SIB, with the potential to seriously limit opportunities for active engagement and quality of life, it has received little attention from researchers. The scale of this neglect is indicated by the fact that Hagopian and his colleagues (Hagopian et al., 2015, 2017, 2018), in their research into treatment outcomes for people engaging in SIB maintained by automatic reinforcement, have been unable to identify a sufficient number of reported cases of such SIB accompanied by SR to make it possible to include this subtype of SIB in their analyses. Little is known about the causation of SR and less about its development. Oliver and his colleagues (Oliver et al., 2003; Richards et al., 2017) have made the interesting suggestion that SR may often commence in the form of use of other people or their clothing as self-restraint and then develop into other forms, and clinical case reports suggest that for some people SR may have been encouraged by parents in early childhood as a way of controlling SIB. At the moment however, these suggestions remain interesting speculations. There are only a few studies which have reported successful intervention with SR, and most of these have focused on a specific type of SR in which objects other than the person's own clothing or body are used to achieve self-restraint. Research into SR may perhaps have been inhibited by the fact that it has proven difficult to analyze using the EFA methodology which has become a hallmark of applied behavioral research. A better understanding of the causal dynamics of the behavior, and research into treatment options for the many people who self-restrain using their own bodies or clothing, is urgently needed.

7.7 Case Study

Pauline G

Pauline G is 40 years old and has a severe intellectual disability and has been diagnosed with an autism spectrum condition. Pauline is independent in basic self-care skills but needs support with many activities of daily living. She understands simple requests accompanied by manual sign language, and uses a small number of signs herself, but has no other expressive form of communication. She engages in episodes of self injury in which she hits her face and head, sometimes to the point of causing bruising, and also bangs her head on hard surfaces. During these episodes Pauline cries and appears to be extremely distressed. Pauline has lived in a community residential service for nearly 20 years. For most of this time, her self-injurious behavior (SIB) has been managed by either taking Pauline to her room when she starts to self-injure or if that is not possible by other people leaving the room in which Pauline is engaging in the behavior. The rationale for this approach is that Pauline calms and ceases to engage in self-injury more rapidly if left alone. Pauline also engages in two forms of self-restraint. One of these, if she is wearing suitable clothing, involves placing her arms up inside the body of her sweater or other top, while the second involves holding on to small objects such as the tops from plastic bottles. Pauline is able to participate in many activities while keeping these items in her hands, and episodes of SIB occur almost exclusively when she drops or loses these items. At any one time, she normally has two specific items which she is using to self-restrain. Although these do change over time, if Pauline drops one of her items, she wants to retrieve that specific item; even a very similar item, if new to her, will not be immediately effective in enabling her to self-restrain. Pauline normally goes to sleep holding her self-restraint items, and the only situations in which she is reliably able to let go of the items without engaging in SIB are when she is in the bath or when she is swimming, which is probably her favorite activity.

Pauline's most recent annual review meeting happened to take place a few days after she had experienced a particularly severe and extended episode of SIB following one of her regular visits to a horse riding center. Pauline lost two small plastic figures which were her currently preferred means of self-restraint. The staff supporting her had eventually been able to persuade her to accept two similar figures as self-restraint materials, but had been unable to do so until they had returned to the house where Pauline lived, by which time she had very badly bruised one side of her face. These events prompted much discussion at the review meeting regarding the risks of relying too much on Pauline's self-restraint to control her SIB, and the meeting formally requested the manager of the residential service to make a referral concerning Pauline's SIB to the local clinical psychology service.

Reviewing records from Pauline's previous contacts with the clinical psychology service, the psychologist who received the referral noted that following a previous referral 3 years earlier, a colleague had conducted a quite extensive assessment including completion of a Functional Assessment Interview (FAI) with Pauline's named "keyworker" at the residential service and several hours of direct observation. These efforts had however provided only limited useful information. The FAI had led to the conclusion that Pauline engaged in SIB when she dropped or mislaid her self-restraint objects, although sometimes when this occurred she would switch to self-restraining by putting her hands up her top. The almost invariable consequence of Pauline engaging in SIB was reported to be that the staff supporting her ceased all attempts to engage her in the current activity and attempted to calm her, usually by trying to find her self-restraint objects or offering her alternatives. The previously involved psychologist, having concluded that Pauline did not have capacity to give informed consent for further assessment, had engaged in consultations with Pauline's parents and staff of the residential service as to whether further assessment procedures would be in her best interests. She had concluded that to undertake some direct observation of Pauline's behavior would be in her best interests, whereas to carry out an experimental functional analysis (EFA) would not. She had recorded in her notes that this was because of the increased risk of Pauline harming herself entailed in the EFA procedure. In the course of 4 h of direct observation however, the previously involved psychologist had seen only one incident in which Pauline engaged in SIB. Her observations were nevertheless of some interest.

She had been observing while Pauline was being supported in preparing a meal. At the time Pauline was whisking eggs to make an omelette while simultaneously holding a plastic bottle top (her preferred self-restraint items at the time) in each hand, when she dropped one of the bottle tops, which fell to the floor and unfortunately bounced into a small gap between two cupboards. Pauline immediately dropped the whisk from her right hand (which had dropped the top) and released the mixing bowl from her left, and attempted to place her hands up her sweater, but was prevented from easily doing so by the apron she was wearing. She then started to slap her face and the side of her head very hard with her right hand. The member of staff supporting her had managed to retrieve the bottle top from the floor and offered it to Pauline, who however continued to self-injure, only calming when the member of staff eventually managed to remove Pauline's apron so that she could self-restrain using her jumper. The previously involved psychologist had recommended attempting to substitute objects less easily mislaid for Pauline's self-restraint objects, but it appeared that owing to staffing changes in both the residential and clinical psychology departments, this suggestion had not been taken forward.

Following an initial meeting with Pauline, which led her to the conclusion that Pauline did not have the capacity to give informed consent to further assessment, the newly involved clinical psychologist considered that repeating previously completed assessments would not, at that stage, be in Pauline's best interests. She did however think that it would be helpful to Pauline to carry out a brief assessment to determine whether any factors not identified by the previous assessment were now maintaining Pauline's SIB. When she met with Pauline's current keyworker, in the course of an initial clinical interview, she therefore completed a Questions About Behavioural Function (QABF) assessment with her concerning Pauline's head-hitting. The resulting QABF subscale severity scores were one for the attention subscale, seven for the escape subscale, four for the non-social subscale, one for the physical subscale, and eight for the tangible subscale, suggesting that Pauline's SIB was maintained by escape from task demands and obtaining tangibles. On the basis of the overall clinical interview and the information from her predecessor's assessment, the clinical psychologist was however skeptical regarding the possibility that socially mediated reinforcement processes were important in maintaining Pauline's SIB. Her head-hitting and other SIB certainly appeared to be more likely to occur when she was being asked to participate in activities, but it appeared possible that this was simply because such situations increased the probability that she would drop her self-restraint objects. Similarly, endorsement of statements suggesting that Pauline engaged in SIB in order to obtain tangibles appeared to refer primarily to situations where she self-injured while trying to recover self-restraint objects which she had dropped. Also, Pauline's keyworker mentioned that although Pauline often started to self-injure when she dropped one or both of her self-restraint objects, sometimes she would continue to self-injure even when support workers immediately gave the objects back to Pauline. It was, her keyworker said, as though Pauline could not stop the behavior once it had started.

Having reviewed this information, the clinical psychologist saw little reason to doubt that her predecessor's recommendation remained the most practicable approach to reducing the frequency with which Pauline engaged in SIB and considered that it would be in Pauline's best interests to pursue the previously recommended intervention. Serendipitously, Pauline's currently preferred self-restraint items were two large beads from a creative crafts set which she had been given as a birthday present. The clinical psychologist suggested that Pauline's keyworker could work with Pauline to progressively string additional beads to the ones Pauline was using to self-restrain, eventually developing these into bracelets which Pauline could wear. This process was successfully completed within 2 weeks. Pauline's keyworker also helped Pauline to make two further sets of bracelets and managed to persuade her to change the bracelets she was wearing, so that a spare pair which Pauline would accept as a working means of self-restraint was readily available if she accidentally lost or broke a bracelet she was wearing. Following 3 months in which Pauline had worn the bracelets every day and rarely self-injured, the clinical psychologist closed the case.

Eight months later, the psychologist was surprised to receive a further referral regarding Pauline's self-injury. Telephoning the residential home, she was told that Pauline had been engaging in extensive self-injury for several weeks. The bracelets no longer appeared to function as an effective form of self-restraint, although Pauline was sometimes self-restraining by putting her hands and lower arms up the front of her sweater. The staff member who spoke to the clinical psychologist also told her that Pauline had been crying a lot and generally seemed distressed and unhappy following a series of changes in her life. Her grandfather, who used to visit her each month, had died. As a result of his death, Pauline's grandmother, who had been diagnosed with vascular dementia several years previously, and required extensive support in activities of daily living, had moved to live with Pauline's parents. This in turn had impacted on their relationship with Pauline. Previously her parents had visited her, together, twice a week, taking her out on at least one of these visits. Since they had become carers for Pauline's grandmother however, one of them would stay at home while the other visited Pauline. At first they had also reduced their visits to one a week, but seeing how unhappy Pauline had become, they were again trying to manage to fit in a second visit. Her parents were however no longer taking Pauline out, as they felt unable to cope with her SIB without help from the residential service staff. In fact, Pauline's normal routines had been further disrupted by the fact that the residential staff had also temporarily stopped taking Pauline out shopping, to the riding center, or swimming, because her SIB was so difficult to manage in busy public places. The clinical psychologist asked if she could make an appointment to speak with Pauline's keyworker, but was told that she had moved to another job. The psychologist therefore arranged to meet with the home manager to discuss short-term plans for the management of Pauline's SIB. She anticipated that a period of focus on minimizing the harm that Pauline was causing herself, reassuring and supporting the staff working with her, and trying to restore as much as possible of Pauline's previous activities would probably be the immediate priorities for her involvement.

References

Ball, T. S., Sibbach, L., Jones, R., Steele, B., & Frazier, L. (1975). An accelerometer-activated device to control assaultive and self-destructive behaviors in retardates. *Journal of Behavior Therapy and Experimental Psychiatry, 6*(3), 223–228. https://doi.org/10.1016/0005-7916(75)90104-4

Banda, D. R., McAfee, J. K., & Hart, S. L. (2012). Decreasing self-injurious behavior and fading self-restraint in a student with autism and Tourette syndrome. *Behavioral Interventions, 27*(3), 164–174. https://doi.org/10.1002/bin.1344

Christie, R., Bay, C., Kaufman, I. A., Bakay, B., Borden, M., & Nyhan, W. L. (1982). Lesch-Nyhan disease: Clinical experience with nineteen patients. *Developmental Medicine and Child Neurology, 24*(3), 293–306. https://doi.org/10.1111/j.1469-8749.1982.tb13621.x

Derby, K. M., Fisher, W. W., & Piazza, C. C. (1996). The effects of contingent and noncontingent attention on self-injury and self-restraint. *Journal of Applied Behavior Analysis, 29*(1), 107–110. https://doi.org/10.1901/jaba.1996.29-107

Favell, J. E., McGimsey, J. F., & Jones, M. L. (1978). The use of physical restraint in the treatment of self-injury and as positive reinforcement. *Journal of Applied Behavior Analysis, 11*(2), 225–241. https://doi.org/10.1901/jaba.1978.11-225

Fisher, W. W., Grace, N. C., & Murphy, C. (1996). Further analysis of the relationship between self-injury and self-restraint. *Journal of Applied Behavior Analysis, 29*(1), 103–106. https://doi.org/10.1901/jaba.1996.29-103

Fisher, W. W., & Iwata, B. A. (1996). On the function of self-restraint and its relationship to self-injury. *Journal of Applied Behavior Analysis, 29*(1), 93–98. https://doi.org/10.1901/jaba.1996.29-93

Forman, D., Hall, S., & Oliver, C. (2002). Descriptive analysis of self-injurious behaviour and self-restraint. *Journal of Applied Research in Intellectual Disabilities, 15*(1), 1–7. https://doi.org/10.1046/j.1360-2322.2001.00091.x

Fovel, J. T., Lash, P. S., Barron, D. A., Jr., & Roberts, M. S. (1989). A survey of self-restraint, self-injury, and other maladaptive behaviors in an institutionalized retarded population. *Research in Developmental Disabilities, 10*(4), 377–382. https://doi.org/10.1016/0891-4222(89)90038-3

Foxx, R. M., & Dufrense, D. (1984). "Harry": The use of physical restraint as a reinforcer, timeout from restraint, and fading restraint in treating a self-injurious man. *Analysis and Intervention in Developmental Disabilities, 4*(1), 1–13. https://doi.org/10.1016/0270-4684(84)90014-4

Hagopian, L. P., Rooker, G. W., & Yenokyan, G. (2018). Identifying predictive behavioral markers: A demonstration using automatically reinforced self-injurious behavior. *Journal of Applied Behavior Analysis, 51*(3), 443–465. https://doi.org/10.1002/jaba.477

Hagopian, L. P., Rooker, G. W., & Zarcone, J. R. (2015). Delineating subtypes of self-injurious behavior maintained by automatic reinforcement. *Journal of Applied Behavior Analysis, 48*(3), 523–543. https://doi.org/10.1002/jaba.236

Hagopian, L. P., Rooker, G. W., Zarcone, J. R., Bonner, A. C., & Arevalo, A. R. (2017). Further analysis of subtypes of automatically reinforced SIB: A replication and quantitative analysis of published datasets. *Journal of Applied Behavior Analysis, 50*(1), 48–66. https://doi.org/10.1002/jaba.368

Hyman, P., Oliver, C., & Hall, S. (2002). Self-injurious behavior, self-restraint, and compulsive behaviors in Cornelia de Lange syndrome. *American Journal on Mental Retardation, 107*(2), 146–154 + 156–157. https://doi.org/10.1352/0895-8017(2002)107<0146:SIBSRA>2.0.CO;2

Isley, E. M., Kartsonis, C., McCurley, C. M., Eager Weisz, K., & Roberts, M. S. (1991). Self-restraint: A review of etiology and applications in mentally retarded adults with self-injury. *Research in Developmental Disabilities, 12*(1), 87–95. https://doi.org/10.1016/0891-4222(91)90024-M

Iwata, B. A., Dorsey, M. F., Slifer, K. J., Bauman, K. E., & Richman, G. S. (1982). Toward a functional analysis of self-injury. *Analysis and Intervention in Developmental Disabilities, 2*, 3–20. https://doi.org/10.1016/0270-4684(82)90003-9

King, B. H. (1993). Self-injury by people with mental retardation: A compulsive behavior hypothesis. *American Journal of Mental Retardation, 98*(1), 93–112.

Lerman, D. C., Iwata, B. A., Smith, R. G., & Vollmer, T. R. (1994). Restraint fading and the development of alternative behaviour in the treatment of self-restraint and self-injury. *Journal of Intellectual Disability Research, 38*(2), 135–148. https://doi.org/10.1111/j.1365-2788.1994.tb00369.x

Lovaas, O. I., & Simmons, J. Q. (1969). Manipulation of self-destruction in three retarded children. *Journal of Applied Behavior Analysis, 2*(3), 143–157. https://doi.org/10.1901/jaba.1969.2-143

Myers, J. J., Jr., & Deibert, A. N. (1971). Reduction of self-abusive behavior in a blind child by using a feeding response. *Journal of Behavior Therapy and Experimental Psychiatry, 2*(2), 141–144. https://doi.org/10.1016/0005-7916(71)90030-9

Nyhan, W. L. (1976). Behavior in the Lesch-Nyhan syndrome. *Journal of Autism and Childhood Schizophrenia, 6*(3), 235–252. https://doi.org/10.1007/BF01543464

Oliver, C., Murphy, G., Hall, S., Arron, K., & Leggett, J. (2003). Phenomenology of self-restraint. *American Journal on Mental Retardation, 108*(2), 71–81 + 144. https://doi.org/10.1352/0895-8017(2003)108<0071:POSR>2.0.CO;2

Pace, G. M., Iwata, B. A., Edwards, G. L., & McCosh, K. C. (1986). Stimulus fading and transfer in the treatment of self-restraint and self-injurious behavior. *Journal of Applied Behavior Analysis, 19*(4), 381–389. https://doi.org/10.1901/jaba.1986.19-381

Powell, S. B., Bodfish, J. W., Parker, D., Crawford, T. W., & Lewis, M. H. (1996). Self-restraint and self-injury: Occurrence and motivational significance. *American Journal of Mental Retardation, 101*(1), 41–48.

Powers, K. V., Roane, H. S., & Kelley, M. E. (2007). Treatment of self-restraint associated with the application of protective equipment. *Journal of Applied Behavior Analysis, 40*(3), 577–581. https://doi.org/10.1901/jaba.2007.40-577

Rapp, J. T., & Miltenberger, R. G. (2000). Self-restraint and self-injury: A demonstration of separate functions and response classes. *Behavioral Interventions, 15*(1), 37–51. https://doi.org/10.1002/(SICI)1099-078X(200001/03)15:1<37::AID-BIN40>3.0.CO;2-5

Richards, C., Davies, L., & Oliver, C. (2017). Predictors of self-injurious behavior and self-restraint in autism spectrum disorder: Towards a hypothesis of impaired behavioral control. *Journal of Autism and Developmental Disorders, 47*(3), 701–713. https://doi.org/10.1007/s10803-016-3000-5

Rojahn, J. (1986). Self-injurious and stereotypic behavior of noninstitutionalized mentally retarded people: Prevalence and classification. *American Journal of Mental Deficiency, 91*(3), 268–276.

Rojahn, J., Mulick, J. A., McCoy, D., & Schroeder, S. R. (1978). Setting effects, adaptive clothing, and the modification of head banging and self-restraint in two profoundly retarded adults. *Behavioural Analysis and Modification, 2*(3), 185–196. Reprinted in Murphy, G., & Wilson, B. (Eds.), *Self-injurious behaviour: A collection of published papers on prevalence, causes, and treatment in people who are mentally handicapped or autistic* (pp. 409–416). Kidderminster: British Institute of Mental Handicap

Rooker, G. W., & Roscoe, E. M. (2005). Functional analysis of self-injurious behavior and its relation to self-restraint. *Journal of Applied Behavior Analysis, 38*(4), 537–542. https://doi.org/10.1901/jaba.2005.12-05

Scheithauer, M., O'Connor, J., & Toby, L. M. (2015). Assessment of self-restraint using a functional analysis of self-injury. *Journal of Applied Behavior Analysis, 48*(4), 907–911. https://doi.org/10.1002/jaba.230

Shear, C. S., Nyhan, W. L., Kirman, B. H., & Stern, J. (1971). Self-mutilative behavior as a feature of the de Lange syndrome. *The Journal of Pediatrics, 78*(3), 506–509. https://doi.org/10.1016/S0022-3476(71)80236-6

Silverman, K., Watanabe, K., Marshall, A. M., & Baer, D. M. (1984). Reducing self-injury and corresponding self-restraint through the strategic use of protective clothing. *Journal of Applied Behavior Analysis, 17*(4), 545–552. https://doi.org/10.1901/jaba.1984.17-545

Smith, R. G., Iwata, B. A., Vollmer, T. R., & Pace, G. M. (1992). On the relationship between self-injurious behavior and self-restraint. *Journal of Applied Behavior Analysis, 25*(2), 433–445. https://doi.org/10.1901/jaba.1992.25-433

Smith, R. G., Lerman, D. C., & Iwata, B. A. (1996). Self-restraint as positive reinforcement for self-injurious behavior. *Journal of Applied Behavior Analysis, 29*(1), 99–102. https://doi.org/10.1901/jaba.1996.29-99

Vollmer, T. R., & Vorndran, C. M. (1998). Assessment of self-injurious behavior maintained by access to self-restraint materials. *Journal of Applied Behavior Analysis, 31*(4), 647–650. https://doi.org/10.1901/jaba.1998.31-647

Chapter 8
Self-Injurious Behavior in Persons with Autism Spectrum Conditions

8.1 Introduction

Changes in diagnostic practice have resulted in significant increases in the number of people diagnosed with autism spectrum conditions (ASCs) and in estimates of the proportion so diagnosed who have intellectual quotients (IQs) within the normal range (Rydzewska et al., 2019). While ASCs have been identified as a risk factor for SIB in people with intellectual disabilities (IDs), high rates of self-harm are also reported by people with ASCs without IDs. There are reasons to believe that the factors related to the development of SIB in people with ASCs may differ somewhat from those associated with SIB in people with IDs. Some studies of SIB in young children with ASCs (e.g., Soke et al., 2018) have found a positive relationship between child IQ and current SIB, a finding strikingly different from the association of SIB with lower ability usually found in studies involving people with IDs. This chapter provides a critical overview of research into factors which may, at each stage in the development of SIB, contribute to the elevated risk of developing and maintaining SIB experienced by people with ASCs. The chapter also describes the phenomenology of self-harm in intellectually able people with ASCs and implications for assessment and treatment of SIB experienced by people with ASCs and ID.

F. Furniss, A. B. Biswas, *Self-Injurious Behavior in Individuals with Neurodevelopmental Conditions*, Autism and Child Psychopathology Series,
https://doi.org/10.1007/978-3-030-36016-0_8

8.2 Emergence of Self-Injurious Behavior

8.2.1 Sensitivity to Events Eliciting Initial Self-Injurious Responses

As noted in Chap. 2, it appears probable that the increased risk for SIB experienced by people with ASCs is associated with some specific aspects of the phenotype of ASCs rather than with the overall diagnosis, and several recent studies involving children with ASCs (or at risk for developing ASCs) have attempted to delineate specific associations. In these studies (described in greater detail in Chap. 2), atypical sensory processing, insistence on sameness, social communication and functioning, and anxiety have emerged as significant correlates of SIB (Dempsey, Dempsey, Guffey, Minard, & Goin-Kochel, 2016; Duerden et al., 2012; Soke et al., 2017, 2018). Few studies however have reported on factors associated with the initial emergence of SIB, owing to the relatively low numbers of incident cases of SIB in even the larger studies. In children with IDs however, Davies and Oliver (2016) have reported that baseline levels of repetitive and restricted behaviors and interests predicted emergence of SIB at follow-up 15–18 months later.

Consideration of the possible roles of these factors in the emergence of SIB is complicated by the possibility that several may be highly correlated. Both developmental and functional imaging studies suggest that insistence on sameness constitutes a subtype of repetitive and restricted behaviors (RRBs) distinct from repetitive sensory and motor behaviors (Barrett, Uljarević, Jones, & Leekam, 2018; Traynor et al., 2018; Uljarević et al., 2017). In older children, insistence on sameness, atypical sensory processing, and anxiety appear to be closely related (Black et al., 2017; Russell, Frost, & Ingersoll, 2019). In older children, insistence on sameness is also sometimes argued to represent a mechanism for coping with anxiety. If the situations which initially evoke SIB are typically frustration and rapid situational transitions (Berkson, 2002), it can however readily be understood how limited social communication and functioning could increase the probability of frustration in interactions with caregivers and insistence on sameness could increase the aversiveness of rapid situational transitions. Sensory hypersensitivity might further exacerbate the aversiveness of rapid transitions by effectively amplifying the magnitudes of changes in stimulation during transitions. Alternatively, or additionally, sensory hypersensitivity might intensify the experience of pain and/or discomfort arising from medical conditions, which are suspected to be among the aversive experiences which might elicit early SIB (Petty, Bacarese-Hamilton, Davies, & Oliver, 2014). A recent study of young children (mean age 3.9 years) who were being evaluated for possible developmental difficulties found that parent-completed ratings of their children's pain-related behaviors over a period of a week were higher for children who engaged in SIB than for those who did not (Courtemanche, Black, & Reese, 2016). These differences may however relate to differences in pain-related events rather than in heightened sensitivity to pain, since Courtemanche and Black (2016) found no differences in pain reports concerning children with and without an ASC.

8.2.2 Sensitivity to Pavlovian Conditioning of Behavior Elicited by Aversive Events

In the model of development of SIB presented in Chap. 3, the early development of SIB involves not only elicitation of self-injurious behavior by aversive experiences but also a process of Pavlovian conditioning which results in the behavior being evoked by a range of stimuli associated with the originally eliciting experiences. A major factor influencing the probability of such conditioning is child temperament. The variability observed, from early infancy, in the readiness and intensity of children's emotional responses to stimuli, interest in social interaction, level of motor activity, attention, and other characteristics, has often been interpreted as reflecting variability in neurobiological regulatory mechanisms with putative high genetic heritability and described as temperament (Rothbart, 2007). Temperament itself is presumed to provide the basis for the development of personality as the child interacts with the social and material world and simultaneously develops increasingly complex motor, cognitive, and emotional capacities for such interaction (Tackett, 2006). In children without neurodevelopmental conditions (NDCs), low levels of a trait generally labelled "effortful control," comprising the ability to modulate emotion and/or maintain goal-directed behavior despite emotional challenge (Kochanska, Murray, & Harlan, 2000), emerge as a clear correlate of a variety of internalizing and externalizing psychopathologies (Nigg, 2006). High levels of a second temperamental trait, variously called "emotionality" or "negative affectivity," which involves high reactivity and sensitivity to aversive situations or emotions, may however also increase risk for emotional and behavioral difficulties.

Recent research has shown that temperamental differences between children who are at familial high risk for developing an ASC, those who later develop an ASC, and children without NDCs can be detected in the first 2 years of life. Clifford, Hudry, Elsabbagh, Charman, and Johnson (2013) showed that children at risk for developing an ASC showed reduced effortful control at ages 14 and 24 months, and children later diagnosed with an ASC showed higher negative affectivity during their second year of life, by comparison with children without ASCs. For children with ASCs, parental reports concerning younger children suggest that compared with children without NDCs, those with ASCs show lower adaptability and persistence and lower effortful control but often do not show higher negative affectivity (Adamek et al., 2011; Garon et al., 2009; Hepburn & Stone, 2006). Failures to find differences at the level of overarching temperamental factors may however result from patterns of difference in subscale scores. Macari, Koller, Campbell, and Chawarska (2017), for example, showed that toddlers with ASCs scored significantly lower than toddlers without NDCs on all five of the subscales measuring aspects of effortful control used in their study (and lower than toddlers with developmental delay on four of these), while of the five subscales assessing aspects of negative affectivity, the toddlers with ASCs scored lower than those without NDCs only on the subscale assessing soothability. Studies including older children have found higher levels of negative affectivity in children with ASCs than in children without NDCs, but have but disagreed as to whether effortful control is lower in children with ASCs (de Pauw, Mervielde, Van Leeuwen, & De Clercq, 2011; Samyn, Roeyers, & Bijttebier, 2011; Schwartz et al., 2009). In children with ASCs, internalizing problems are associated with negative affectivity, while studies differ as to whether effortful control is negatively correlated with such problems within groups of children with ASCs, but concur that it correlates with this factor in combined groups of children with and without ASCs (de Pauw et al., 2011; Schwartz et al., 2009). This pattern of results may indicate that although there are systematic differences in temperament between children with ASCs and those without NDCs, the relationships between temperament and emotional and behavioral difficulties are similar in children with and without ASCs. Burrows, Usher, Schwartz, Mundy, and Henderson (2016) reported an interesting study in which intellectually able children and teenagers with ASCs (with verbal IQ over 70) completed self-report measures of temperament, while their parents completed measures of the young people's internalizing and externalizing emotional and behavioral difficulties. The young people with ASCs reported higher levels of negative affectivity than a comparison group of young people without NDCs, but the two groups did not differ in self-reported effortful control. Across all participants in the study, higher levels of negative affectivity, and lower levels of effortful control, were associated with levels of both internalizing and externalizing difficulties; these relationships were not however significantly affected by group membership.

Although the relationship between negative affectivity and emotional and behavioral difficulties has been established both for children with ASCs and those without NDCs, the possible relationship between temperament and the development of SIB does not appear to have been specifically examined in children with IDs or ASCs. A number of points of indirect evidence may however suggest a role for elevated negative affectivity in the Pavlovian conditioning of reactions toward aversive stimuli which we propose to be an important dynamic in the early development of SIB. Firstly, individuals high in negative emotionality show increased sensitivity to stimuli associated with aversive stimulation and frustrative nonreward (Gray, 1976), providing a basis for the generalization to such stimuli of the ability to elicit SIB. Secondly, children with Down syndrome display lower levels of negative emotionality than typically developing children (Gartstein, Marmion, & Swanson, 2006; Nygaard, Smith, & Torgersen, 2002), and having Down syndrome appears to protect against the development of SIB (Cooper et al., 2009). Although there is less evidence to suggest a specific role for reduced effortful control in the development of SIB, other than its general relationship with emotional and behavioral difficulties in children with or without ASCs, a study of older teenagers and young adults with ASCs has found that anxiety is associated with insistence on sameness, that both anxiety and insistence on sameness are associated with lower levels of effortful control, and that the two relationships between anxiety with effortful control and with insistence on sameness are both mediated by the other factor (Uljarević, Richdale, Evans, Cai, & Leekam, 2017). If insistence on sameness increases the aversiveness of transitions to children with ASCs, therefore, aspects of temperament may mediate the emotional consequences of experiencing such events.

8.3 Development of Operant (Goal-Directed) Functions of Self-Injurious Behavior

There would appear to be no reason to suppose that the risk of transition from emergent to operant or goal-directed SIB should be fundamentally different for people with ASCs compared with people with other NDCs. Additional risk might however be conferred if people with ASCs, already at risk for other reasons, are motivated to engage in SIB by a broader range of consequences than people with other NDCs. Reese, Richman, Belmont, and Morse (2005) used the Functional Assessment Interview (O'Neill et al., 1997) to identify functions of challenging behavior in children with developmental disabilities with and without ASCs and categorized the functions of the problem behaviors into three "standard" functions (gain attention, escape demand, or gain tangible item), and three hypothesized "autism-specific" functions (e.g., escape sensory stimulation). Reese et al. (2005) found that the challenging behaviors of the non-autistic children were typically reinforced by attention, task avoidance, or tangibles, but for boys, (although not for girls), with ASCs, challenging behaviors more often had the function of enabling engagement in repetitive behavior (e.g., by gaining/maintaining access to items used in such behaviors) or avoiding idiosyncratically aversive stimuli.

Studies employing more extensive assessment methods including descriptive antecedent-behavior-consequence assessment or brief or standard experimental functional analyses (EFAs) (Derby et al., 1992; Iwata, Dorsey, Slifer, Bauman, & Richman, 1982) have however produced conflicting results regarding the extent to which the functions of challenging behaviors including SIB may differ between persons with ASCs and those with other developmental disabilities. Love, Carr, and LeBlanc (2009) reviewed data from 32 functional assessments of problem behavior in children with ASCs aged from 2 to 12 years and found that in most cases (88%) problem behavior was assessed as having a social function, consistent with results from earlier studies involving participants with varied developmental disabilities (e.g., Asmus et al., 2004; Derby et al., 1992; Iwata et al., 1994; Kurtz et al., 2003). Love et al. (2009) did find however that a greater proportion of their participants (45%) were identified as showing behaviors controlled by more than one type of reinforcement than had typically been reported in previous studies. O'Reilly et al. (2010) in contrast conducted EFAs with ten children with ASCs aged from 4 to 8 years and found results consistent with functions of gaining access to tangibles and demand avoidance in two cases and largely undifferentiated patterns of responding across conditions for the remaining eight. A study involving preschoolers with fragile X syndrome, a neurodevelopmental condition strongly associated with features of ASCs, reported that out of 12 functional assessments of the challenging behaviors of the children, 11 identified a clear function or functions of the behavior (Machalicek et al., 2014). Working with older children with fragile X syndrome, Kurtz, Chin, Robinson, O'Connor, and Hagopian (2015) reported that clear functions of challenging behavior were identified in seven out of nine children on initial assessment, with functions being identified for the other two children after further individualized assessment. Both studies reported however that escape (from task demands or social interaction) and access to tangibles were more commonly identified as the reinforcer maintaining challenging behavior than access to social interaction.

Although people with ASCs therefore probably engage in challenging behavior, including SIB, which is maintained by a pattern of consequences rather different from that usually seen with people with IDs of heterogeneous origin, it is doubtful whether the range of consequences maintaining challenging behavior is broader for people with ASCs. Of course, the probability of SIB (or other challenging behaviors) acquiring operant functions will depend not only on the consequences maintaining those behaviors but on the person's ability to obtain those outcomes by other means. Love et al. (2009) argued, for example, that their findings of frequent social functions for challenging behaviors in children with ASCs might be expected given the impairments in social and communicative skills associated with autism.

8.4 The Transition from Operant (Goal-Directed) to Habitual/Impulsive Self-Injurious Behavior

Although the evidence is limited, and some of it is indirect, it is likely that the severity of characteristics of ASC is a predictor of persistence of SIB and other behavioral difficulties. Baghdadli et al. (2008) and Rattaz, Michelon, and Baghdadli (2015) reported that for their group of children with ASCs, severity of signs of ASCs assessed at mean age 4.9 years predicted presence of SIB at 3-year follow-up conducted when the children were between 5 and 10 years of age and a high score on a measure of SIB in adolescence (mean age 15 years). Emerson et al. (2001) collected information on 95 people with IDs out of a total of 127 identified in a total population study 7 years previously as presenting severe SIB and found that 67 (71%) still showed serious SIB. A diagnosis of autism at the time of the original study was associated with presence of SIB at follow-up, but autism diagnosis was not identified as a predictor of persistent SIB in a logistic regression analysis. Cooper et al. (2009) followed up 34 adults with IDs out of a group of 50 identified as presenting SIB in a total population study 2 years previously and found that 21 (62%) continued to engage in SIB. Melville et al. (2008), using the same dataset, examined changes in mental ill-health (including engaging in challenging behaviors) in adults with IDs and a diagnosis of autism and a control group of participants without ASCs who were matched (on a two-to-one basis) to each participant with autism for gender, ability level, age (to within 5 years), and presence vs. absence of Down syndrome. Over a period of 2 years, 12 (37.5%) of the 32 control participants initially identified as presenting challenging behavior ceased to do so, whereas only 1 (5.9%) of the 17 people with autism presenting challenging behavior ceased to do so.

Whether or not the severity of features of an ASC predicts persistence of SIB, the behavior does appear to be highly persistent in people with ASCs who begin to engage in it. In a cross-sectional study, Esbensen, Seltzer, Lam, and Bodfish (2009) found that although various types of repetitive and restricted behaviors appeared to reduce with age in people with ASCs, the differences in restricted interests and stereotyped behavior across age groups were greater than those for ritualistic/sameness and compulsive behaviors and SIB. In a naturalistic, retrospective review of changes with age in adults with ASCs supported by a community services agency, Wise, Smith, and Rabins (2017) found that over a mean time period of 25 years, the prevalence of SIB (and many other challenging behaviors) had significantly reduced, but at the most recent time point, SIB was the most common challenging behavior experienced.

Although direct evidence on this point is lacking, it seems possible that the persistence of SIB in people with ASCs may be associated with development of the behavior to one of the more advanced stages, i.e., habitual/impulsive, stereotyped, or compulsive SIB. The association between impulsivity and persistence of SIB observed by Richards, Moss, Nelson, and Oliver (2016) in their 3-year follow-up of young people with ASCs may therefore reflect a transition from goal-directed to habitual/impulsive control of the behavior facilitated by high levels of impulsivity in people with ASCs. Other characteristics and experiences commonly experienced by people with ASCs might however be additional drivers of this process. In animal models of SIB, social stress (Muehlmann et al., 2012) and innate responsivity to stress (Muehlmann, Wilkinson, & Devine, 2011) are associated with emergence of SIB in vulnerable individuals, and chronic stress has been identified as a factor promoting the transition from goal-directed to habitual/impulsive control of behavior (Everitt & Robbins, 2016). People with ASCs are both exposed to high levels of stressors and self-report high levels of experienced stress. In children, having an ASC is associated with enhanced risk of experiencing levels of adverse childhood experiences (such as family income insufficiency, parental divorce or separation, death of a parent, witnessing domestic violence) known to have adverse effects on physical and mental well-being in adulthood in the general population (Berg, Shiu, Acharya, Stolbach, & Msall, 2016). Children with ASCs are also more likely to experience bullying by peers than children without ASCs (Hoover & Kaufman, 2018). Adults with ASCs, but without IDs, report experiencing more stressful life events, and higher levels of perceived stress, than adults without NDCs (Bishop-Fitzpatrick, Minshew, Mazefsky, & Eack, 2017; Hirvikoski & Blomqvist, 2015). Adults with ASCs are similarly rated by clinical researchers as showing more signs of stress than adults without NDCs (Bishop-Fitzpatrick, Mazefsky, Minshew, & Eack, 2015). Adults with ASCs and IDs experience higher levels of stress from a number of sources than adults with IDs alone (Gillott & Standen, 2007).

In addition to experiencing more stressors, and experiencing more subjective stress, than people without ASCs, it is also possible that people with ASCs differ from those without ASCs in their physiological responses to stressful experiences. In a systematic review of studies of physiological reactivity to stimuli in people with ASCs, which included studies using measures of autonomic nervous system activity such as heart rate and heart rate variability, and measures related to activity of the limbic-hypothalamic-pituitary-adrenal axis such as salivary cortisol levels, Lydon et al. (2016) identified 17 controlled studies of reactions to social stimuli, 7 controlled studies of reactions to emotional stimuli, and 16 controlled studies of reactions to overtly stressful stimuli and situations. The control groups whose reactions were compared to those of children and adults with ASCs were generally comprised of "typically developing" individuals. Lydon et al. (2016) reported that one or more of the responses of people with ASCs differed from those of control participants in 12 of the 17 studies employing social stimuli, in 4 of the 7 studies using emotional stimuli, and in 10 of the 14 studies with stressful stimuli or experiences. With regard to baseline measures of arousal, across multiple measures, participants with ASCs were generally found either not to differ from control participants or to have higher levels of arousal (Lydon et al., 2016). Lydon et al. (2016) commented on the variability in findings across studies, even where the participants involved, stimuli and physiological measures used, and study procedures, appeared to be highly similar, concluding that heterogeneity among people with ASCs in terms of physiological processes was a potential explanation for this pattern of results. This heterogeneity may relate to a developmental process in which initially reduced responsivity to specific stimuli or experiences (e.g., social stress) changes toward a more developmentally conventional pattern with maturity (Taylor, Muscatello, & Corbett, 2018). Although studies comparing groups of people with ASCs and those without NDCs on measures of response to stressful (and other) stimuli have produced mixed results, these individual differences in activation in the autonomic nervous system and limbic-hypothalamic-pituitary-adrenal axis may be important in shifting control of SIB from predominantly goal-directed to predominantly habitual/impulsive control. In children without NDCs, sympathetic under-arousal has been associated with conduct problems (Cappadocia, Desrocher, Pepler, & Schroeder, 2009). Baker et al. (2018) showed that when children with ASCs (with ages ranging from 4 to 11 and estimated IQs from 47 to 139) engaged in various play, problem-solving, and compliance tasks with their primary caregivers, level of sympathetic arousal during compliance tasks (as assessed by nonspecific skin conductance responses) was inversely associated with parent-completed assessments of the child's externalizing behavior problems. During problem-solving tasks, the relationship between sympathetic arousal and parent-assessed level of behavioral difficulties was moderated by the quality of support the caregiver provided to the child during the task.

In summary, people with ASCs experience high levels of adverse events and high levels of perceived stress which may drive the development of SIB from primarily goal-directed to primarily habitual (stimulus-response) control. The evidence regarding the response of people with ASCs to stressful experiences suggests that there may be considerable inter-individual differences in responsivity, possibly related to developmental processes. For those with lower levels of arousal in response to challenging events, this lowered responsiveness may also contribute to the evolution from goal-directed to habitual/impulsive control of SIB. We will return to this apparently paradoxical suggestion in Sect. 8.7.

8.5 Further Evolution of Self-Injurious Behavior into Stereotyped and Compulsive Forms in People with Autism Spectrum Conditions

8.5.1 Evolution into Stereotyped Self-Injurious Behavior

A diagnosis of an ASC is associated with increased prevalence and/or severity of stereotyped behaviors (STBs), even by comparison with people with severe IDs without ASCs (Bodfish, Symons, Parker, & Lewis, 2000). In the operant model which proposes that SIB develops from early repetitive behaviors through a process of shaping by socially or automatically mediated reinforcement (Guess & Carr, 1991; Kennedy, 2002), this might be accounted for in terms of individuals with ASCs being particularly likely to engage in STBs, and/or engaging in a greater number of STBs, which can then be shaped into SIB. It might also be the case however that once SIB is established in the behavioral repertoire of a person with an ASC, the processes which increase the probability of people with ASCs engaging in non-injurious STBs progressively acquire increased control of the SIB, driving its evolution into a stereotyped form of the behavior. In factor analyses of relevant descriptive assessments, SIB and other stereotyped movements usually emerge as separate factors. Lam and Aman (2007) had 307 caregivers of persons with ASCs complete the Repetitive Behavior Scale-Revised (Bodfish et al., 2000). Factor analysis of the data yielded a five-factor solution, with a "self-injurious behavior" factor distinct from factors representing "ritualistic/sameness," "stereotypic," and "compulsive" behaviors and "restricted interests." Brinkley et al. (2007) conducted factor analyses of scores on the Aberrant Behavior Checklist (ABC; Aman, Singh, Stewart, & Field, 1985) of 275 individuals with ASCs. In the total sample, a three-item SIB factor emerged in addition to a stereotypy factor; in a subsample of 59 individuals with more severe SIB however these items loaded onto a factor otherwise reflecting stereotypy. These studies provide results consistent with the possibility that people with ASCs initially develop SIB which is at first influenced by processes other than those which drive STBs, but that as the SIB develops in severity it increasingly comes under the control of the processes maintaining other STBs.

The development and maintenance of STBs is believed to involve disturbances in the normal pattern of interactions between the "direct" and "indirect" pathways in the cortico-striato-thalamo-cortical motor loop (Muehlmann & Lewis, 2012). As was described in Chap. 3, the striatal "medium spiny neurons" (MSNs) which express D_1 dopamine receptors and A_1 adenosine receptors and use the neuropeptides dynorphin and substance P as cotransmitters with γ-aminobutyric acid (GABA) project directly to the internal globus pallidus and to the pars reticulata of the substantia nigra, from where further inhibitory GABAergic fibers connect to nuclei within the thalamus. Those striatal MSNs which express D_2 dopamine receptors and A_2 adenosine receptors and use the neuropeptide enkephalin as a cotransmitter with GABA, are connected to the thalamus via the indirect pathway. These MSNs project to the external globus pallidus, from where an inhibitory GABAergic projection runs to the subthalamic nucleus, which itself directs excitatory glutamatergic projections to the internal globus pallidus and to the pars reticulata of the substantia nigra, thus rejoining the "direct" pathway (Crossman & Neary, 2019; Muehlmann & Lewis, 2012). In normal functioning, the basal ganglia are believed to maintain a selected behavior via the direct pathway, while the indirect pathway inhibits competing actions. A shift in the balance in activity between the pathways from the indirect to the direct pathway is believed to induce stereotypies, while a shift in relative activity from the direct to the indirect pathway will reduce them (Langen, Kas, Staal, van Engeland, & Durston, 2011).

People with ASCs however experience a number of restricted and repetitive behaviors, not only motor STBs, and other circuits may be involved in the maintenance of such behaviors. As was discussed in Chap. 3, striatal structures are believed to be key components in multiple, intercommunicating, but functionally distinct, corticostriatal circuits involving links with specific cortical areas including sensory and motor cortex, dorsolateral prefrontal cortex, and anterior cingulate and orbitofrontal cortex (Fig. 8.1). Transdiagnostic models of RRBs (e.g., Langen, Durston, Kas, van Engeland, & Staal, 2011) suggest that disruption in each of these loops may contribute to the development and maintenance of RRBs. Disruption of the "associative" circuit involving the dorsolateral prefrontal cortex may, for example, contribute to STB by impairing those aspects of "executive function" which involve selecting between response alternatives on the basis of their dynamically changing

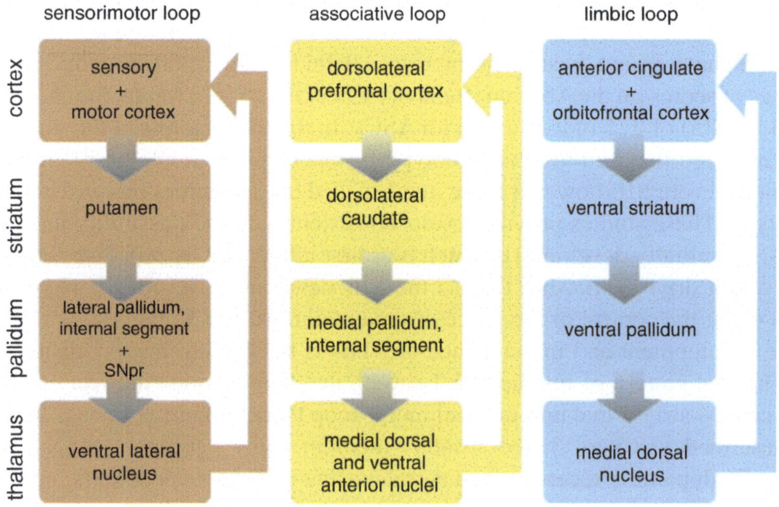

Fig. 8.1 Parallel corticostriatal macro-circuits with their main input, relay, and output regions. Abnormal repetition of behavior can result from damage to any of the corticostriatal circuits, where the exact location of the disruption (i.e., which loop is involved) determines what type of repetitive behavior is seen. *SNpr* substantia nigra pars reticulata. (Reproduced with permission of Elsevier from Langen, M., Kas, M. J. H., Staal, W. G., van Engeland, H., & Durston, S. (2011). The neurobiology of repetitive behavior: Of mice... *Neuroscience and Biobehavioral Reviews, 35*(3), 345–355. © 2010 Elsevier Ltd)

consequences, potentially leading to one response alternative being repeated despite its no longer achieving a desired goal. These difficulties may be observed as perseverative responses in situations involving reversal learning (e.g., Tanimura, Yang, & Lewis, 2008). In a study involving 17 adults with ASCs and with performance IQs of 70 or more, Lopez, Lincoln, Ozonoff, and Lai (2005) found that measures of RRBs were correlated with measures of perseveration and (poorer) response inhibition and working memory.

There is some evidence from volumetric magnetic resonance imaging (MRI) studies linking atypical development of components of the cortico-striato-thalamo-cortical motor loop with RRBs in people with ASCs. Hollander et al. (2005) examined correlations between the volume of the putamen, which receives the greater part of projections from motor cortex to the striatum, and measures of repetitive behaviors, in 17 adults with ASCs. Volume of the putamen showed substantial correlations with measures of repetitive behavior, which however did not achieve significance with a required probability value adjusted for multiple analyses. Langen et al. (2014) showed that growth in putamen volume in 49 children with ASCs was significantly associated with scores on a measure of insistence on sameness. The measure of insistence on sameness was taken at the time of the first MRI scan of putamen volume, so the association was presumably due to the developmental process involved rather than the actual increase in putamen volume. There is substantially more evidence for an association between RRBs and volume, or growth rate, of the caudate nucleus, the striatal structure receiving the greater part of projections to the striatum from areas of association cortex (Wilkes & Lewis, 2018). In general, greater caudate volume, or higher caudate growth rate, has been found to be associated with levels of RRB (Wilkes & Lewis, 2018). Qiu et al. (2016) assessed young children with ASCs at 2.5 years of age and followed them up after 2 years, comparing them with a group of children with developmental delay, but without ASCs, who were matched to the ASC group on age, gender balance, and developmental and intelligence quotients. The children with ASCs had greater caudate volume at initial assessment and greater growth of the caudate at follow-up. Change scores on measures of "higher-order" RRBs correlated negatively with degree of growth in right caudate nucleus volume. This apparent contradiction with the results of earlier studies may relate to the fact that Qiu et al. (2016) examined changes in RRBs, while other studies (e.g., Langen et al., 2014) have correlated changes in caudate volume with RRB scores measured at the time of the initial MRI scan. In a cross-sectional study of age and brain development in 99 people with ASCs, and a control group of "typically developing" participants matched for age, gender balance, and IQ, Langen et al. (2009) found that after controlling for total brain volume, there was an effect of group on volumes of the caudate, putamen, and nucleus accumbens, with each of these structures larger in people with ASCs. A significant group by age interaction was also found for caudate volume, reflecting the fact that caudate volume was related positively to age in participants with ASCs, but negatively with age in the control group. Voxel-based morphometry suggested that changes in the striatum were localized to the head of the caudate nucleus. Volume of the caudate, but not the putamen or nucleus accumbens, was positively correlated with a measure of insistence on sameness, although supplementary analyses suggested that this relationship was greater for younger participants.

Recent studies have begun to use resting-state functional magnetic resonance imaging (rs-fMRI) to examine connectivity between the striatum and cortical areas and relationships with measures of RRBs. Functional MRI evaluates levels of neuronal activity within an area of the brain by detecting the displacement of deoxygenated by oxygenated blood which occurs as blood flow to the area increases. Oxyhemoglobin is diamagnetic, interacting only weakly with magnetic fields, whereas deoxyhemoglobin is paramagnetic, interacting strongly with any external field and creating localized variations in the field which can be detected by appropriate MRI techniques. Following adjustments for overall blood volume, cerebral blood flow, and cerebral oxygen metabolic rates (Wilkes & Lewis, 2018), the blood-oxygen-level dependent (BOLD) contrast can be used to estimate levels of neuronal activation. In rs-fMRI, the method is used to detect coherence in patterns of activation in different areas, from which functional connectivity between the areas is inferred (Wilkes & Lewis, 2018). Abbott et al. (2018) examined intrinsic functional connectivity (iFC) of corticostriatal circuitry in 50 children and teenagers with ASCs and 52 "typically developing" control participants and obtained measures of RRBs for 36 and 34 members of these groups, respectively. Participants with ASCs were subdivided into "high RRB" (n = 17) and "low RRB" (n = 19) subgroups, while 1 participant from the control group with an unusually high RRB score was excluded from subgroup analyses. Comparisons of indices of corticostriatal connectivity within frontoparietal (cognitive/associative), motor, and limbic circuits, and ratios of connectivity between the circuits, showed significantly lower connectivity in the ASC "high RRB" subgroup relative to the control group for right frontoparietal and bilateral motor circuit indices, but higher connectivity for the right limbic index. The ASC "high RRB" subgroup also showed lower right frontoparietal/limbic and bilateral motor/limbic ratios compared to the control group. Differences between the two ASC subgroups were also found, with the ASC "high RRB" subgroup showing lower right frontoparietal and right motor indices, and right frontoparietal/limbic and right motor/limbic ratios, by comparison with the "low RRB" subgroup. Correlations across all participants between corticostriatal connectivity indices and ratios and scores on the Repetitive Behavior Scale-Revised (RBS-R), (Bodfish et al., 2000) showed that right hemisphere frontoparietal/limbic and motor/limbic ratios were negatively correlated with total scores on the RBS-R, with lower connectivity of frontoparietal and motor relative to limbic circuits associated with greater severity of RRBs. Examination of subscale scores on the RBS-R showed negative correlations for the right frontoparietal/limbic connectivity ratio with RBS-R stereotypic, compulsive, and restricted interests subscale scores and negative correlations for the right motor/limbic connectivity ratio with RBS-R self-injurious, stereotypic, and ritualistic/sameness subscales scores; only connectivity ratios which were correlated with overall RBS-R score were used in correlations with subscales. Abbott et al.'s (2018) results thus suggest that a lower ratio of right corticostriatal connectivity in the associative/cognitive loop relative to the limbic loop is associated with motor stereotypy, compulsive behaviors, and restricted interests, whereas lower right corticostriatal connectivity in the motor loop relative to the limbic group is associated with motor stereotypy, SIB, and ritualistic/insistence on sameness behaviors.

In a similar rs-fMRI study involving older children and young adults, 30 with ASCs and 32 "typically developing," Traynor et al. (2018) found that by comparison with the control group, the participants with ASCs showed marked over-connectivity of the left thalamus with several sensory processing areas of the cortex including the bilateral primary somatosensory cortex, left auditory cortex, left premotor cortex, left superior temporal gyrus, and right insular cortex. The participants with ASCs also showed over-connectivity of the left putamen with the right fusiform gyrus and left primary somatosensory cortex and of the right globus pallidus with left primary motor cortex. With regard to RRBs, total RBS-R score within the group of participants with ASCs was positively correlated with connectivity between the left primary visual cortex (V1) and the right inferior frontal gyrus, pars orbitalis, while scores on a factor derived from the RBS-R scores with a high loading from insistence on sameness correlated positively with connectivity between the right inferior parietal lobe and the right inferior frontal gyrus, pars triangularis.

Although they concur in finding evidence for disrupted corticostriatal connectivity in people with ASCs, interpretation of the contrasting patterns of results from these studies is difficult. Differences in studies between patterns of results may relate to the complexities of correcting for possible confounding factors in BOLD measurements (Wilkes & Lewis, 2018) and developmental processes resulting in changes in patterns of connectivity with age (Traynor et al., 2018). As mentioned by both Abbott et al. (2018) and Traynor et al. (2018), and important in the present context, the requirement to remain still during rs-fMRI makes it likely that participants in these studies experience relatively low severity RRBs, as illustrated by the low mean RBS-R scores for Traynor et al.'s participants. Taken together, however, the results of these studies suggest that RRBs in people with ASCs are influenced by interactions between multiple corticostriatal circuits, including the associative/cognitive and limbic loops as well as the motor loop, and that connectivity of cortical areas involved in inhibitory control and monitoring of salient cues associated with changes in response-consequence relationships also influence these behaviors.

Evidence for the possible relevance of disruption of the "associative" circuit involving the dorsolateral prefrontal cortex in causation of RRBs was provided by a study of the relationship between reversal learning and RRBs by D'Cruz et al. (2013). In this study, the participants were 41 children, teenagers and young adults with ASCs and IQs of 70 or over, together with a group of 37 "typically developing" control participants matched with the ASC group for age, intelligence, and gender balance. Following pretraining to give participants experience with the probabilistic contingencies, and reversal of contingencies, to be used in the study, participants learned to choose the correct stimulus location from a pair of locations to win points. When they reached a criterion of eight correct responses within ten consecutive trials, the rewarded stimulus location was immediately changed without any warning to the participants. Both prior to and following reversal, feedback and points were provided on an 80:20 probabilistic schedule, with 80% of correct choices and 20%

of incorrect choices randomly reinforced. Participants with and without ASCs performed comparably during initial learning. Following reversal, participants with ASCs switched from the previously correct choice to the newly correct choice as rapidly as the control participants, i.e., made no greater number of "perseverative errors." Participants with ASCs however then reverted more frequently to the previously correct response than control participants ("regressive errors") and made more regressive errors immediately following the omission of reinforcement of the newly correct response. For participants with ASCs, numbers of regressive errors were significantly correlated with independently ascertained RBS-R total scores and other measures of RRBs, but not with ratings of social or communicative abilities. The dissociation in the performance of participants with ASCs between perseverative and regressive errors suggests involvement of the associative/cognitive corticostriatal loop. Although the performance with continuous reinforcement was not tested, the results of D'Cruz et al. also suggest that inconsistent schedules of reinforcement may differentially impact on people with ASCs, impairing adaptive responses to contingency changes. D'Cruz, Mosconi, Ragozzino, Cook, and Sweeney (2016) addressed this issue in a study in which participants with and without ASCs engaged in similar reversal learning tasks under conditions of continuous and probabilistic reinforcement, while functional MRI (fMRI) data were simultaneously acquired. In both a two-choice reversal learning task with continuous reinforcement and a four-choice task with probabilistic reinforcement following reversals, participants with ASCs performed as well as control participants in terms of both perseverative and regressive errors. In the two-choice task, the experience of non-reinforcement at the point of reversal was associated with significant activation (as compared with the level of activation recorded when expected reinforcement occurred) bilaterally in the primary visual cortex for control participants, while those with ASCs showed significant activation in left motor cingulate cortex and left premotor cortex and bilaterally in the posterior parietal cortex. However, there were no significant between-group differences in activation patterns. In the four-choice task with probabilistic reinforcement, by contrast, the experience of reversal was associated with significantly greater activation for control participants than those with ASCs bilaterally in the thalamus, motor, cognitive, and affective subdivisions of the anterior cingulate cortex, premotor cortex, pre-supplementary motor area, posterior parietal cortex, and precuneus and also in the right lateral extrastriate cortex, left dorsolateral prefrontal cortex, and right ventral striatum. Taken together, the results of these studies suggest that for typically developing participants, the experience of unexpected non-reinforcement triggers activity in cortical areas concerned with attention (posterior parietal cortex and precuneus), motor planning (pre-supplementary motor area and motor cingulate cortex), inhibition of currently prepotent responses (dorsolateral prefrontal cortex), action selection in the face of competing attentional demands, and performance monitoring (cognitive division of the anterior cingulate cortex) (D'Cruz et al., 2016). People with ASCs may not show this complex pattern of responses because of diminished responsivity to unexpected non-reinforcement in limbic corticostriatal circuits involving the ventral striatum, anterior cingulate cortex, and orbitofrontal cortex, which in typically developing individuals trigger the complex of activity necessary to modify ongoing responding. D'Cruz et al.'s (2013) findings suggest that this diminished response to changes in reinforcement contingencies may be related to the development and maintenance of RRBs.

In summary therefore, there is evidence from volumetric studies of atypical development of striatal structures in people with ASCs, with some evidence that such atypical development is associated with engagement in RRBs. Resting-state fMRI studies further suggest that people with ASCs experience patterns of activity in corticostriatal circuits which differ from those in "typically developing" persons, although the evidence relating such differential patterning of activity to levels of RRBs is limited. People with ASCs find it difficult to adjust their responding to changes in reinforcement contingencies in situations where reinforcement is probabilistic, and this difficulty also appears to relate to engagement in RRBs.

These findings clearly suggest the involvement of multiple corticostriatal pathways in the causation of RRBs in people with ASCs, but do not necessarily implicate imbalances in activity between the direct and indirect corticostriatal pathways in this causation. Some evidence for this possibility has however been found in animal models of RRBs. Representing a mouse model of RRBs, C58 mice engage in high rate motor stereotypies. They also however show reversal learning which is unimpaired when responding is continuously reinforced, but impaired under probabilistic contingencies of reinforcement (Whitehouse, Curry-Pochy, Shafer, Rudy, & Lewis, 2017). Lewis et al. (2018) found that in C58 mice, neuronal metabolic activity in the subthalamic nucleus, a key component in indirect (and "hyperdirect") corticostriatal circuits, was diminished in C58 mice by comparison with mice not prone to engagement in similar stereotypies. Lewis, Rajpal, and Muehlmann (2019) have further shown that a combination of adenosine A_1 and A_{2A} receptor agonists which are known to increase the firing frequency of dorsal striatal neurons in the indirect pathway of the basal ganglia reduced repetitive behavior, although A_1 and A_{2A} agonists given in isolation each failed to do so, suggesting that the effect of the drug combination may be due to rebalancing of direct and indirect pathway interaction.

Although the enhanced risk for SIB in people with ASCs may therefore be due to early RRBs evolving into SIB, an alternative hypothesis is that functional disruption of several corticostriatal circuits in people with ASCs increases the potential for any behavior pattern, once established, to become stereotypically expressed. This tendency toward stereotypy probably involves imbalances in activity between the direct and indirect pathways in the motor and associative/cognitive and possibly also in the limbic, corticostriatal pathways. These imbalances affect the normal regulation of motor behavior but also impact on the person's ability to adjust responding adaptively when contingencies of reinforcement change, resulting in repetition of behaviors which are no longer functional. As with the shift from goal-directed to habitual/impulsive control of behavior, inconsistency in schedules of reinforcement appears to constitute a significant environmental driver of the evolution toward stereotypy in responding. Attentional difficulties which limit awareness of cues signalling changes in reinforcement schedules, and imbalances of activity in the limbic corticostriatal loop affecting adjustment to changing motivational conditions, may also contribute toward stereotypy.

8.5.2 Evolution of Compulsive Self-Injurious Behavior from Habitual/Impulsive Forms

The evolution of habitual/impulsive behavior into compulsive forms which persist despite severe negative consequences is less well understood than the change in predominance from goal-directed to habitual control. As was mentioned in Chap. 2, individual vulnerability seems to be important, with impulsivity (including increased discounting of delayed reinforcement), anxiety, and novelty-seeking putative risk factors for developing compulsivity (Everitt & Robbins, 2016). The role of impulsivity in the development of SIB in people with ASCs was discussed in Sect. 8.4, and here we focus on the role of anxiety, while arousal modulation (which may be related to novelty-seeking) is discussed in Sect. 8.7.

The high prevalence of anxiety at clinically significant levels among people with ASCs is well-established (Kent & Simonoff, 2017), as is the substantial overlap in findings from neurobiological studies of people with ASCs and those with anxiety disorders. For both groups, the amygdala, prefrontal cortex (PFC), and amygdala/PFC connectivity have received much attention (Herrington, Parma, & Miller, 2017). The separation of obsessive/compulsive disorder (OCD) from the anxiety disorders in the *Diagnostic and Statistical Manual of Mental Disorders* of the American Psychiatric Association (DSM-5) reflects however the difficulties in understanding how anxiety contributes to compulsivity in behavior. The suggestion that engaging in compulsive behaviors serves to reduce anxiety in people with OCD has been challenged by findings including the lack of impact on symptoms of OCD of non-serotonergic anxiolytic medications such as benzodiazepines (Robbins, Vaghi, & Banca, 2019). In people with ASCs, anxiety has been found to be associated with SIB, and with insistence on sameness and ritualistic behaviors, but not with compulsive behaviors, when the expected correlations between measures of different aspects of RRBs are controlled for (Factor, Condy, Farley, & Scarpa, 2016; Lidstone et al., 2014; Russell et al., 2019; Stratis & Lecavalier, 2013).

Where studies find no association between anxiety and compulsive behaviors, this may be because the assessments used, e.g., the RBS-R, index compulsivity by behaviors topographically resembling those seen in OCD, e.g., arranging/ordering items, washing or cleaning, or checking behaviors. In people diagnosed with OCD, being prevented from engaging in these behaviors typically leads to at least a short-term increase in anxiety. In some people with ASCs however, these behaviors may be performed without the experience of increased anxiety on their interruption. The degree of compulsivity attached to the performance of any behavior may alternatively be viewed in terms of the person's reaction when their engagement in that behavior is interrupted.

In OCD, compulsive behaviors may develop from avoidance behaviors (Robbins et al., 2019), and "compulsive" SIB may be functionally, rather than topographically, analogous to these behaviors. People with ASCs have usually been found to perform similarly to individuals without ASCs on simple Pavlovian discriminated fear conditioning in which one stimulus (CS+) is associated with an aversive unconditional stimulus (UCS), whereas another stimulus (CS−) occurs without the UCS (South, Larson, White, Dana, & Crowley, 2011), although their performance may be impaired if the CS+ is presented in the course of a more complex series of stimuli (Powell, Travers, Klinger, & Klinger, 2016). People with ASCs however show delayed learning relative to people without NDCs during reversal learning in which, following initial learning under conditions of partial reinforcement (i.e., the CS+ is sometimes, but not always, paired with the UCS), the previous CS− is presented as the new CS+, while the previous CS+ is no longer paired with the UCS (South, Newton, & Chamberlain, 2012). An earlier study by Gaigg and Bowler (2007), which also used partial reinforcement during acquisition, had also found that adults with ASCs learned to respond to CS+ presentations but showed attenuated differentiation of autonomic responding between (unreinforced) presentations of the CS+ and CS−.

Top et al. (2016) used fMRI to examine activity in brain regions believed to be involved in fear responding, while 20 adults with ASCs and 19 age-matched control participants without NDCs participated in learning and extinction phases of Pavlovian fear conditioning, again with partial reinforcement during initial fear conditioning. After initial learning and extinction on day 1 of the study, participants returned approximately 24 h later for further extinction trials. During initial fear conditioning, all brain regions of interest (right and left amygdala, right and left anterior insula, right and left medial orbitofrontal cortex, bilateral dorsal anterior cingulate cortex, and right, but not left, hippocampus) showed significantly greater response to threat (CS+) than safe (CS−) conditions. The group of participants with ASCs however showed a significantly decreased differential response to threat versus safe cues in right amygdala during the initial fear acquisition phase, showing no significant difference in response to threat and safety cues. In the first set of extinction trials on the second day, in which participants presumably had no clear expectations regarding the conditions they would encounter, both groups showed greater responses in insula and anterior cingulate cortex to CS+ vs. CS− presentations. In the left amygdala, however, the participants with ASCs showed no differentiation in responding to threat and safety cues, whereas control participants showed significantly higher response to threat vs. safety cues.

As Top et al. (2016) noted, their findings relate to the difference between responding to the CS+ (threat signal) and CS− (safety signal), and this pattern of results could arise through several processes. The central amygdala is generally regarded as playing a key role in the acquisition and expression of fear, while the anterior cingulate cortex (ACC) is active in regulating the expression of learned fear, and fMRI studies show activation of both areas in human fear learning and expression. Fear extinction is not however a simple process of weakening of previously learned patterns within these structures, but an active process, involving the basolateral complex of the amygdala, the hippocampus, and the infralimbic region of the medial prefrontal cortex (Milad, Rosenbaum, & Simon, 2014). Interactions between these structures ensure that when a cue (CS+) which previously elicited fear has been extinguished, its presentation within the context in which extinction occurred leads to activation of inhibitory neurons in the basolateral amygdala which inhibit output neurons in the central amygdala, stopping the expression of fear; if the previously extinguished cue is experienced in a different context however, inhibition of the central amygdala does not occur, leading to reinstatement of fear responding (Milad et al., 2014). The results of Top et al. (2016) might therefore result from a situation of chronic overactivity in the central amygdala of persons with ASCs, which presumably would be associated with increased fear responding to all stimuli, reducing differentiation between responding to CS+ and CS− cues. Alternatively, reduced inhibition of fear responding by the ACC and prefrontal areas linked with it could lead to a heightened, generalized perception of threat irrespective of the stimulus context. Finally, the simplest account would involve attenuation of the response of the amygdala in fear conditioning (Top et al., 2016).

Another possible explanation for the reduced differentiation in responding to threat and safety cues in people with ASCs concerns the cognitive/associative processes involved in monitoring changes in the expected consequences of alternative actions in response to cues as their motivational history changes. The ventromedial prefrontal cortex (vmPFC) appears to play a key role in this process, and activity in the vmPFC correlates with subjective valence of stimuli presented for both "typically developing" people and those with ASCs, although in the latter case only for non-social stimuli (Kishida et al., 2019). The vmPFC is involved in revaluation of both positive and aversive stimuli, and Milad et al. (2013) found that people without NDCs, but with OCD, showed reduced vmPFC activity (compared with control participants) in the later stages of fear extinction, in which however they showed extinction of fear responding comparable with that of control participants. During a later "extinction recall" test however the participants with OCD again showed reduced vmPFC activation and also increased fear responding to the extinguished stimuli. A similar study, using partial reinforcement, studied fear reversal learning, in which following initial fear acquisition the previous CS− is presented as the new CS+, while the previous CS+ is no longer paired with the UCS (Apergis-Schoute et al., 2017). It was found that although people with OCD showed successful initial fear conditioning, their differentiation of threat and safety signals after reversal was impaired by comparison with that of control participants. Detailed examination of vmPFC activity and differential responding to CS+ and CS− stimuli throughout the study led Apergis-Schoute et al. to conclude that the fear learning of participants with OCD was based on learning the predictive value of the CS+, but not that of the CS−. During reversal learning, participants with OCD learned the association between the new CS+ and shock but showed impaired learning of the association between the new CS− and safety, reducing differentiation in responding between the stimuli, with the impairment due to hyperactivation of the vmPFC throughout the process.

Taken together, these findings suggest that although people with ASCs appear to learn associations between stimuli and situations and aversive events in the same way as people without NDCs, their fear and anxiety may not abate in the usual way when the situation or stimulus is no longer accompanied by the aversive event. This effect is more likely to occur when the original association between the stimulus or situation and aversive experience was probabilistic rather than consistent. This specific pattern of learning may be underpinned by generally high levels of activation in fear-relevant brain networks limiting the possible range of magnitude of difference between responses to different stimuli or to reduced levels of activation in these networks similarly reducing the magnitude of between-stimulus differentiation. Alternatively, findings from OCD research suggest that people without ASCs who also experience high levels of anxiety and threat may do so because the vmPFC effectively tracks associations between stimuli and occurrence, but not absence, of aversive events. Whatever the mechanism, the long-term consequences of these processes are likely to include a heightened overall perception of threat and difficulty in extinguishing associations between stimuli or situations and previously associated aversive events. If SIB has originally had the function of avoiding or escaping from aversive experiences and has then become elicited by S-R processes in response to stimuli associated with those events, these processes will lead to SIB which occurs in response to a wide variety of events or situations and which will be particularly difficult to reduce even if those stimuli are no longer associated with the original aversive experiences.

The possibility that compulsive avoidance responding, including SIB, may result from effective vmPFC mediated tracking of the association between events and aversive outcomes, but inefficient tracking of the associations between "safety signals" and the absence of aversive consequences, has particularly challenging implications for intervention. In Chap. 6, we suggested that in cases where people experience "generalized habitual" SIB, a possible intervention is to introduce them to a "safe situation" in which they can experience an environment free from the aversive experiences which initially motivated their SIB and then to use stimuli associated with the safe environment as "safety signals" to indicate the ongoing absence of the aversive experience as the person enters other environments. The effectiveness of such intervention will obviously be jeopardized if the person's ability to associate stimuli with absence of aversive events is compromised.

8.6 Additional Risk for Self-Injurious Behavior in Persons with Autism Spectrum Conditions: Summary

From the foregoing overview, it can be seen that people with ASCs are likely to be at high risk both for the initial emergence of SIB and at each stage in its possible progression to more severe and difficult-to-treat forms (see Table 8.1).

Table 8.1 Possible additional risks for SIB in persons with ASCs

Stage of development of SIB	Possible additional risk factors for people with ASCs
Emergent	– Sensory sensitivity – Insistence on sameness – Temperament (↑ negative affectivity, possible ↓ effortful control)
Operant/goal-directed	– Difficulties in communication and socialization
Habitual/impulsive	– Increased exposure to adverse events – Increased perceived stress – Possible atypicality of physiological stress response
Stereotyped	– Atypical development of structures in striatum – Atypical corticostriatal functional connectivity – ↑ response persistence in response to contingency change (especially with probabilistic reinforcement)
Compulsive	– Possible overall increase in perception of threat – Impaired extinction of conditioned fear – Possible difficulty in tracking of "safety signals"

Evidence for these sources of increased risk have included epidemiological, developmental, psychological, clinical, neuroimaging, and experimental studies. Research into SIB in people with ASCs has however recently begun to include adults with ASCs but without IDs, who are able to offer individual perspectives on the phenomenology and function of SIB. In addition to their direct value in illuminating the phenomenology and functions of SIB in those more able adults who provide this information, these perspectives may aid insight into the causes of SIB in younger children with ASCs and adults with severe IDs, and we turn next to a brief examination of research to date on these issues.

8.7 Self-Injurious Behavior in Adults with Autism Spectrum Conditions but Without Intellectual Disabilities

It is sometimes argued that the SIB engaged in by adults with ASCs but without IDs (hereafter: autistic adults) is fundamentally different from that engaged in by people with IDs (Matson & Turygin, 2012; Moseley, Gregory, Smith, Allison, & Baron-Cohen, 2019). Here however we will take a more empirical view, comparing the phenomenology of SIB in these groups, and hence will continue to use the term SIB in referring to self-harming behaviors in both groups. We will outline what is known about the expressed experience of autistic adults who engage in SIB and compare key aspects of the phenomenology of SIB in people with and without IDs.

Until very recently, research into SIB in autistic adults has been concerned with the behavior primarily insofar as it may be a risk marker for suicidality (Cassidy, Bradley, Shaw, & Baron-Cohen, 2018). However, a small number of studies have now gathered information concerning the phenomenology of, and risk markers for, SIB in sufficient detail to enable comparison of aspects of the behavior in autistic adults and those with IDs in addition to ASCs. All of these studies to date have used the Non-Suicidal Self-Injury Assessment Tool (NSSI-AT; Whitlock, Exner-Cortens, & Purington, 2014), an instrument for assessing lifetime non-suicidal self-injury (NSSI) in non-clinical populations. The NSSI-AT comprises 12 modules, the first of which is intended to identify respondents who engage in SIB. Respondents are asked whether they have ever engaged in any of 16 specified topographies of SIB (plus an "other" option) with the intention of hurting themselves. The listed topographies include some which are frequently observed in people with IDs and ASCs (e.g., self-scratching/pinching, self-hitting, and self-biting) together with others (e.g., carving words or symbols into the skin, burning oneself) which are rarely observed in those with IDs and ASCs. The NSSI-AT can be completed in paper form but was designed as a web-based instrument in which access to areas of the assessment depends on prior responses. In the web-based form, only respondents who endorse having engaged in SIB, for example, are taken to later questions (Whitlock et al., 2014). The next module of the NSSI-AT assesses self-reported functions of SIB, categorized as managing depressive or dissociated emotional states (affective imbalance-low pressure), management of agitation or high-energy affective states (affective imbalance-high pressure), social communication, self-punishment or as a way to avoid engaging in other, more damaging behaviors (self-retribution and deterrence), and sensation-seeking. Each function is assessed by three or four questions. At this stage in the NSSI-AT, respondents who report engaging in SIB solely as a way of attempting, or preparing to attempt, suicide are "skipped out" of further questions. Later modules in the NSSI-AT concern the frequency with which respondents engage in SIB, time since the last episode, etc., the age at which SIB began, wound locations, respondents' initial motivations for engaging in SIB, severity of injuries caused, and other issues including experience of treatment services and personal reflections. Test-retest reliabilities (kappa or intraclass correlation coefficient) in a small sample of college students were 0.7 or greater for key NSSI-AT scores (presence of any NSSI, age at first incident, function of behavior, etc.), with the exception of number of wound locations, for which the ICC was 0.63 (Whitlock et al., 2014).

In a study by Maddox, Trubanova, and White (2017), 42 autistic adults (21 of whom reported that they engaged in SIB), and 42 college students who reported engaging in SIB, completed the NSSI-AT and other measures. All autistic participants had at least successfully completed high school. Gender balance (with autistic participants not engaging in SIB more likely to be men), age (with college students younger than autistic participants), and place of residence differed between groups. As noted, 50% of autistic participants reported engaging in SIB. For autistic participants, gender was associated with engagement in SIB, with women disproportionately over-represented among those who engaged in SIB. Endorsement of avoidance of suicide as a function of SIB was associated with autism, being endorsed by 9 of the 21 autistic adults who engaged in SIB, but only 5 of the 42 control participants. The self-injuring groups did not differ on any other measure from the NSSI-AT. Within the autistic self-injuring group, a measure of difficulty in regulating emotion was positively associated with score for sensation-seeking function of SIB on the

NSSI-AT. Cassidy et al. (2018), in a study of risk markers for suicidality in autistic adults, found that 65% of a group of autistic adults who reported having received an ASC diagnosis from a trained clinician reported lifetime SIB and replicated Maddox et al.'s finding of an association between SIB and female gender.

In the largest study to date of SIB in autistic adults, Moseley et al. (2019) presented information gathered from 103 autistic adults who responded to an online advertisement, including information from the NSSI-AT and other measures. Of the participants, 49 were classified as "current self-harmers," 27 as "historic self-harmers," and 27 as "non-self-harmers," based on their responses to the NSSI-AT. The three groups did not differ significantly on age, and gender distribution was not associated with group membership. Additional psychiatric comorbidity and use of psychotropic medication were associated with group membership, with the proportion of people with comorbidities lower among the non-self-harmers than in the two self-harming groups, and the use of medication more common among the current self-harmers than in the other two groups.

With regard to topographies of SIB, the most frequently reported was self-scratching or pinching (reported by 72.4% of those who self-injured), followed by self-cutting (reported by 50%), hitting objects (reported by 44.6%), self-hitting (also reported by 44.6%), and self-biting (41.2%). The most frequently reported target body sites were the arms (targeted by 61.8%), hands (targeted by 58.1%), head (targeted by 47.4%), wrists (targeted by 42.5%), and face (targeted by 35.1%). As is obvious from these figures, people who engaged in SIB frequently engaged in multiple topographies at several sites. The relative importance of alternative functions of SIB was evaluated by examining the mean number of NSSI-AT statements endorsed for each function. Interpretation of these results is slightly complicated, because the number of items available to endorse varies across functions. It appears clear however that the two functions concerned with managing affective balance were most frequently identified by participants as functions of their SIB, followed by self-punishment/deterrence and sensation-seeking, with social communication least frequently mentioned. Regression analyses using individual variables as predictors showed that scores on measures of alexithymia, depression, anxiety, and sensory sensitivity were each able to individually differentiate non-self-harmers from one or both of the self-harming groups. However, none of these factors emerged as a significant predictor of group membership when all were included in a regression analysis (Moseley et al., 2019).

These fascinating studies suggest a more nuanced interpretation of the relationships between SIB in autistic adults, neurotypical adults, and people with IDs together with ASCs. In many respects, the self-harming behavior engaged in by autistic adults cannot be differentiated from that engaged in by neurotypical individuals but differs from that experienced by those with ASCs and IDs. Maddox et al. (2017), for example, reported a mean age of commencement of SIB of 12.7 years for autistic participants and 13.19 years for the control group of college students. Moseley et al. (2019) similarly reported a mean age of commencement of 15.1 years in autistic people, while SIB typically emerges in the first few years of life for children with ASCs accompanied by IDs. The self-reported functions of SIB in autistic adults, which predominantly concern regulation of emotional states, also appear to correspond closely to those reported by neurotypical individuals (Maddox et al., 2017), while the social/communicative functions often identified as the functions of SIB in people with IDs are much less endorsed as such by autistic adults.

In some respects however, there are also similarities between the SIB shown by people with IDs and ASCs and autistic adults. The proportion of autistic adults who report engaging or having engaged in SIB appears to be between 50 and 65%; prevalence for children and adults with IDs and ASCs has been reported to be 50% (Richards, Oliver, Nelson, & Moss, 2012), and figures close to 50% have been reported for groups of children and adults with ASCs which probably included many with IDs (Richards, Davies, & Oliver, 2017). With regard to topographies of SIB, the two most frequently reported by autistic adults in the studies of Maddox et al. (2017) and Moseley et al. (2019), self-scratching or pinching (reported by over 70% of people who engaged in SIB in both studies) and self-cutting (reported by over 30% in both studies) are found much less frequently in studies including participants with IDs (Richards et al., 2012, 2017). For some other topographies, however, prevalences in people with ASCs with and without IDs are much closer. If one assumes an overall prevalence rate of 50% for SIB in autistic adults, then the overall prevalences for self-hitting and self-biting in autistic adults are between 11.9% and 22.3% and between 16.65% and 20.6%, respectively (Maddox et al., 2017; Moseley et al., 2019). The corresponding figures from studies involving people with ASCs and IDs range from 24.5 to 29.5 and 15.7 to 18.8%, respectively (Richards et al., 2012, 2017). With regard to the functions of behavior, the accounts of autistic adults most frequently describe control of affective states, while social/communicative functions are most frequently identified for persons with IDs and ASCs. For both groups, however, sensation-seeking (or positive automatic reinforcement) is identified as a function of the behavior in a substantial minority of cases.

These comparisons are complicated by the fact that studies involving participants with and without IDs have used different assessments of SIB, and by the fact that effective sample selection will often have been made by parents or other caregivers in the case of people with IDs, and by the research participants themselves in studies involving autistic adults. It seems possible however that there are some common elements in the development of SIB in people with IDs and ASCs and autistic adults, with the latter group showing an increased range of forms and functions of the behavior, and with some functions much reduced in relative importance, but with residual similarities which indicate some commonality in development. This possibility has implications for assessment and treatment of SIB, not only in autistic adults but also in people with IDs and ASCs. Modification of affective state is reported by autistic adults to be an important function of SIB. If there is some degree of continuity in the processes maintaining SIB in autistic adults and those who also have severe intellectual disabilities, similar processes may also have a role in maintaining SIB in the latter group. Although direct evidence on this issue is limited, it may be that one function of SIB is to increase arousal level when it is unpleasantly low. Lydon, Healy, and Dwyer (2013) monitored the heart rate of three children with ASCs and examined changes in heart rate before, during, and following episodes of SIB and other challenging behaviors and found preliminary evidence for increases in heart rate during and/or after episodes of SIB. Although multiple explanations of these findings are possible, they are consistent with the possibility that the children engaged in SIB in order to increase levels of arousal. In a larger study, Nuske et al. (2019) found heart rate increases immediately preceding episodes of challenging behavior in children with ASCs, possibly indicating that these children are reacting to stress by engaging in challenging behavior, but consistent also with the increase in heart rate being associated with preparation to engage in the behavior. A related but alternative possibility is that people with ASCs may engage in activities, possibly including SIB, which maintain high levels of arousal which have resulted from a previous activity (Hoch, Moore, McComas, & Symons, 2010).

8.8 Self-Injurious Behavior in People with Autism Spectrum Conditions: Implications for Assessment and Treatment

People with ASCs are at particularly high risk for developing SIB. It appears probable that they are also at increased risk for persistence of SIB once established, possibly due to an increased probability of SIB progressing to habitual/impulsive, stereotyped, or compulsive stages. For young children with ASCs, sensory sensitivity, insistence on sameness, and elevated negative affectivity (and possibly reduced effortful control) in temperament are all probable risk markers for emergence of SIB and should be considered as such during clinical assessment. The probability of SIB acquiring operant functions is likely to be increased in children with ASCs by difficulties in communication and socialization, and interventions focused on the development of communication skills should be a priority both in terms of primary prevention of SIB and for treatment of SIB once established.

People with ASCs who have an extended history of engaging in SIB will probably have been exposed to or affected by several factors which increase the risk of SIB progressing to stages in which operant control plays a reduced role in maintaining the behavior. Exposure to adverse life events, subjective stress, and heightened threat perception are among such factors and should be considered during clinical assessment. Although the principal options for intervention with SIB in which habitual (S-R) processes play an important role, or in which compulsivity is salient, will continue to be graduated exposure, possibly accompanied in the latter case by interventions to reduce arousal level, challenges such as reduced effectiveness of safety signals should be expected and anticipated by measures such as further enhancing the salience of such signals.

References

Abbott, A. E., Linke, A. C., Nair, A., Jahedi, A., Alba, L. A., Keown, C. L., ... Müller, R. A. (2018). Repetitive behaviors in autism are linked to imbalance of corticostriatal connectivity: A functional connectivity MRI study. *Social Cognitive and Affective Neuroscience, 13*(1), 32–42. https://doi.org/10.1093/scan/nsx129

Adamek, L., Nichols, S., Tetenbaum, S. P., Bregman, J., Ponzio, C. A., & Carr, E. G. (2011). Individual temperament and problem behavior in children with autism spectrum disorders. *Focus on Autism and Other Developmental Disabilities, 26*(3), 173–183. https://doi.org/10.1177/1088357611405041

Aman, M. G., Singh, N. N., Stewart, A. W., & Field, C. J. (1985). The Aberrant Behavior Checklist: A behavior rating scale for the assessment of treatment effects. *American Journal of Mental Deficiency, 89*(5), 485–491.

Apergis-Schoute, A. M., Gillan, C. M., Fineberg, N. A., Fernandez-Egea, E., Sahakian, B. J., & Robbins, T. W. (2017). Neural basis of impaired safety signaling in obsessive compulsive disorder. *Proceedings of the National Academy of Sciences of the United States of America, 114*(12), 3216–3221. https://doi.org/10.1073/pnas.1609194114

Asmus, J. M., Ringdahl, J. E., Sellers, J. A., Call, N. A., Andelman, M. S., & Wacker, D. P. (2004). Use of a short-term inpatient model to evaluate aberrant behavior: Outcome data summaries from 1996 to 2001. *Journal of Applied Behavior Analysis, 37*(3), 283–304. https://doi.org/10.1901/jaba.2004.37-283

Baghdadli, A., Picot, M. C., Pry, R., Michelon, C., Burzstejn, C., Lazartigues, A., & Aussilloux, C. (2008). What factors are related to a negative outcome of self-injurious behaviour during childhood in pervasive developmental disorders? *Journal of Applied Research in Intellectual Disabilities, 21*(2), 142–149. https://doi.org/10.1111/j.1468-3148.2007.00389.x

Baker, J. K., Fenning, R. M., Erath, S. A., Baucom, B. R., Moffitt, J., & Howland, M. A. (2018). Sympathetic under-arousal and externalizing behavior problems in children with autism spectrum disorder. *Journal of Abnormal Child Psychology, 46*(4), 895–906. https://doi.org/10.1007/s10802-017-0332-3

Barrett, S. L., Uljarević, M., Jones, C. R. G., & Leekam, S. R. (2018). Assessing subtypes of restricted and repetitive behaviour using the Adult Repetitive Behaviour Questionnaire-2 in autistic adults. *Molecular Autism, 9*(1), 58. https://doi.org/10.1186/s13229-018-0242-4

Berg, K. L., Shiu, C. A., Acharya, K., Stolbach, B. C., & Msall, M. E. (2016). Disparities in adversity among children with autism spectrum disorder: A population-based study. *Developmental Medicine and Child Neurology, 58*(11), 1124–1131. https://doi.org/10.1111/dmcn.13161

Berkson, G. (2002). Early development of stereotyped and self-injurious behaviors: II. age trends. *American Journal on Mental Retardation, 107*(6), 468–477 + 493. https://doi.org/10.1352/0895-8017(2002)107<0468:EDOSAS>2.0.CO;2

Bishop-Fitzpatrick, L., Mazefsky, C. A., Minshew, N. J., & Eack, S. M. (2015). The relationship between stress and social functioning in adults with autism spectrum disorder and without intellectual disability. *Autism Research, 8*(2), 164–173. https://doi.org/10.1002/aur.1433

Bishop-Fitzpatrick, L., Minshew, N. J., Mazefsky, C. A., & Eack, S. M. (2017). Perception of life as stressful, not biological response to stress, is associated with greater social disability in adults with autism spectrum disorder. *Journal of Autism and Developmental Disorders, 47*(1), 1–16. https://doi.org/10.1007/s10803-016-2910-6

Black, K. R., Stevenson, R. A., Segers, M., Ncube, B. L., Sun, S. Z., Philipp-Muller, A., ... Ferber, S. (2017). Linking anxiety and insistence on sameness in autistic children: The role of sensory hypersensitivity. *Journal of Autism and Developmental Disorders, 47*(8), 2459–2470. https://doi.org/10.1007/s10803-017-3161-x

Bodfish, J. W., Symons, F. J., Parker, D. E., & Lewis, M. H. (2000). Varieties of repetitive behavior in autism: Comparisons to mental retardation. *Journal of Autism and Developmental Disorders, 30*(3), 237–243. https://doi.org/10.1023/A:1005596502855

Brinkley, J., Nations, L., Abramson, R. K., Hall, A., Wright, H. H., Gabriels, R., ... Cuccaro, M. L. (2007). Factor analysis of the Aberrant Behavior Checklist in individuals with autism spectrum disorders. *Journal of Autism and Developmental Disorders, 37*(10), 1949–1959. https://doi.org/10.1007/s10803-006-0327-3

Burrows, C. A., Usher, L. V., Schwartz, C. B., Mundy, P. C., & Henderson, H. A. (2016). Supporting the spectrum hypothesis: Self-reported temperament in children and adolescents with high functioning autism. *Journal of Autism and Developmental Disorders, 46*(4), 1184–1195. https://doi.org/10.1007/s10803-015-2653-9

Cappadocia, M. C., Desrocher, M., Pepler, D., & Schroeder, J. H. (2009). Contextualizing the neurobiology of conduct disorder in an emotion dysregulation framework. *Clinical Psychology Review, 29*(6), 506–518. https://doi.org/10.1016/j.cpr.2009.06.001

Cassidy, S., Bradley, L., Shaw, R., & Baron-Cohen, S. (2018). Risk markers for suicidality in autistic adults. *Molecular Autism, 9*(1), 42. https://doi.org/10.1186/s13229-018-0226-4

Clifford, S. M., Hudry, K., Elsabbagh, M., Charman, T., & Johnson, M. H. (2013). Temperament in the first 2 years of life in infants at high-risk for autism spectrum disorders. *Journal of Autism and Developmental Disorders, 43*(3), 673–686. https://doi.org/10.1007/s10803-012-1612-y

Cooper, S.-A., Smiley, E., Allan, L. M., Jackson, A., Finlayson, J., Mantry, D., & Morrison, J. (2009). Adults with intellectual disabilities: Prevalence, incidence and remission of self-injurious behaviour, and related factors. *Journal of Intellectual Disability Research, 53*(3), 200–216. https://doi.org/10.1111/j.1365-2788.2008.01060.x

Courtemanche, A. B., & Black, W. R. (2016). Everyday expressions of pain in children with and without autism spectrum disorder. *Research in Autism Spectrum Disorders, 26*, 65–70. https://doi.org/10.1016/j.rasd.2016.02.010

Courtemanche, A. B., Black, W. R., & Reese, R. M. (2016). The relationship between pain, self-injury, and other problem behaviors in young children with autism and other developmental disabilities. *American Journal on Intellectual and Developmental Disabilities, 121*(3), 194–203. https://doi.org/10.1352/1944-7558-121.3.194

Crossman, A. R., & Neary, D. (2019). *Neuroanatomy: An illustrated colour text.* Amsterdam: Elsevier.

D'Cruz, A.-M., Mosconi, M. W., Ragozzino, M. E., Cook, E. H., & Sweeney, J. A. (2016). Alterations in the functional neural circuitry supporting flexible choice behavior in autism spectrum disorders. *Translational Psychiatry, 6*(10), e916. https://doi.org/10.1038/tp.2016.161

D'Cruz, A.-M., Ragozzino, M. E., Mosconi, M. W., Shrestha, S., Cook, E. H., & Sweeney, J. A. (2013). Reduced behavioral flexibility in autism spectrum disorders. *Neuropsychology, 27*(2), 152–160. https://doi.org/10.1037/a0031721

Davies, L. E., & Oliver, C. (2016). Self-injury, aggression and destruction in children with severe intellectual disability: Incidence, persistence and novel, predictive behavioural risk markers. *Research in Developmental Disabilities, 49–50*, 291–301. https://doi.org/10.1016/j.ridd.2015.12.003

De Pauw, S. S. W., Mervielde, I., Van Leeuwen, K. G., & De Clercq, B. J. (2011). How temperament and personality contribute to the maladjustment of children with autism. *Journal of Autism and Developmental Disorders, 41*(2), 196–212. https://doi.org/10.1007/s10803-010-1043-6

Dempsey, J., Dempsey, A. G., Guffey, D., Minard, C. G., & Goin-Kochel, R. P. (2016). Brief report: Further examination of self-injurious behaviors in children and adolescents with autism spectrum disorders. *Journal of Autism and Developmental Disorders, 46*(5), 1872–1879. https://doi.org/10.1007/s10803-016-2704-x

Derby, K. M., Wacker, D. P., Sasso, G., Steege, M., Northup, J., Cigrand, K., & Asmus, J. (1992). Brief functional assessment techniques to evaluate aberrant behavior in an outpatient setting: A summary of 79 cases. *Journal of Applied Behavior Analysis, 25*(3), 713–721. https://doi.org/10.1901/jaba.1992.25-713

Duerden, E. G., Oatley, H. K., Mak-Fan, K. M., McGrath, P. A., Taylor, M. J., Szatmari, P., & Roberts, S. W. (2012). Risk factors associated with self-injurious behaviors in children and adolescents with autism spectrum disorders. *Journal of Autism and Developmental Disorders, 42*(11), 2460–2470. https://doi.org/10.1007/s10803-012-1497-9

Emerson, E., Kiernan, C., Alborz, A., Reeves, D., Mason, H., Swarbrick, R., … Hatton, C. (2001). Predicting the persistence of severe self-injurious behavior. *Research in Developmental Disabilities, 22*(1), 67–75. https://doi.org/10.1016/S0891-4222(00)00062-7

Esbensen, A. J., Seltzer, M. M., Lam, K. S. L., & Bodfish, J. W. (2009). Age-related differences in restricted repetitive behaviors in autism spectrum disorders. *Journal of Autism and Developmental Disorders, 39*(1), 57–66. https://doi.org/10.1007/s10803-008-0599-x

Everitt, B. J., & Robbins, T. W. (2016). Drug addiction: Updating actions to habits to compulsions ten years on. *Annual Review of Psychology, 67*, 23–50. https://doi.org/10.1146/annurev-psych-122414-033457

Factor, R. S., Condy, E. E., Farley, J. P., & Scarpa, A. (2016). Brief report: Insistence on sameness, anxiety, and social motivation in children with autism spectrum disorder. *Journal of Autism and Developmental Disorders, 46*(7), 2548–2554. https://doi.org/10.1007/s10803-016-2781-x

Gaigg, S. B., & Bowler, D. M. (2007). Differential fear conditioning in Asperger's syndrome: Implications for an amygdala theory of autism. *Neuropsychologia, 45*(9), 2125–2134. https://doi.org/10.1016/j.neuropsychologia.2007.01.012

Garon, N., Bryson, S. E., Zwaigenbaum, L., Smith, I. M., Brian, J., Roberts, W., & Szatmari, P. (2009). Temperament and its relationship to autistic symptoms in a high-risk infant sib cohort. *Journal of Abnormal Child Psychology, 37*(1), 59–78. https://doi.org/10.1007/s10802-008-9258-0

Gartstein, M. A., Marmion, J., & Swanson, H. L. (2006). Infant temperament: An evaluation of children with Down syndrome. *Journal of Reproductive and Infant Psychology, 24*(1), 31–41. https://doi.org/10.1080/02646830500475237

Gillott, A., & Standen, P. J. (2007). Levels of anxiety and sources of stress in adults with autism. *Journal of Intellectual Disabilities, 11*(4), 359–370. https://doi.org/10.1177/1744629507083585

Gray, J. A. (1976). The behavioural inhibition system: A possible substrate for anxiety. In M. P. Feldman & A. Broadhurst (Eds.), *Theoretical and experimental bases of the behaviour therapies* (pp. 3–41). London: Wiley.

Guess, D., & Carr, E. (1991). Emergence and maintenance of stereotypy and self-injury. *American Journal on Mental Retardation, 96*(3), 299–319.

Hepburn, S. L., & Stone, W. L. (2006). Using Carey temperament scales to assess behavioral style in children with autism spectrum disorders. *Journal of Autism and Developmental Disorders, 36*(5), 637–642. https://doi.org/10.1007/s10803-006-0110-5

Herrington, J. D., Parma, V., & Miller, J. S. (2017). Neurobiological mechanisms of anxiety in ASD. In C. M. Kerns, P. Renno, E. A. Storch, P. C. Kendall, & J. J. Wood (Eds.), *Anxiety in children and adolescents with autism spectrum disorder: Evidence-based assessment and treatment* (pp. 55–77). Amsterdam: Elsevier. https://doi.org/10.1016/B978-0-12-805122-1.00004-1

Hirvikoski, T., & Blomqvist, M. (2015). High self-perceived stress and poor coping in intellectually able adults with autism spectrum disorder. *Autism, 19*(6), 752–757. https://doi.org/10.1177/1362361314543530

Hoch, J., Moore, T., McComas, J., & Symons, F. J. (2010). Arousal and activity choice in autism: A single-case assessment integrating autonomic and behavioral analysis. *Journal of Applied Biobehavioral Research, 15*(3), 119–133. https://doi.org/10.1111/j.1751-9861.2010.00056.x

Hollander, E., Anagnostou, E., Chaplin, W., Esposito, K., Haznedar, M. M., Licalzi, E., … Buchsbaum, M. (2005). Striatal volume on magnetic resonance imaging and repetitive behaviors in autism. *Biological Psychiatry, 58*(3), 226–232. https://doi.org/10.1016/j.biopsych.2005.03.040

Hoover, D. W., & Kaufman, J. (2018). Adverse childhood experiences in children with autism spectrum disorder. *Current Opinion in Psychiatry, 31*(2), 128–132. https://doi.org/10.1097/YCO.0000000000000390

Iwata, B. A., Dorsey, M. F., Slifer, K. J., Bauman, K. E., & Richman, G. S. (1982). Toward a functional analysis of self-injury. *Analysis and Intervention in Developmental Disabilities, 2*, 3–20. https://doi.org/10.1016/0270-4684(82)90003-9

Iwata, B. A., Pace, G. M., Dorsey, M. F., Zarcone, J. R., Vollmer, T. R., Smith, R. G., … Willis, K. D. (1994). The functions of self-injurious behavior: An experimental-epidemiological analysis. *Journal of Applied Behavior Analysis, 27*(2), 215–240. https://doi.org/10.1901/jaba.1994.27-215

Kennedy, C. H. (2002). Evolution of stereotypy into self-injury. In S. R. Schroeder, M. L. Oster-Granite, & T. Thompson (Eds.), *Self-injurious behavior: Gene-brain-behavior relationships* (pp. 133–143). Washington, DC: American Psychological Association.

Kent, R., & Simonoff, E. (2017). Prevalence of anxiety in autism spectrum disorders. In C. M. Kerns, P. Renno, E. A. Storch, P. C. Kendall, & J. J. Wood (Eds.), *Anxiety in children and adolescents with autism spectrum disorder: Evidence-based assessment and treatment* (pp. 5–32). Amsterdam: Elsevier. https://doi.org/10.1016/B978-0-12-805122-1.00002-8

Kishida, K. T., De Asis-Cruz, J., Treadwell-Deering, D., Liebenow, B., Beauchamp, M. S., & Montague, P. R. (2019). Diminished single-stimulus response in vmPFC to favorite people in children diagnosed with autism spectrum disorder. *Biological Psychology, 145*, 174–184. https://doi.org/10.1016/j.biopsycho.2019.04.009

Kochanska, G., Murray, K. T., & Harlan, E. T. (2000). Effortful control in early childhood: Continuity and change, antecedents, and implications for social development. *Developmental Psychology, 36*(2), 220–232. https://doi.org/10.1037/0012-1649.36.2.220

Kurtz, P. F., Chin, M. D., Huete, J. M., Tarbox, R. S. F., O'Connor, J. T., Paclawskyj, T. R., & Rush, K. S. (2003). Functional analysis and treatment of self-injurious behavior in young children: A summary of 30 cases. *Journal of Applied Behavior Analysis, 36*, 205–219. https://doi.org/10.1901/jaba.2003.36-205

Kurtz, P. F., Chin, M. D., Robinson, A. N., O'Connor, J. T., & Hagopian, L. P. (2015). Functional analysis and treatment of problem behavior exhibited by children with fragile X syndrome. *Research in Developmental Disabilities, 43–44*, 150–166. https://doi.org/10.1016/j.ridd.2015.06.010

Lam, K. S. L., & Aman, M. G. (2007). The Repetitive Behavior Scale-revised: Independent validation in individuals with autism spectrum disorders. *Journal of Autism and Developmental Disorders, 37*(5), 855–866. https://doi.org/10.1007/s10803-006-0213-z

Langen, M., Bos, D., Noordermeer, S. D. S., Nederveen, H., Van Engeland, H., & Durston, S. (2014). Changes in the development of striatum are involved in repetitive behavior in autism. *Biological Psychiatry, 76*(5), 405–411. https://doi.org/10.1016/j.biopsych.2013.08.013

Langen, M., Durston, S., Kas, M. J. H., van Engeland, H., & Staal, W. G. (2011). The neurobiology of repetitive behavior: ...and men. *Neuroscience and Biobehavioral Reviews, 35*(3), 356–365. https://doi.org/10.1016/j.neubiorev.2010.02.005

Langen, M., Kas, M. J. H., Staal, W. G., van Engeland, H., & Durston, S. (2011). The neurobiology of repetitive behavior: Of mice⋯. *Neuroscience and Biobehavioral Reviews, 35*(3), 345–355. https://doi.org/10.1016/j.neubiorev.2010.02.004

Langen, M., Schnack, H. G., Nederveen, H., Bos, D., Lahuis, B. E., de Jonge, M. V., … Durston, S. (2009). Changes in the developmental trajectories of striatum in autism. *Biological Psychiatry, 66*(4), 327–333. https://doi.org/10.1016/j.biopsych.2009.03.017

Lewis, M. H., Lindenmaier, Z., Boswell, K., Edington, G., King, M. A., & Muehlmann, A. M. (2018). Subthalamic nucleus pathology contributes to repetitive behavior expression and is reversed by environmental enrichment. *Genes, Brain and Behavior, 17*(8), e12468. https://doi.org/10.1111/gbb.12468

Lewis, M. H., Rajpal, H., & Muehlmann, A. M. (2019). Reduction of repetitive behavior by co-administration of adenosine receptor agonists in C58 mice. *Pharmacology Biochemistry and Behavior, 181*, 110–116. https://doi.org/10.1016/j.pbb.2019.04.006

Lidstone, J., Uljarević, M., Sullivan, J., Rodgers, J., McConachie, H., Freeston, M., … Leekam, S. (2014). Relations among restricted and repetitive behaviors, anxiety and sensory features in children with autism spectrum disorders. *Research in Autism Spectrum Disorders, 8*(2), 82–92. https://doi.org/10.1016/j.rasd.2013.10.001

Lopez, B. R., Lincoln, A. J., Ozonoff, S., & Lai, Z. (2005). Examining the relationship between executive functions and restricted, repetitive symptoms of autistic disorder. *Journal of Autism and Developmental Disorders, 35*(4), 445–460. https://doi.org/10.1007/s10803-005-5035-x

Love, J. R., Carr, J. E., & LeBlanc, L. A. (2009). Functional assessment of problem behavior in children with autism spectrum disorders: A summary of 32 outpatient cases. *Journal of Autism and Developmental Disorders, 39*(2), 363–372. https://doi.org/10.1007/s10803-008-0633-z

Lydon, S., Healy, O., & Dwyer, M. (2013). An examination of heart rate during challenging behavior in autism spectrum disorder. *Journal of Developmental and Physical Disabilities, 25*(1), 149–170. https://doi.org/10.1007/s10882-012-9324-y

Lydon, S., Healy, O., Reed, P., Mulhern, T., Hughes, B. M., & Goodwin, M. S. (2016). A systematic review of physiological reactivity to stimuli in autism. *Developmental Neurorehabilitation, 19*(6), 335–355. https://doi.org/10.3109/17518423.2014.971975

Macari, S. L., Koller, J., Campbell, D. J., & Chawarska, K. (2017). Temperamental markers in toddlers with autism spectrum disorder. *Journal of Child Psychology and Psychiatry and Allied Disciplines, 58*(7), 819–828. https://doi.org/10.1111/jcpp.12710

Machalicek, W., McDuffie, A., Oakes, A., Ma, M., Thurman, A. J., Rispoli, M. J., & Abbeduto, L. (2014). Examining the operant function of challenging behavior in young males with fragile X syndrome: A summary of 12 cases. *Research in Developmental Disabilities, 35*(7), 1694–1704. https://doi.org/10.1016/j.ridd.2014.03.014

Maddox, B. B., Trubanova, A., & White, S. W. (2017). Untended wounds: Non-suicidal self-injury in adults with autism spectrum disorder. *Autism, 21*(4), 412–422. https://doi.org/10.1177/1362361316644731

Matson, J. L., & Turygin, N. C. (2012). How do researchers define self-injurious behavior? *Research in Developmental Disabilities, 33*(4), 1021–1026. https://doi.org/10.1016/j.ridd.2012.01.009

Melville, C. A., Cooper, S.-A., Morrison, J., Smiley, E., Allan, L., Jackson, A., … Mantry, D. (2008). The prevalence and incidence of mental ill-health in adults with autism and intellectual disabilities. *Journal of Autism and Developmental Disorders, 38*(9), 1676–1688. https://doi.org/10.1007/s10803-008-0549-7

Milad, M. R., Furtak, S. C., Greenberg, J. L., Keshaviah, A., Im, J. J., Falkenstein, M. J., … Wilhelm, S. (2013). Deficits in conditioned fear extinction in obsessive-compulsive disorder and neurobiological changes in the fear circuit. *JAMA Psychiatry, 70*(6), 608–618. https://doi.org/10.1001/jamapsychiatry.2013.914

Milad, M. R., Rosenbaum, B. L., & Simon, N. M. (2014). Neuroscience of fear extinction: Implications for assessment and treatment of fear-based and anxiety related disorders. *Behaviour Research and Therapy, 62*, 17–23. https://doi.org/10.1016/j.brat.2014.08.006

Moseley, R. L., Gregory, N. J., Smith, P., Allison, C., & Baron-Cohen, S. (2019). A 'choice', an 'addiction', a way 'out of the lost': Exploring self-injury in autistic people without intellectual disability. *Molecular Autism, 10*(1), 18. https://doi.org/10.1186/s13229-019-0267-3

Muehlmann, A. M., Kies, S. D., Turner, C. A., Wolfman, S., Lewis, M. H., & Devine, D. P. (2012). Self-injurious behaviour: Limbic dysregulation and stress effects in an animal model. *Journal of Intellectual Disability Research, 56*(5), 490–500. https://doi.org/10.1111/j.1365-2788.2011.01485.x

Muehlmann, A. M., & Lewis, M. H. (2012). Abnormal repetitive behaviours: Shared phenomenology and pathophysiology. *Journal of Intellectual Disability Research, 56*(5), 427–440. https://doi.org/10.1111/j.1365-2788.2011.01519.x

Muehlmann, A. M., Wilkinson, J. A., & Devine, D. P. (2011). Individual differences in vulnerability for self-injurious behavior: Studies using an animal model. *Behavioural Brain Research, 217*(1), 148–154. https://doi.org/10.1016/j.bbr.2010.10.012

Nigg, J. T. (2006). Temperament and developmental psychopathology. *Journal of Child Psychology and Psychiatry and Allied Disciplines, 47*(3–4), 395–422. https://doi.org/10.1111/j.1469-7610.2006.01612.x

Nuske, H. J., Finkel, E., Hedley, D., Parma, V., Tomczuk, L., Pellecchia, M., … Dissanayake, C. (2019). Heart rate increase predicts challenging behavior episodes in preschoolers with autism. *Stress, 22*(3), 303–311. https://doi.org/10.1080/10253890.2019.1572744

Nygaard, E., Smith, L., & Torgersen, A. M. (2002). Temperament in children with Down syndrome and in prematurely born children. *Scandinavian Journal of Psychology, 43*(1), 61–71. https://doi.org/10.1111/1467-9450.00269

O'Neill, R. E., Horner, R. H., Albin, R. W., Sprague, J. R., Storey, K., & Newton, J. S. (1997). *Functional assessment and program development for problem behavior: A practical handbook* (2nd ed.). Pacific Grove, CA: Brooks/Cole.

O'Reilly, M., Rispoli, M., Davis, T., Machalicek, W., Lang, R., Sigafoos, J., ... Didden, R. (2010). Functional analysis of challenging behavior in children with autism spectrum disorders: A summary of 10 cases. *Research in Autism Spectrum Disorders, 4*(1), 1–10. https://doi.org/10.1016/j.rasd.2009.07.001

Petty, J. L., Bacarese-Hamilton, M., Davies, L. E., & Oliver, C. (2014). Correlates of self-injurious, aggressive and destructive behaviour in children under five who are at risk of developmental delay. *Research in Developmental Disabilities, 35*(1), 36–45. https://doi.org/10.1016/j.ridd.2013.10.019

Powell, P. S., Travers, B. G., Klinger, L. G., & Klinger, M. R. (2016). Difficulties with multisensory fear conditioning in individuals with autism spectrum disorder. *Research in Autism Spectrum Disorders, 25*, 137–146. https://doi.org/10.1016/j.rasd.2016.02.008

Qiu, T., Chang, C., Li, Y., Qian, L., Xiao, C. Y., Xiao, T., ... Ke, X. (2016). Two years changes in the development of caudate nucleus are involved in restricted repetitive behaviors in 2-5-year-old children with autism spectrum disorder. *Developmental Cognitive Neuroscience, 19*, 137–143. https://doi.org/10.1016/j.dcn.2016.02.010

Rattaz, C., Michelon, C., & Baghdadli, A. (2015). Symptom severity as a risk factor for self-injurious behaviours in adolescents with autism spectrum disorders. *Journal of Intellectual Disability Research, 59*(8), 730–740. https://doi.org/10.1111/jir.12177

Reese, R. M., Richman, D. M., Belmont, J. M., & Morse, P. (2005). Functional characteristics of disruptive behavior in developmentally disabled children with and without autism. *Journal of Autism and Developmental Disorders, 35*(4), 419–428. https://doi.org/10.1007/s10803-005-5032-0

Richards, C., Davies, L., & Oliver, C. (2017). Predictors of self-injurious behavior and self-restraint in autism spectrum disorder: Towards a hypothesis of impaired behavioral control. *Journal of Autism and Developmental Disorders, 47*(3), 701–713. https://doi.org/10.1007/s10803-016-3000-5

Richards, C., Moss, J., Nelson, L., & Oliver, C. (2016). Persistence of self-injurious behaviour in autism spectrum disorder over 3 years: A prospective cohort study of risk markers. *Journal of Neurodevelopmental Disorders, 8*(1), 21. https://doi.org/10.1186/s11689-016-9153-x

Richards, C., Oliver, C., Nelson, L., & Moss, J. (2012). Self-injurious behaviour in individuals with autism spectrum disorder and intellectual disability. *Journal of Intellectual Disability Research, 56*(5), 476–489. https://doi.org/10.1111/j.1365-2788.2012.01537.x

Robbins, T. W., Vaghi, M. M., & Banca, P. (2019). Obsessive-compulsive disorder: Puzzles and prospects. *Neuron, 102*(1), 27–47. https://doi.org/10.1016/j.neuron.2019.01.046

Rothbart, M. K. (2007). Temperament, development, and personality. *Current Directions in Psychological Science, 16*(4), 207–212. https://doi.org/10.1111/j.1467-8721.2007.00505.x

Russell, K. M., Frost, K. M., & Ingersoll, B. (2019). The relationship between subtypes of repetitive behaviors and anxiety in children with autism spectrum disorder. *Research in Autism Spectrum Disorders, 62*, 48–54. https://doi.org/10.1016/j.rasd.2019.03.006

Rydzewska, E., Hughes-McCormack, L. A., Gillberg, C., Henderson, A., MacIntyre, C., Rintoul, J., & Cooper, S.-A. (2019). Prevalence of sensory impairments, physical and intellectual disabilities, and mental health in children and young people with self/proxy-reported autism: Observational study of a whole country population. *Autism, 23*(5), 1201–1209. https://doi.org/10.1177/1362361318791279

Samyn, V., Roeyers, H., & Bijttebier, P. (2011). Effortful control in typically developing boys and in boys with ADHD or autism spectrum disorder. *Research in Developmental Disabilities, 32*(2), 483–490. https://doi.org/10.1016/j.ridd.2010.12.038

Schwartz, C. B., Henderson, H. A., Inge, A. P., Zahka, N. E., Coman, D. C., Kojkowski, N. M., ... Mundy, P. C. (2009). Temperament as a predictor of symptomotology and adaptive functioning in adolescents with high-functioning autism. *Journal of Autism and Developmental Disorders, 39*(6), 842–855. https://doi.org/10.1007/s10803-009-0690-y

Soke, G. N., Rosenberg, S. A., Hamman, R. F., Fingerlin, T., Rosenberg, C. R., Carpenter, L., … DiGuiseppi, C. (2017). Factors associated with self-injurious behaviors in children with autism spectrum disorder: Findings from two large national samples. *Journal of Autism and Developmental Disorders, 47*(2), 285–296. https://doi.org/10.1007/s10803-016-2951-x

Soke, G. N., Rosenberg, S. A., Rosenberg, C. R., Vasa, R. A., Lee, L. C., & DiGuiseppi, C. (2018). Self-injurious behaviors in children with autism spectrum disorder enrolled in the Study to Explore Early Development. *Autism, 22*(5), 625–635. https://doi.org/10.1177/1362361316689330

South, M., Larson, M. J., White, S. E., Dana, J., & Crowley, M. J. (2011). Better fear conditioning is associated with reduced symptom severity in autism spectrum disorders. *Autism Research, 4*(6), 412–421. https://doi.org/10.1002/aur.221

South, M., Newton, T., & Chamberlain, P. D. (2012). Delayed reversal learning and association with repetitive behavior in autism spectrum disorders. *Autism Research, 5*(6), 398–406. https://doi.org/10.1002/aur.1255

Stratis, E. A., & Lecavalier, L. (2013). Restricted and repetitive behaviors and psychiatric symptoms in youth with autism spectrum disorders. *Research in Autism Spectrum Disorders, 7*(6), 757–766. https://doi.org/10.1016/j.rasd.2013.02.017

Tackett, J. L. (2006). Evaluating models of the personality-psychopathology relationship in children and adolescents. *Clinical Psychology Review, 26*(5), 584–599. https://doi.org/10.1016/j.cpr.2006.04.003

Tanimura, Y., Yang, M. C., & Lewis, M. H. (2008). Procedural learning and cognitive flexibility in a mouse model of restricted, repetitive behaviour. *Behavioural Brain Research, 189*(2), 250–256. https://doi.org/10.1016/j.bbr.2008.01.001

Taylor, J. L., Muscatello, R. A., & Corbett, B. A. (2018). Differences in anticipatory versus reactive stress to social evaluative threat in adults versus adolescents with autism. *Autism Research, 11*(9), 1276–1285. https://doi.org/10.1002/aur.1998

Top, D. N., Stephenson, K. G., Doxey, C. R., Crowley, M. J., Kirwan, C. B., & South, M. (2016). Atypical amygdala response to fear conditioning in autism spectrum disorder. *Biological Psychiatry: Cognitive Neuroscience and Neuroimaging, 1*(4), 308–315. https://doi.org/10.1016/j.bpsc.2016.01.008

Traynor, J. M., Doyle-Thomas, K. A. R., Hanford, L. C., Foster, N. E., Tryfon, A., Hyde, K. L., … Hall, G. B. C. (2018). Indices of repetitive behaviour are correlated with patterns of intrinsic functional connectivity in youth with autism spectrum disorder. *Brain Research, 1685*, 79–90. https://doi.org/10.1016/j.brainres.2018.02.009

Uljarević, M., Arnott, B., Carrington, S. J., Meins, E., Fernyhough, C., McConachie, H., … Leekam, S. R. (2017). Development of restricted and repetitive behaviors from 15 to 77 months: Stability of two distinct subtypes? *Developmental Psychology, 53*(10), 1859–1868. https://doi.org/10.1037/dev0000324

Uljarević, M., Richdale, A. L., Evans, D. W., Cai, R. Y., & Leekam, S. R. (2017). Interrelationship between insistence on sameness, effortful control and anxiety in adolescents and young adults with autism spectrum disorder (ASD). *Molecular Autism, 8*(1), 36. https://doi.org/10.1186/s13229-017-0158-4

Whitehouse, C. M., Curry-Pochy, L. S., Shafer, R., Rudy, J., & Lewis, M. H. (2017). Reversal learning in C58 mice: Modeling higher order repetitive behavior. *Behavioural Brain Research, 332*, 372–378. https://doi.org/10.1016/j.bbr.2017.06.014

Whitlock, J., Exner-Cortens, D., & Purington, A. (2014). Assessment of nonsuicidal self-injury: Development and initial validation of the non-suicidal self-injury-assessment tool (NSSI-AT). *Psychological Assessment, 26*(3), 935–946. https://doi.org/10.1037/a0036611

Wilkes, B. J., & Lewis, M. H. (2018). The neural circuitry of restricted repetitive behavior: Magnetic resonance imaging in neurodevelopmental disorders and animal models. *Neuroscience and Biobehavioral Reviews, 92*, 152–171. https://doi.org/10.1016/j.neubiorev.2018.05.022

Wise, E. A., Smith, M. D., & Rabins, P. V. (2017). Aging and autism spectrum disorder: A naturalistic, longitudinal study of the comorbidities and behavioral and neuropsychiatric symptoms in adults with ASD. *Journal of Autism and Developmental Disorders, 47*(6), 1708–1715. https://doi.org/10.1007/s10803-017-3095-3

Chapter 9
Current Developments and Future Prospects for Prevention and Treatment of Self-Injurious Behavior

9.1 Introduction

In this chapter we outline some current and possible future directions in research into self-injurious behavior (SIB) and their potential to guide innovation in prevention and treatment. It is however highly probable that the current pace of developments in the field of genetics will rapidly render some of our predictions obsolete. Only a decade ago, it was still widely believed that the primary benefit to be gained from identifying the genetic correlates of syndromes associated with developmental disabilities would be to eventually increase the possibility of rational pharmacotherapy. Although such hopes are still very much alive, our developing understanding of the complexity of the cascade of consequences resulting from some single gene mutations, such as that causing Rett syndrome, has led to renewed consideration of genome editing, messenger RNA (mRNA) editing, or mRNA therapy, as viable treatment options (Katz et al., 2016). With due respect for this rapidly evolving context for any discussion regarding interventions for people with neurodevelopmental conditions (NDCs), this chapter will focus on three areas of current development with possible future promise. The first concerns possibilities for primary and secondary prevention of the development and maintenance of chronic SIB by intervention in early childhood. The second is work toward identification of cross-syndrome processes in the neurobiology of genetic syndromes associated with SIB, which may have potential to contribute to the building of a more robust foundation for stratified pharmacotherapy. The third area considered in this chapter is current basic research in learning processes which may increase the effectiveness and robustness of behavioral interventions for SIB.

F. Furniss, A. B. Biswas, *Self-Injurious Behavior in Individuals with Neurodevelopmental Conditions*, Autism and Child Psychopathology Series,
https://doi.org/10.1007/978-3-030-36016-0_9

9.2 Primary and Secondary Prevention of Self-Injurious Behavior

As was discussed in Chap. 6, the potential for behavioral interventions to prevent the initial emergence of SIB, or to prevent its progression to more severe and treatment-resistant forms, has been widely discussed. There has however been little progress in translating the discussion of such possibilities into effective preventative programs. Such translation will require the identification of effective interventions and their development into forms (e.g., manualized treatments) in which they can be implemented by relevant clinical professionals. Effective prevention will further require the ability to identify which members of the population of people with NDCs are at high risk of developing SIB and delivery of the effective intervention in a form which is safe and acceptable to the people concerned and their families. The high prevalence of SIB (from around 10% to over 50%) in young children with neurodevelopmental conditions, together with the young age at which the behavior develops (often 12–24 months; see Chap. 2), presents challenges for any program of prevention.

Effective identification of children with NDCs who are at high risk of developing SIB poses a number of difficulties. For children with some genetic syndromes (e.g., Lesch-Nyhan syndrome and Smith-Magenis syndrome), risk is known to be extremely high, and in others (e.g., fragile X syndrome), it is certainly elevated. In terms of the child's condition, however, the presence of marked features of an autism spectrum condition (ASC) is currently the risk factor which impacts on the greatest number of children. The presence of an ASC may however not be suspected, much less diagnosed, by the age at which SIB typically emerges.

Childhood temperament can be reliably measured at an age before overt behavioral difficulties begin to emerge, and temperamental factors have recently been investigated as possible markers for ASC among infants at familial high risk for the condition (Pijl et al., 2019) and as possible markers for later emergence of attention deficit hyperactivity disorder (ADHD) symptoms in young children (Willoughby, Gottfredson, & Stifter, 2017). These investigations have demonstrated the existence of group-level differences in temperament between infants who were later diagnosed with ASCs and those who later were identified as typically developing (Pijl et al., 2019) and associations between temperament and later ADHD symptoms in children (Willoughby et al., 2017). The latter finding is of relevance given that overactivity, impulsivity, and attentional difficulties have been found to be associated with SIB in a number of NDCs including ASCs, Cornelia de Lange syndrome, fragile X syndrome, Lowe syndrome, and Prader-Willi syndrome, as well as in people with intellectual disabilities (IDs) of heterogeneous origin (Arron, Oliver, Moss, Berg, & Burbidge, 2011; Collacott, Cooper, Branford, & McGrother, 1998; Cooper et al., 2009; Davies & Oliver, 2016; Richman et al., 2013; Rojahn, Matson, Naglieri, & Mayville, 2004; Tsiouris, Kim, Brown, & Cohen, 2011). Both Pijl et al. (2019) and Willoughby et al. (2017) however reported that the predictive power of temperament was insufficient to use assessment of temperament as a clinically useful marker of risk for individual children. Nevertheless, Pijl et al. (2019) noted that temperament could be used to predict later absence of features of ASC in high-risk infants, and Willoughby et al. (2017) suggested that temperamental features might be sufficiently predictive of later ADHD to be useful in targeting early intervention. Temperament may therefore warrant further investigation as a possible early marker for the emergence of SIB.

Rather than focusing on individual child characteristics however, primary prevention might possibly be best targeted according to perinatal or postnatal complications around the birth of the child (Soke et al., 2018), family socioeconomic disadvantage (SED) (Soke et al., 2017), or assessments of family process (Chadwick, Kusel, & Cuddy, 2008). Given the association of family SED with child mental health difficulties (Midouhas, Yogaratnam, Flouri, & Charman, 2013), and the enhanced risk for children with ASCs of experiencing potentially damaging levels of adverse childhood experiences including family income insufficiency (Berg, Shiu, Acharya, Stolbach, & Msall, 2016), social factors rather than individual child characteristics might provide the most useful basis for targeting of primary prevention interventions including parent training such as that described by Fodstad, Kirsch, Faidley, and Bauer (2018).

Given our current state of knowledge, it is likely however that preventative efforts will be concentrated on secondary prevention aimed at reducing, or limiting the development of, SIB once it has emerged. The child's ability, and especially communicative ability, severity of restricted and repetitive behaviors (RRBs), and other signs of ASCs, and the level of concern expressed by teachers regarding the child's SIB are potentially useful indicators for particular concern regarding the possibility of SIB becoming persistent (Baghdadli et al., 2008; Davies & Oliver, 2016; Dimian et al., 2017; Rattaz, Michelon, & Baghdadli, 2015).

Although it is generally agreed that behavioral interventions have a key role to play in such secondary prevention, it is equally widely agreed that progress in embedding these in routine clinical practice has been limited (Oliver, Licence, & Richards, 2017). One barrier to the widespread adoption of these interventions is that until recently much applied behavior analytic research has been primarily devoted to investigating the effects of individual treatment components such as noncontingent reinforcement (NCR) and functional communication training (FCT) on specific behaviors, such as SIB, in cases where these behaviors are maintained by a single source of reinforcement. Self-injurious behavior however commonly co-occurs with many other behavioral difficulties, including aggression directed toward other people, and may have multiple maintaining consequences. In addition, clinical intervention often involves attempting to bring problems under some degree of control as rapidly as possible. This often involves implementing a package comprising multiple interventions introduced simultaneously, rather than one at a time. Behavioral intervention has therefore often require clinicians to use the research literature as a general guide to develop an effective intervention for the individual case.

In recent years however, there has been a greater focus in applied behavior analytic research on developing and evaluating interventions which can be directly applied in family and other settings. Hanley, Jin, Vanselow, and Hanratty (2014) evaluated a procedure for functional analysis of challenging behaviors such as SIB which uses an approach which is tailored to the individual engaging in the behavior and the context in which it occurs. This interview-informed, synthesized contingency analysis (IISCA) uses an interview with caregivers or other informants, and where necessary a brief period of observation, to identify situations in which challenging behavior occurs, reinforcers which may be maintaining the behavior, and specific materials or items which may be significant for the individual, in order to design an experimental functional analysis (EFA) specific to the individual. A single test condition, incorporating the presence of the reinforcement contingency which is hypothesized to maintain the challenging behavior, is designed for each person, together with a control condition which is identical except that the reinforcement contingency is omitted. The specific materials and social interactions modelled in the analysis are those which caregivers report as evoking or possibly maintaining the challenging behavior, and if it is hypothesized that multiple consequences maintain the behavior, these are simultaneously included in the analysis. The results of the IISCA are then used to develop an intervention individualized to the person concerned and their everyday social context. Hanley et al. (2014) reported the use of this approach with three children with ASCs. A function was identified for the challenging behavior(s) of each child, and individualized treatment packages were developed, comprising functional communication training, increasing the complexity of the child's communicative response, and techniques to help each child tolerate denials and delays in reinforcement, including building longer chains of behavior to obtain reinforcement. Finally, the intervention was extended from the outpatient clinic to situations more closely resembling the child's everyday environment, usually by firstly directly supervising the parents or other caregivers in implementing the intervention in the outpatient clinic, followed by implementation in other settings and in the child's home. The assessment and intervention lasted between 8 and 14 weeks and required 22–23 one-hour outpatient appointments. For each child, challenging behaviors were reduced to zero or near-zero levels, with only occasional occurrences even during the treatment extension phase, while use of functional communication and tolerance of delays and denials of reinforcement were shown to increase. The parents of the children reported high levels of satisfaction with the assessment procedures, the recommended interventions, and the improvements shown by their children. Jessel, Ingvarsson, Metras, Kirk, and Whipple (2018) reported outcomes for 25 children, most of whom had ASCs, and whose challenging behaviors were believed to be socially reinforced, using the IISCA approach. For ten of the children, the challenging behaviors were reported to include SIB. Jessel et al. (2018) again provided assessment and intervention on an outpatient basis, but this time based on a process in which the children attended the outpatient clinic for 7 h per day, 5 days a week, for 2 weeks. Assessment was completed and intervention commenced in the first week, and parents were trained to implement the intervention in the second week. The IISCA identified the function of the challenging behavior(s) for each child, and interventions based on FCT followed by reinforcement schedule thinning resulted in reductions in challenging behavior of

90% or greater for each child. Parents again reported high levels of satisfaction with the assessment and intervention process.

These evaluations of IISCA-based interventions suggest that they are effective and acceptable to parents and require between 30 and 70 h of therapy. The long-term sustainability of these interventions however remains to be demonstrated. Lucyshyn et al. (2015) addressed this issue, noting that to be truly sustainable, behavioral interventions need to remain effective and acceptable to families over periods of years following the completion of initial intensive therapy. Lucyshyn et al.'s (2015) response to this challenge was to work collaboratively with families to achieve meaningful changes in children's behavior and participation in meaningful household routines, an approach which they labelled "family-centered positive behavior support" (fcPBS).

The fcPBS approach, similar to the IISCA-based intervention approach, uses multicomponent interventions based on initial functional assessment. Rather than developing a general intervention, however, the fcPBS approach structures interventions around regular routines in family life, including home routines such as getting ready for school, mealtimes and the child's bedtime, and community-based routines such as grocery shopping or eating out. Lucyshyn et al. (2015), working together with parents, developed positive behavior support (PBS) plans for each routine (although plans might be similar across routines). For each routine, parents were initially trained to implement the plan by therapists modelling the behavior support strategies and coaching the parents in their use. Further support was provided by meetings with parents in which plan strategies were discussed and role-played, and solutions to problems were identified. In cases where parents and children appeared to be locked into existing coercive interactions, therapists directly initiated use of the plan with the child for the first one or two routines. This initial training required a mean of 76.6 sessions per family, comprising a mean of 102.7 h of intervention over a mean period of 107.4 weeks.

When the child's behavior had improved to the point where challenging behavior was occurring in less than 10% of observation intervals, and the child was participating constructively in the routine for approximately 80% of the steps involved, "maintenance support" commenced. Maintenance support involved providing parents with limited coaching during routines, with feedback after routines were completed. Parents were encouraged to generate their own solutions to any problems which occurred and to generalize the use of support plans to settings other than those where they had been directly trained. Maintenance support per family totalled 32.4 h on average, distributed in a mean of 39.3 sessions over a mean period of 113.3 weeks. During the intervention, additional support for parents (e.g., mindfulness training) was organized as necessary.

Lucyshyn et al. (2015) enrolled 12 families into their study, 2 of whom withdrew in the second year. The 12 children (8 boys and 4 girls) had ASCs and/or IDs and engaged in challenging behaviors including non-compliance, physical aggression, and destructive behaviors. The support plans concerned a total of 36 family routines, and follow-ups were completed between 11 and 24 months after the end of the intervention for 8 of the 10 families who had completed initial intervention and maintenance support. At baseline, the ten children who completed the intervention were engaging in challenging behaviors for between 26.6 and 70.3% of 10-s observation intervals (mean 51.2%) and were constructively participating in between 18.3 and 49.4% of routine steps (mean 30.8%). At follow-up the eight children for whom data were obtained were engaging in challenging behaviors for between 0.1 and 7.6% of observation intervals (mean 3.0%) and were participating in between 82.4 and 100% of routine steps (mean 92.4%). Some parents reported some negative side effects of the intervention, such as siblings of the participating children being upset at receiving less attention from their parents than they previously had, but overall parents rated the procedures of the intervention and its results as both acceptable and important to them. By comparison with baseline measures, mothers of the children involved reported significant improvements in family quality of life and reduced parenting stress during intervention and follow-up, and fathers also reported reduced parenting stress (Lucyshyn, Miller, Cheremshynski, Lohrmann, & Zumbo, 2018).

Taken together, the studies of Hanley et al. (2014), Jessel et al. (2018), and Lucyshyn et al. (2015) provide convincing demonstrations that synthesized, multicomponent behavioral interventions based on functional assessment can reduce the challenging behaviors, including SIB, of children with ASCs and other developmental disabilities and that these improvements can be maintained for up to 2 years following intervention. There are a number of limitations to these studies, including the fact that none of the children who participated in the study of Lucyshyn et al. (2015) were reported to engage in SIB. These two strands of work strongly suggest however that effective behavioral intervention for challenging behaviors such as SIB will require use of multicomponent synthesized interventions based on functional assessment, initial implementation of the intervention by professional therapists (where necessary), modelling and coaching to support parents or other caregivers in implementing the intervention, and support for problem-solving, maintenance, and generalization thereafter. They also suggest that such interventions require somewhere between 20 and 130 h of therapeutic input over periods of up to 4 years.

Lucyshyn et al. (2015) suggested that the length of time required for intervention in their study was partly due to the requirements of their experimental design and suggested that attempts at replication should use more time-efficient designs. Clearly, the utility of these interventions for secondary prevention of chronic SIB would be increased if the duration of the initial intervention could be reduced. Hanley et al. (2014) and Jessel, Hanley, Ghaemmaghami, and Metras (2019) have reported preliminary data on outcomes for interventions developed using an abbreviated IISCA process. These interventions still however require considerable time input from professional staff to implement interventions initially, model these to parents, and provide ongoing support. Further work is needed both to further evaluate their effectiveness and to examine how they can be delivered within existing service frameworks (Oliver et al., 2017).

9.3 Cross-Syndrome Processes in the Neurobiology of Genetic Syndromes Associated with Self-Injurious Behavior

As copy number variants and other genetic changes of possible causal significance continue to be detected in people with IDs and ASCs who engage in SIB (e.g., Shirley et al., 2016), the probability that different cases of SIB may share some common mechanisms which could be modified by a single intervention might seem to be reducing. As the causation of various neurodevelopmental conditions is coming to be understood in more detail however, the possibility of identifying commonalities in causal processes also increases. The drive to delineate brain circuits related to complex behavior patterns across syndromes has been strengthened by the Research Domain Criteria (RDoC) initiative of the US National Institute of Mental Health (Cuthbert, 2015). One key strategy of research inspired by the RDoC project is to identify endophenotypes (such as deficits in working memory, attention, and sensory processing), and their neural correlates, which may underpin symptom expression across conditions (Kas et al., 2019). Within research in neurodevelopmental conditions, therefore, an existing foundation of behavioral research into specific behavior patterns such as SIB is being complemented by attempts in biological research to move beyond a focus on individual syndromes to identifying brain circuits or processes and their behavioral correlates across multiple syndromes. The approach is seen as critical to informing translational research in animal models and stimulating new drug development (Cuthbert, 2019).

In 2003, Rubenstein and Merzenich published a highly influential paper suggesting that many of the features of ASCs could be understood as resulting from an overall imbalance between excitatory and inhibitory processes in the brain, impacting on neural systems underpinning sensory processing, memory, and social and emotional behaviors. Currently, substantial interest is focused on the possibility of an impairment in inhibitory processes, with research examining both functional connectivity in relevant networks (Voorhies et al., 2018) and synaptic development and functioning in γ-aminobutyric acid (GABA)ergic cortical and hippocampal interneurons. A large number of genes encoding products involved in inhibitory synapse function have been associated with various NDCs (and/or animal models of these conditions), including some specifically associated with SIB, such as ASCs and Rett syndrome (Rodriguez, Joya, & Hines, 2018). In the case of ASCs, the protein products involved include trans-synaptic adhesion molecules, synaptic scaffolding proteins, and synaptic signalling proteins, including various subunits of the $GABA_A$ receptor. In the case of Rett syndrome, as was described in greater detail in Chap. 3, it has been shown that loss of methyl-CpG-binding protein 2 (MeCP2) in GABAergic inhibitory neurons throughout the brain causes mice to develop many features related to the human Rett syndrome phenotype, while loss of MeCP2 from a subset of forebrain GABAergic neurons only leads to various behavioral abnormalities, although these do not include SIB (Chao et al., 2010). Additionally, it has been found that removal of MeCP2 from the parvalbumin-positive class of

GABAergic inhibitory neurons led to motor, sensory, fear conditioning, and social deficits, while mice lacking MeCP2 in the somatostatin-positive class of GABAergic inhibitory neurons developed seizures and stereotyped behaviors (Ito-Ishida, Ure, Chen, Swann, & Zoghbi, 2015).

Deficits in inhibitory signalling, or imbalance between excitatory and inhibitory processes, could therefore contribute to diverse difficulties across several NDCs (Rodriguez et al., 2018). In response to this possibility, drugs modulating GABAergic function by various mechanisms have been tested in animal models of various NDCs, with mixed but potentially promising results (Braat & Kooy, 2015). A recent review of clinical trials of various GABA modulators with children, adolescents, and young adults (Brondino et al., 2016) concluded however that despite some promising results, the limited amount and quality of the available evidence, with relatively small open-label trials predominating, did not justify suggesting the use of these drugs with people with ASCs. A recent review of relevant work with murine models of ASC also noted the difficulties which had been experienced in translating positive results from preclinical work into effective clinical trials (Golden, Buxbaum, & De Rubeis, 2018). However, further trials of GABA modulators are underway, fragile X syndrome (FXS) being one focus of ongoing interest (Benke & Möhler, 2018). A recent double-blind crossover trial of ganaxolone, a positive allosteric modulator of $GABA_A$ receptors, involving children with FXS, showed no therapeutic differences between placebo and ganaxolone phases in clinical ratings of the children and on various measures of anxiety, mood, and behavior (Ligsay et al., 2017). Post hoc analyses focusing on participants with higher anxiety, and separately on those with lower ability, suggested however that ganaxolone use improved anxiety in the former, and attention and other measures in the latter, subgroups. It has been suggested that heterogeneity in trial participants may be one of the reasons that trials to date of GABA modulators have produced rather disappointing results (Brondino et al., 2016), but tightening participation criteria while recruiting sufficient trial participants will be a significant challenge for many of the NDCs.

One aim of the RDoC project is facilitation of bidirectional translation between animal studies and clinical trials. "Back-translation" is particularly important when drugs, often designed to be highly selective for specific receptors, produce positive results in relevant animal models but then fail to do so in human clinical trials. A major obstacle in back-translation is that basic research with human participants aimed at understanding the reasons why preclinically effective interventions have failed in human trials has been stifled by a lack of brain receptor-selective compounds approved for human use (Nutt, Robbins, & Hayes, 2018). Initiatives are now underway to address this problem, with availability for approved research of a selective dopamine D_1 receptor antagonist expected to be one initial outcome (Nutt et al., 2018). Hopefully such initiatives will enable closure of the loop between preclinical and clinical research envisioned by the RDoC project (Cuthbert, 2019).

9.4 Basic Research in Learning Processes Informing Development of Behavioral Interventions

In behavioral research, as in neurobiological research, there has been a recent flowering of basic and translational research relevant to intervention with SIB and other challenging behaviors. In the case of behavioral research, these developments have been stimulated by the difficulties experienced in maintaining the effectiveness of behavioral interventions over long periods, or in other words by the problem of relapse. As was briefly mentioned in Chap. 6, the reappearance of SIB following apparently successful behavioral treatment has been conceptualized as falling into several categories. In the first, "reinstatement," SIB which at one time has been reinforced, and then extinguished, reappears when response-independent reinforcers are encountered at a later time. In the second category of relapse, "renewal," SIB is reinforced in one situation (e.g., a person's family home), extinguished in a second situation (e.g., an inpatient treatment unit), and reappears when the person returns to the original situation, or moves to a third situation (e.g., a community residential service). These situations are respectively referred to as "ABA" and "ABC" forms of renewal, with letters representing the sequence of contexts involved. Finally, in the third category of relapse, "resurgence," during the phase in which SIB is extinguished, reinforcement is provided instead for an alternative behavior (i.e., functional communication training or differential reinforcement of alternative behavior), and in the third phase, both SIB and the alternative behavior are placed on extinction. Each type of "relapse" can be reliably modelled in non-problematic behaviors in nonhuman animals by arranging the appropriate changes in reinforcement contingencies and stimulus contexts (Kuroda, Mizutani, Cançado, & Podlesnik, 2017), and basic and translational research into these processes has the potential to improve the robustness of behavioral interventions for SIB.

In basic behavioral research, reinstatement and renewal have been accounted for by behavioral momentum theory (BMT: see Nevin et al., 2017, for a succinct overview of the theory and its applications). A central tenet of BMT is that the change in response rate in the face of a disruptive change in the environment (e.g., extinction) depends both on the severity of the disruption and on the rate or amount of reinforcement obtained during responding prior to the disruption. The most straightforward implication of BMT for behavioral treatment of SIB, where the "disruption" involved is a behavioral intervention and the behavior is SIB which is placed on extinction as part of the intervention, is that the greater the reinforcement which has been obtained while SIB was being reinforced, the more resistant it will be to change. BMT proposes that resistance to change results from the association of the rate or amount of reinforcement with the stimulus context. Critically, the key variable is proposed to be the rate or amount of reinforcement received, not simply the rate or amount of reinforcement which is contingent on the SIB or other behavior concerned. Thus, if the behavior is being reinforced, provision of additional reinforcers noncontingent on behavior, e.g., on a fixed-time (FT) or variable-time (VT) schedule, will also strengthen the persistence of the behavior. This corollary of

BMT therefore may have unfortunate implications for the long-term use of noncontingent reinforcement (NCR: see Chap. 6) to reduce SIB in everyday environments where it might reasonably be expected that carers or other persons may occasionally provide reinforcement for SIB. In such a situation, BMT predicts that although the NCR intervention may reduce the occurrence of SIB in the short term, the provision of reinforcers in the NCR schedule together with the occasional reinforcement of SIB by carers will increase the long-term persistence of the behavior. If the intervention ends or its quality is seriously degraded with the passage of time since its inception, the persistence of SIB in the long term might thus be enhanced rather than weakened (DeLeon, Gregory, & St. Peter, 2013).

In a series of three experiments with pigeons, Podlesnik and Shahan (2009) showed that the association of the rate or amount of reinforcement with the stimulus context, even when some of that reinforcement is response-independent, contributes to all three categories of relapse. Pigeons were trained to respond for food on the same reinforcement schedule in two alternating contexts. In one context, additional food was given response-independently. Consistent with the predictions of BMT, initial responding was lower, but resistance to extinction was higher, in the context in which additional food had been provided. Further, the relative relapse of responding associated with modelling of reinstatement, resurgence, and renewal situations was greater in the context associated with higher overall reinforcement. In a clinical study with seven children with ASCs and limited means of communication, who engaged in SIB, aggressive, and disruptive behaviors, Fisher et al. (2019) measured baseline levels of the challenging behaviors when they were reinforced under two differing schedules of reinforcement associated with different contextual stimuli. Fisher et al. (2019) then implemented FCT, with extinction of challenging behavior, in each context until the children's levels of challenging behavior had reduced by least 85% from baseline levels for two consecutive sessions. Brief extinction challenges were then implemented, again in both contexts, in which neither challenging behavior nor the communicative responses which had been taught during FCT were reinforced. Fisher et al. observed resurgence of the children's challenging behaviors for four of the seven children, and as would be predicted by BMT, the magnitude of the resurgence was generally greater in the context which during baseline had been associated with a richer schedule of reinforcement.

Fisher et al.'s (2019) findings that not all the children showed resurgence of challenging behavior following extinction challenges after FCT indicate that there is still much to be learned regarding the conditions under which relapse does and does not occur. In applied research and clinical work, especially when it involves potentially immediately harmful behaviors such as SIB, the necessity to minimize treatment relapse effects limits the ability of researchers to fully evaluate factors affecting its occurrence. Although the origins of BMT were in basic research with nonhuman animals, its application to the understanding of treatment relapse has also therefore stimulated translational research involving children with ASCs as research participants. Translational research in which arbitrary, non-harmful responses are reinforced and then extinguished enables researchers to vary parameters affecting "relapse" without placing participants at risk of harm. Liggett, Nastri, and Podlesnik

(2018), for example, working with three children with ASCs, taught the children a simple response (placing a ball in a Montessori "object permanence" box), using preferred food items as reinforcers. After the response had been established and maintained on a variable-ratio 2 schedule (i.e., the response was reinforced on average once out of every two times that the child placed the ball in the box), the response was placed on extinction, while a highly preferred toy was introduced, to model an intervention using extinction of a target response together with noncontingent availability of a reinforcer. When the children were reliably playing with the toy and no longer performing the arbitrary target response, challenges simulating conditions which typically lead to reinstatement and resurgence were presented. To model conditions predicted to result in reinstatement, food items were made available response-independently, while the children's preferred toys remained available. To model conditions predicted to result in resurgence, the preferred toys were placed out of the children's reach. A combined challenge in which the edibles were presented noncontingently with the toys out of the children's reach was also evaluated. In each of these conditions, the arbitrary response was no longer being reinforced. Liggett et al. (2018) showed that "relapse" of the ball-in-the-box response occurred under all three challenge conditions, but also that this effect was generally greater when both challenges were in effect. Their results suggest therefore that post-treatment situations in which an alternative source of reinforcement ceases to be available while the original reinforcer for a challenging behavior is occasionally presented will produce both reinstatement and resurgence effects. Together these will produce a greater return of the challenging behavior than would result from either in isolation. Further translational studies have investigated how the contextual changes which can result in renewal can also exacerbate resurgence. Renewal effects can be observed in "ABA" and "ABC" forms, but may also be seen when a reinforced response is first established and then extinguished in the same setting, but then re-emerges in a different setting, or when contextual features of the original setting change (AAB renewal: Cohenour, Volkert, & Allen, 2018). Although the attention of practitioners was originally drawn to the role of renewal during relapse which occurs when people return to "home" environments following successful behavioral intervention in specialist services, renewal effects can also be observed with stimulus changes, including changes to the social context, which occur while other features of the situation remain unchanged (Browning & Shahan, 2018). Podlesnik et al. (2019) carried out a series of translational experiments examining the interaction between resurgence (i.e., relapse when an "alternative" behavior ceases to be reinforced) and context changes associated with the transition from reinforcement to extinction. It was found that resurgence effects were generally greater when extinction of the alternative behavior was implemented on return to the environment in which the original "challenging" behavior had been reinforced (ABA context change) than when it occurred in the context in which "treatment" (extinction of the original behavior and reinforcement of the alternative) had taken place (ABB context change), suggesting that resurgence is exacerbated when it occurs under conditions which would be expected to result in renewal.

Translational research has also begun to explore conditions under which resurgence might be minimized. Some potential strategies for reducing the probability of resurgence of SIB were discussed in Chap. 6. Recently, Craig, Cunningham, Sweeney, Shahan, and Nevin (2018) compared an analogue of differential reinforcement of alternative behavior (DRA), i.e., extinction of a previously reinforced target response together with reinforcement of an alternative response, with a differential reinforcement of other behavior (DRO)-DRA procedure in which access to the DRA schedule was dependent on the participating pigeons not engaging in the target behavior for a specified period of time. Craig et al. (2018) showed that although the target behavior extinguished more rapidly with the standard DRA procedure, during an extinction challenge when neither target nor alternative behaviors were reinforced, resurgence of the original target behavior was less following the DRO-DRA procedure than following standard DRA.

BMT does not successfully predict all aspects of resurgence and related phenomena, and alternatives have been proposed which suggest that resurgence can be accounted for by decreases in the value of a more recently reinforced alternative behavior relative to that of an originally reinforced challenging behavior (Greer & Shahan, 2019). Others however consider that despite its predictive limitations, the demonstrated utility of BMT in suggesting ways in which reinstatement and resurgence effects can be minimized supports its ongoing utility as a framework for translational research into these questions (Fisher et al., 2018). One key problem for BMT is however its explanation of reinstatement. BMT proposes that reinstatement effects arise from Pavlovian stimulus-response associations between the reinforcer itself and the originally learned response, leading to presentation of the reinforcer evoking the response. Reinstatement effects are thus proposed to be an exemplar of the more general process of Pavlovian-to-instrumental transfer (PIT). The process differs from antecedent stimulus control of behavior, which operant theory defines as an ability to evoke behavior which is dependent on presence of the stimulus being correlated with reinforcement of the behavior. Assuming that the stimulus continues to be present when the behavior is then placed on extinction, stimulus control of the behavior will be reduced simultaneously with extinction of the behavior. If a stimulus has come to evoke the behavior through Pavlovian processes, by contrast, its ability to evoke the behavior will be unaffected by the change in reinforcement contingencies, hence enabling it to evoke the behavior even if the behavior itself has been extinguished.

Although this discussion has focused mainly on issues relating to relapse following treatment, BMT assumes that PIT processes are more generally involved in increasing the resistance of behavior to any kind of disruption, including extinction. Testing this proposal directly is obviously difficult because the behavior cannot be reinforced in the absence of the reinforcing stimulus. A potential indication of the relevance of PIT in explaining resistance to extinction can however be obtained by pairing a further stimulus (acting as a Pavlovian conditional stimulus or CS) with a potential operant reinforcer in Pavlovian conditioning in advance of operant training, then using the potential reinforcer to establish an operant response with the CS absent, and then extinguishing that response in the presence of the Pavlovian CS. On the prediction from BMT, the presence of the CS should increase resistance to extinction of the response. Comparisons of rates of extinction in the presence of CSs associated with differential rates of response-independent reinforcer presentation prior to operant training do not however show differential resistance to extinction in the presence of those stimuli, indicating the need for an alternative or more complete account of the processes underlying reinstatement (Nevin et al., 2017).

Further insight into processes involved in relapse following successful treatment may be provided from recent research into anxiety disorders, where similar relapse is a significant problem following successful treatment using progressive exposure, showing parallels with difficulties in treating habitual/impulsive SIB by progressive exposure with reinforcement. Contemporary conceptualizations of the extinction of fear learning emphasize that extinction is an active process in which fear responses in previously fear-evoking situations are actively inhibited rather than simply weakened. Extinction learning can thus be thought of as involving the acquisition of new memories, which themselves will be retrieved context-dependently. The neural substrates of these processes involve a complex network of structures including the prefrontal cortex, amygdala, and hippocampus together with a number of other areas including the ventrolateral periaqueductal gray, bed nucleus of the stria terminalis, ventral tegmental area, and striatum (Singewald & Holmes, 2019). As an active learning process, extinction, like initial response acquisition, is context dependent (Bouton, 2019). Response renewal in an ABA context sequence can readily be understood within a straightforward operant model. When a response which has been learned in one context and then extinguished in another reappears when a person returns to the original situation, discriminative stimuli originally controlling the response in the first context, not having been present during extinction, will have retained the ability to elicit the behavior when the person returns to their home setting. This model however does not effectively account for the renewal which is seen in an ABC context series where a person moves to a new situation following successful treatment. Such renewal can however readily be explained if the extinction of SIB is understood as an active learning process which is itself context dependent. If the environmental cues associated with extinction learning are absent from the third context, but some of the cues which originally elicited SIB are present, renewal of the SIB will occur. These insights have straightforward implications for arranging treatments in such a way as to reduce the probability of such renewal. Conducting treatment involving extinction of the problematic response (whether fear or SIB) in multiple contexts will increase the probability that any new situation will share at least some features with a context in which extinction has taken place. Basic and translational studies have shown that extinction in multiple contexts reduces ABC renewal and that extended extinction in multiple contexts also reduces ABA renewal (Bernal-Gamboa, Nieto, & Uengoer, 2017; Krisch, Bandarian-Balooch, & Neumann, 2018; Olatunji, Tomarken, Wentworth, & Fritzsche, 2017). Organizing intervention in multiple contexts with a behavior such as SIB, and working with people for whom progressive exposure has to be provided in vivo, clearly poses ethical and logistical questions beyond those involved in treatment of fear in neurotypical individuals. It may however be critical to achieving reductions in SIB which will be maintained across the multiple contexts of everyday life.

9.5 Future Prospects for Prevention and Treatment of Self-Injurious Behavior

Chaney (2013) describes the use of protective equipment, such as padded gloves, to prevent people from hurting themselves in the psychiatric hospitals of the 1880s. Our understanding of the processes involved in the development and maintenance of SIB has developed enormously since those times, but many people with NDCs still rely on such measures. In this chapter we have reviewed recent developments in interventions which have substantial potential for helping people to avoid the development of persistent SIB, or to reduce it once it has become established, with consequential improvements in their quality of life.

With respect to primary and secondary prevention of SIB, effective interventions are available, and further progress will depend on the development of services to provide these supports for young children with NDCs (Oliver et al., 2017). Such services will need to be directed to those most needing them, and here the current focus on psychological characteristics of the individual child, although it has advanced our understanding of the factors involved in the development and maintenance of SIB, has yet to provide methods for clinically useful assessment of risk. More research is needed, but a greater focus on known sociodemographic risk markers for childhood emotional and behavioral difficulties might well be helpful.

Although the necessity of a multidisciplinary approach to helping people who engage in SIB is generally accepted (Minshawi, Hurwitz, Morriss, & McDougle, 2015), the conceptual gulf between neuropsychiatric and applied behavior analytic models of SIB has limited progress toward a genuinely integrated approach. Our advancing knowledge of the brain circuits involved in various learning processes should provide a basis for increasingly rapid progress in this area, with the aim of more rationally combining behavioral and pharmacological interventions in situations where both are relevant. A recognition that behavior results from an interaction between neural networks and the environment, and that environmental conditions, including reinforcement contingencies, have long-term as well as short-term effects on neural circuits, will be essential to progress. A recent study using resting-state functional magnetic resonance imaging to examine associations between resting-state connectivity and RRBs in young children with high and low familial risk for ASCs at 12 and 24 months of age found associations of functional connectivity between various pairs of networks with ritualistic/sameness, restricted, and stereotyped behaviors, but not with self-injurious behaviors, consistent with the hypothesis that SIB develops through a complex interaction with the environment rather than as a direct consequence of differences in aspects of brain connectivity (McKinnon et al., 2019). There is much progress yet to be made in improving the effectiveness of treatments for SIB, and the increasing emphasis on translational and back-translational research in both biomedical and behavioral research shows encouraging recognition of this issue.

Much biomedical and behavioral research into the self-injury experienced by people with IDs, ASCs, and other NDCs has until recently proceeded in relative isolation from that undertaken into non-suicidal self-injury in people without NDCs. Its isolation from research into problems involving anxiety, attentional difficulties, compulsive behaviors, and other mental health difficulties in the general population has been even greater. Recent research has however made substantial progress toward identifying endophenotypic characteristics, such as impulsivity and insistence on sameness, which increase a person's risk of developing SIB. An increasingly broad range of mental health difficulties are coming to be recognized as neurodevelopmental conditions in which environmental factors interact with development to influence outcome (Cuthbert, 2019). A greater emphasis on transdiagnostic approaches may increase the pace of research relevant to understanding of the endophenotypic characteristics which confer increased risk for possibly diverse negative outcomes across different conditions. These developments promise to substantially increase the pace of development of our understanding of SIB and to benefit the people with NDCs who live with these often highly distressing and damaging behaviors.

References

Arron, K., Oliver, C., Moss, J., Berg, K., & Burbidge, C. (2011). The prevalence and phenomenology of self-injurious and aggressive behaviour in genetic syndromes. *Journal of Intellectual Disability Research, 55*(2), 109–120. https://doi.org/10.1111/j.1365-2788.2010.01337

Baghdadli, A., Picot, M. C., Pry, R., Michelon, C., Burzstejn, C., Lazartigues, A., & Aussilloux, C. (2008). What factors are related to a negative outcome of self-injurious behaviour during childhood in pervasive developmental disorders? *Journal of Applied Research in Intellectual Disabilities, 21*(2), 142–149. https://doi.org/10.1111/j.1468-3148.2007.00389.x

Benke, D., & Möhler, H. (2018). Impact on GABA systems in monogenetic developmental CNS disorders: Clues to symptomatic treatment. *Neuropharmacology, 136*(Part A), 46–55. https://doi.org/10.1016/j.neuropharm.2017.07.030

Berg, K. L., Shiu, C. S., Acharya, K., Stolbach, B. C., & Msall, M. E. (2016). Disparities in adversity among children with autism spectrum disorder: A population-based study. *Developmental Medicine and Child Neurology, 58*(11), 1124–1131. https://doi.org/10.1111/dmcn.13161

Bernal-Gamboa, R., Nieto, J., & Uengoer, M. (2017). Effects of extinction in multiple contexts on renewal of instrumental responses. *Behavioural Processes, 142*, 64–69. https://doi.org/10.1016/j.beproc.2017.06.003

Bouton, M. E. (2019). Extinction of instrumental (operant) learning: Interference, varieties of context, and mechanisms of contextual control. *Psychopharmacology, 236*(1), 7–19. https://doi.org/10.1007/s00213-018-5076-4

Braat, S., & Kooy, R. F. (2015). The $GABA_A$ receptor as a therapeutic target for neurodevelopmental disorders. *Neuron, 86*(5), 1119–1130. https://doi.org/10.1016/j.neuron.2015.03.042

Brondino, N., Fusar-Poli, L., Panisi, C., Damiani, S., Barale, F., & Politi, P. (2016). Pharmacological modulation of GABA function in autism spectrum disorders: A systematic review of human studies. *Journal of Autism and Developmental Disorders, 46*(3), 825–839. https://doi.org/10.1007/s10803-015-2619-y

Browning, K. O., & Shahan, T. A. (2018). Renewal of extinguished operant behavior following changes in social context. *Journal of the Experimental Analysis of Behavior, 110*(3), 430–439. https://doi.org/10.1002/jeab.472

Chadwick, O., Kusel, Y., & Cuddy, M. (2008). Factors associated with the risk of behaviour problems in adolescents with severe intellectual disabilities. *Journal of Intellectual Disability Research, 52*(10), 864–876. https://doi.org/10.1111/j.1365-2788.2008.01102.x

Chaney, S. (2013). *Self-mutilation and psychiatry: Impulse, identity and the unconscious in British explanations of self-inflicted injury, c. 1864 – 1914* (Ph.D. thesis). London: University College London. Retrieved from http://discovery.ucl.ac.uk/view/theses/UCL_Thesis/

Chao, H. T., Chen, H., Samaco, R. C., Xue, M., Chahrour, M., Yoo, J., … Zoghbi, H. Y. (2010). Dysfunction in GABA signalling mediates autism-like stereotypies and Rett syndrome phenotypes. *Nature, 468*(7321), 263–269. https://doi.org/10.1038/nature09582

Cohenour, J. M., Volkert, V. M., & Allen, K. D. (2018). An experimental demonstration of AAB renewal in children with autism spectrum disorder. *Journal of the Experimental Analysis of Behavior, 110*(1), 63–73. https://doi.org/10.1002/jeab.443

Collacott, R. A., Cooper, S.-A., Branford, D., & McGrother, C. (1998). Epidemiology of self-injurious behaviour in adults with learning disabilities. *British Journal of Psychiatry, 173*(5), 428–432. https://doi.org/10.1192/bjp.173.5.428

Cooper, S.-A., Smiley, E., Allan, L. M., Jackson, A., Finlayson, J., Mantry, D., & Morrison, J. (2009). Adults with intellectual disabilities: Prevalence, incidence and remission of self-injurious behaviour, and related factors. *Journal of Intellectual Disability Research, 53*(3), 200–216. https://doi.org/10.1111/j.1365-2788.2008.01060.x

Craig, A. R., Cunningham, P. J., Sweeney, M. M., Shahan, T. A., & Nevin, J. A. (2018). Delivering alternative reinforcement in a distinct context reduces its counter-therapeutic effects on relapse. *Journal of the Experimental Analysis of Behavior, 109*(3), 492–505. https://doi.org/10.1002/jeab.431

Cuthbert, B. N. (2015). Research domain criteria: Toward future psychiatric nosologies. *Dialogues in Clinical Neuroscience, 17*(1), 89–97. Retrieved from https://www.dialogues-cns.org/contents17-1/

Cuthbert, B. N. (2019). The PRISM project: Social withdrawal from an RDoC perspective. *Neuroscience and Biobehavioral Reviews, 97*, 34–37. https://doi.org/10.1016/j.neubiorev.2018.08.006

Davies, L. E., & Oliver, C. (2016). Self-injury, aggression and destruction in children with severe intellectual disability: Incidence, persistence and novel, predictive behavioural risk markers. *Research in Developmental Disabilities, 49–50*, 291–301. https://doi.org/10.1016/j.ridd.2015.12.003

DeLeon, I. G., Gregory, M. K., & St. Peter, C. C. (2013). Recent developments in behavioral intervention informed by basic research. *International Review of Research in Developmental Disabilities, 44*, 213–244. https://doi.org/10.1016/B978-0-12-401662-0.00007-5

Dimian, A. F., Botteron, K. N., Dager, S. R., Elison, J. T., Estes, A. M., Pruett, J. R., … Wolff, J. J. (2017). Potential risk factors for the development of self-injurious behavior among infants at risk for autism spectrum disorder. *Journal of Autism and Developmental Disorders, 47*(5), 1403–1415. https://doi.org/10.1007/s10803-017-3057-9

Fisher, W. W., Greer, B. D., Craig, A. R., Retzlaff, B. J., Fuhrman, A. M., Lichtblau, K. R., & Saini, V. (2018). On the predictive validity of behavioral momentum theory for mitigating resurgence of problem behavior. *Journal of the Experimental Analysis of Behavior, 109*(1), 281–290. https://doi.org/10.1002/jeab.303

Fisher, W. W., Saini, V., Greer, B. D., Sullivan, W. E., Roane, H. S., Fuhrman, A. M., … Kimball, R. T. (2019). Baseline reinforcement rate and resurgence of destructive behavior. *Journal of the Experimental Analysis of Behavior, 111*(1), 75–93. https://doi.org/10.1002/jeab.488

Fodstad, J. C., Kirsch, A., Faidley, M., & Bauer, N. (2018). Demonstration of parent training to address early self-injury in young children with intellectual and developmental delays. *Journal of Autism and Developmental Disorders, 48*(11), 3846–3857. https://doi.org/10.1007/s10803-018-3651-5

Golden, C. E., Buxbaum, J. D., & De Rubeis, S. (2018). Disrupted circuits in mouse models of autism spectrum disorder and intellectual disability. *Current Opinion in Neurobiology, 48*, 106–112. https://doi.org/10.1016/j.conb.2017.11.006

Greer, B. D., & Shahan, T. A. (2019). Resurgence as choice: Implications for promoting durable behavior change. *Journal of Applied Behavior Analysis, 52*(3), 816–846. https://doi.org/10.1002/jaba.573

Hanley, G. P., Jin, C. S., Vanselow, N. R., & Hanratty, L. A. (2014). Producing meaningful improvements in problem behavior of children with autism via synthesized analyses and treatments. *Journal of Applied Behavior Analysis, 47*(1), 16–36. https://doi.org/10.1002/jaba.106

Ito-Ishida, A., Ure, K., Chen, H., Swann, J. W., & Zoghbi, H. Y. (2015). Loss of MeCP2 in parvalbumin-and somatostatin-expressing neurons in mice leads to distinct Rett syndrome-like phenotypes. *Neuron, 88*(4), 651–658. https://doi.org/10.1016/j.neuron.2015.10.029

Jessel, J., Hanley, G. P., Ghaemmaghami, M., & Metras, R. (2019). An evaluation of the single-session interview-informed synthesized contingency analysis. *Behavioral Interventions, 34*(1), 62–78. https://doi.org/10.1002/bin.1650

Jessel, J., Ingvarsson, E. T., Metras, R., Kirk, H., & Whipple, R. (2018). Achieving socially significant reductions in problem behavior following the interview-informed synthesized contingency analysis: A summary of 25 outpatient applications. *Journal of Applied Behavior Analysis, 51*(1), 130–157. https://doi.org/10.1002/jaba.436

Kas, M. J., Penninx, B., Sommer, B., Serretti, A., Arango, C., & Marston, H. (2019). A quantitative approach to neuropsychiatry: The why and the how. *Neuroscience and Biobehavioral Reviews, 97*, 3–9. https://doi.org/10.1016/j.neubiorev.2017.12.008

Katz, D. M., Bird, A., Coenraads, M., Gray, S. J., Menon, D. U., Philpot, B. D., & Tarquinio, D. C. (2016). Rett syndrome: Crossing the threshold to clinical translation. *Trends in Neurosciences, 39*(2), 100–113. https://doi.org/10.1016/j.tins.2015.12.008

Krisch, K. A., Bandarian-Balooch, S., & Neumann, D. L. (2018). Effects of extended extinction and multiple extinction contexts on ABA renewal. *Learning and Motivation, 63*, 1–10. https://doi.org/10.1016/j.lmot.2017.11.001

Kuroda, T., Mizutani, Y., Cançado, C. R. X., & Podlesnik, C. A. (2017). Operant models of relapse in zebrafish (Danio rerio): Resurgence, renewal, and reinstatement. *Behavioural Brain Research, 335*, 215–222. https://doi.org/10.1016/j.bbr.2017.08.023

Liggett, A. P., Nastri, R., & Podlesnik, C. A. (2018). Assessing the combined effects of resurgence and reinstatement in children diagnosed with autism spectrum disorder. *Journal of the Experimental Analysis of Behavior, 109*(2), 408–421. https://doi.org/10.1002/jeab.315

Ligsay, A., Van Dijck, A., Nguyen, D. V., Lozano, R., Chen, Y., Bickel, E. S., … Hagerman, R. J. (2017). A randomized double-blind, placebo-controlled trial of ganaxolone in children and adolescents with fragile X syndrome. *Journal of Neurodevelopmental Disorders, 9*(1). https://doi.org/10.1186/s11689-017-9207-8

Lucyshyn, J. M., Fossett, B., Bakeman, R., Cheremshynski, C., Miller, L., Lohrmann, S., … Irvin, L. K. (2015). Transforming Parent–Child interaction in family routines: Longitudinal analysis with families of children with developmental disabilities. *Journal of Child and Family Studies, 24*(12), 3526–3541. https://doi.org/10.1007/s10826-015-0154-2

Lucyshyn, J. M., Miller, L. D., Cheremshynski, C., Lohrmann, S., & Zumbo, B. D. (2018). Transforming coercive processes in family routines: Family functioning outcomes for families of children with developmental disabilities. *Journal of Child and Family Studies, 27*(9), 2844–2861. https://doi.org/10.1007/s10826-018-1113-5

McKinnon, C. J., Eggebrecht, A. T., Todorov, A., Wolff, J. J., Elison, J. T., Adams, C. M., … Pruett, J. R. (2019). Restricted and repetitive behavior and brain functional connectivity in infants at risk for developing autism spectrum disorder. *Biological Psychiatry: Cognitive Neuroscience and Neuroimaging, 4*(1), 50–61. https://doi.org/10.1016/j.bpsc.2018.09.008

Midouhas, E., Yogaratnam, A., Flouri, E., & Charman, T. (2013). Psychopathology trajectories of children with autism spectrum disorder: The role of family poverty and parenting. *Journal of the American Academy of Child and Adolescent Psychiatry, 52*(10), 1057–1065.e1. https://doi.org/10.1016/j.jaac.2013.07.011

Minshawi, N. F., Hurwitz, S., Morriss, D., & McDougle, C. J. (2015). Multidisciplinary assessment and treatment of self-injurious behavior in autism spectrum disorder and intellectual disability: Integration of psychological and biological theory and approach. *Journal of Autism and Developmental Disorders, 45*(6), 1541–1568. https://doi.org/10.1007/s10803-014-2307-3

Nevin, J. A., Craig, A. R., Cunningham, P. J., Podlesnik, C. A., Shahan, T. A., & Sweeney, M. M. (2017). Quantitative models of persistence and relapse from the perspective of behavioral momentum theory: Fits and misfits. *Behavioural Processes, 141*(Part 1), 92–99. https://doi.org/10.1016/j.beproc.2017.04.016

Nutt, D., Robbins, T., & Hayes, A. (2018). THuNDRous news for human dopamine researchers: A selective dopamine D1 receptor antagonist will soon be available for clinical research. *Journal of Psychopharmacology, 32*(11), 1153–1154. https://doi.org/10.1177/0269881118799380

Olatunji, B. O., Tomarken, A., Wentworth, B., & Fritzsche, L. (2017). Effects of exposure in single and multiple contexts on fear renewal: The moderating role of threat-specific and nonspecific emotionality. *Journal of Behavior Therapy and Experimental Psychiatry, 54*, 270–277. https://doi.org/10.1016/j.jbtep.2016.09.004

Oliver, C., Licence, L., & Richards, C. (2017). Self-injurious behaviour in people with intellectual disability and autism spectrum disorder. *Current Opinion in Psychiatry, 30*(2), 97–101. https://doi.org/10.1097/YCO.0000000000000313

Pijl, M. K. J., Bussu, G., Charman, T., Johnson, M. H., Jones, E. J. H., Pasco, G., … Buitelaar, J. K. (2019). Temperament as an early risk marker for autism spectrum disorders? A longitudinal study of high-risk and low-risk infants. *Journal of Autism and Developmental Disorders, 49*(5), 1825–1836. https://doi.org/10.1007/s10803-018-3855-8

Podlesnik, C. A., Kuroda, T., Jimenez-Gomez, C., Abreu-Rodrigues, J., Cançado, C. R. X., Blackman, A. L., … Teixeira, I. S. C. (2019). Resurgence is greater following a return to the training context than remaining in the extinction context. *Journal of the Experimental Analysis of Behavior, 111*(3), 416–435. https://doi.org/10.1002/jeab.505

Podlesnik, C. A., & Shahan, T. A. (2009). Behavioral momentum and relapse of extinguished operant responding. *Learning and Behavior, 37*(4), 357–364. https://doi.org/10.3758/LB.37.4.357

Rattaz, C., Michelon, C., & Baghdadli, A. (2015). Symptom severity as a risk factor for self-injurious behaviours in adolescents with autism spectrum disorders. *Journal of Intellectual Disability Research, 59*(8), 730–740. https://doi.org/10.1111/jir.12177

Richman, D. M., Barnard-Brak, L., Bosch, A., Thompson, S., Grubb, L., & Abby, L. (2013). Predictors of self-injurious behaviour exhibited by individuals with autism spectrum disorder. *Journal of Intellectual Disability Research, 57*(5), 429–439. https://doi.org/10.1111/j.1365-2788.2012.01628.x

Rodriguez, R. A., Joya, C., & Hines, R. M. (2018). Common ribs of inhibitory synaptic dysfunction in the umbrella of neurodevelopmental disorders. *Frontiers in Molecular Neuroscience, 11*, 132. https://doi.org/10.3389/fnmol.2018.00132

Rojahn, J., Matson, J. L., Naglieri, J. A., & Mayville, E. (2004). Relationships between psychiatric conditions and behavior problems among adults with mental retardation. *American Journal on Mental Retardation, 109*(1), 21–33 + 77. https://doi.org/10.1352/0895-8017(2004)109<21:RBPCAB>2.0.CO;2

Rubenstein, J. L. R., & Merzenich, M. M. (2003). Model of autism: Increased ratio of excitation/inhibition in key neural systems. *Genes, Brain and Behavior, 2*(5), 255–267. https://doi.org/10.1034/j.1601-183X.2003.00037.x

Shirley, M. D., Frelin, L., López, J. S., Jedlicka, A., Dziedzic, A., Frank-Crawford, M. A., … Pevsner, J. (2016). Copy number variants associated with 14 cases of self-injurious behavior. *PLoS One, 11*(3), e0149646. https://doi.org/10.1371/journal.pone.0149646

Singewald, N., & Holmes, A. (2019). Rodent models of impaired fear extinction. *Psychopharmacology, 236*(1), 21–32. https://doi.org/10.1007/s00213-018-5054-x

Soke, G. N., Rosenberg, S. A., Hamman, R. F., Fingerlin, T., Rosenberg, C. R., Carpenter, L., … DiGuiseppi, C. (2017). Factors associated with self-injurious behaviors in children with autism spectrum disorder: Findings from two large national samples. *Journal of Autism and Developmental Disorders, 47*(2), 285–296. https://doi.org/10.1007/s10803-016-2951-x

Soke, G. N., Rosenberg, S. A., Rosenberg, C. R., Vasa, R. A., Lee, L. C., & DiGuiseppi, C. (2018). Self-injurious behaviors in children with autism spectrum disorder enrolled in the study to explore early development. *Autism, 22*(5), 625–635. https://doi.org/10.1177/1362361316689330

Tsiouris, J. A., Kim, S. Y., Brown, W. T., & Cohen, I. L. (2011). Association of aggressive behaviours with psychiatric disorders, age, sex and degree of intellectual disability: A large-scale survey. *Journal of Intellectual Disability Research, 55*(7), 636–649. https://doi.org/10.1111/j.1365-2788.2011.01418.x

Voorhies, W., Dajani, D. R., Vij, S. G., Shankar, S., Turan, T. O., & Uddin, L. Q. (2018). Aberrant functional connectivity of inhibitory control networks in children with autism spectrum disorder. *Autism Research, 11*(11), 1468–1478. https://doi.org/10.1002/aur.2014

Willoughby, M. T., Gottfredson, N. C., & Stifter, C. A. (2017). Observed temperament from ages 6 to 36 months predicts parent- and teacher-reported attention-deficit/hyperactivity disorder symptoms in first grade. *Development and Psychopathology, 29*(1), 107–120. https://doi.org/10.1017/S0954579415001236

Index

F. Furniss, A. B. Biswas, *Self-Injurious Behavior in Individuals with Neurodevelopmental Conditions*, Autism and Child Psychopathology Series,
https://doi.org/10.1007/978-3-030-36016-0

K

L

M

The manufacturer's authorised representative in the EU is Springer Nature Customer Service Centre GmbH, Europaplatz 3, 69115 Heidelberg, Germany. If you have any concerns regarding our products, please contact ProductSafety@springernature.com

Printed and bound by CPI Group (UK) Ltd, Croydon, CR0 4YY
30/09/2026
02225449-0012